Medical Data Mining and Knowledge Discovery

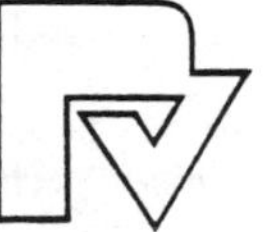

Studies in Fuzziness and Soft Computing

Editor-in-chief
Prof. Janusz Kacprzyk
Systems Research Institute
Polish Academy of Sciences
ul. Newelska 6
01-447 Warsaw, Poland
E-mail: kacprzyk@ibspan.waw.pl
http://www.springer.de/cgi-bin/search_book.pl?series=2941

Vol. 3. A. Geyer-Schulz
Fuzzy Rule-Based Expert Systems and Genetic Machine Learning, 2nd ed. 1996
ISBN 3-7908-0964-0

Vol. 4. T. Onisawa and J. Kacprzyk (Eds.)
Reliability and Safety Analyses under Fuzziness, 1995
ISBN 3-7908-0837-7

Vol. 5. P. Bosc and J. Kacprzyk (Eds.)
Fuzziness in Database Management Systems, 1995
ISBN 3-7908-0858-X

Vol. 6. E.S. Lee and Q. Zhu
Fuzzy and Evidence Reasoning, 1995
ISBN 3-7908-0880-6

Vol. 7. B.A. Juliano and W. Bandler
Tracing Chains-of-Thought, 1996
ISBN 3-7908-0922-5

Vol. 8. F. Herrera and J.L. Verdegay (Eds.)
Genetic Algorithms and Soft Computing, 1996
ISBN 3-7908-0956-X

Vol. 9. M. Sato et al.
Fuzzy Clustering Models and Applications, 1997
ISBN 3-7908-1026-6

Vol. 10. L.C. Jain (Ed.)
Soft Computing Techniques in Knowledge-based Intelligent Engineering Systems, 1997
ISBN 3-7908-1035-5

Vol. 11. W. Mielczarski (Ed.)
Fuzzy Logic Techniques in Power Systems, 1998,
ISBN 3-7908-1044-4

Vol. 12. B. Bouchon-Meunier (Ed.)
Aggregation and Fusion of Imperfect Information, 1998
ISBN 3-7908-1048-7

Vol. 13. E. Orłowska (Ed.)
Incomplete Information: Rough Set Analysis, 1998
ISBN 3-7908-1049-5

Vol. 14. E. Hisdal
Logical Structures for Representation of Knowledge and Uncertainty, 1998
ISBN 3-7908-1056-8

Vol. 15. G.J. Klir and M.J. Wierman
Uncertainty-Based Information, 2nd ed., 1999
ISBN 3-7908-1242-0

Vol. 16. D. Driankov and R. Palm (Eds.)
Advances in Fuzzy Control, 1998
ISBN 3-7908-1090-8

Vol. 17. L. Reznik, V. Dimitrov and J. Kacprzyk (Eds.)
Fuzzy Systems Design, 1998
ISBN 3-7908-1118-1

Vol. 18. L. Polkowski and A. Skowron (Eds.)
Rough Sets in Knowledge Discovery 1, 1998
ISBN 3-7908-1119-X

Vol. 19. L. Polkowski and A. Skowron (Eds.)
Rough Sets in Knowledge Discovery 2, 1998
ISBN 3-7908-1120-3

Vol. 20. J.N. Mordeson and P.S. Nair
Fuzzy Mathematics, 1998
ISBN 3-7908-1121-1

Vol. 21. L.C. Jain and T. Fukuda (Eds.)
Soft Computing for Intelligent Robotic Systems, 1998
ISBN 3-7908-1147-5

Vol. 22. J. Cardoso and H. Camargo (Eds.)
Fuzziness in Petri Nets, 1999
ISBN 3-7908-1158-0

Vol. 23. P.S. Szczepaniak (Ed.)
Computational Intelligence and Applications, 1999
ISBN 3-7908-1161-0

Vol. 24. E. Orłowska (Ed.)
Logic at Work, 1999
ISBN 3-7908-1164-5

Vol. 25. J. Buckley and Th. Feuring
Fuzzy and Neural: Interactions and Applications, 1999
ISBN 3-7908-1170-X

continued on page 497

Krzysztof J. Cios
Editor

Medical Data Mining and Knowledge Discovery

With 98 Figures
and 72 Tables

Physica-Verlag
A Springer-Verlag Company

Professor Krzysztof J. Cios
University of Colorado at Denver
Department of Computer Science and Engineering
1200 Larimer Street
Denver, CO 80217-3364
USA
kcios@carbon.cudenver.edu

ISSN 1434-9922
ISBN 3-7908-1340-0 Physica-Verlag Heidelberg New York

Cataloging-in-Publication Data applied for
Die Deutsche Bibliothek – CIP-Einheitsaufnahme
Medical data mining and knowledge discovery: with 72 tables / Krzysztof J. Cios, ed. – Heidelberg; New York: Physica-Verl., 2001
(Studies in fuzziness and soft computing; Vol. 60)
ISBN 3-7908-1340-0

Physica-Verlag Heidelberg New York
a member of BertelsmannSpringer Science+Business Media GmbH

Printed in Germany

Hardcover Design: Erich Kirchner, Heidelberg

SPIN 10783090 88/2202-5 4 3 2 1 0 – Printed on acid-free paper

to my son Karol

with love

Foreword

Modern medicine generates, almost daily, huge amounts of heterogeneous data. For example, medical data may contain SPECT images, signals like ECG, clinical information like temperature, cholesterol levels, etc., as well as the physician's interpretation. Those who deal with such data understand that there is a widening gap between data collection and data comprehension. Computerized techniques are needed to help humans address this problem. This volume is devoted to the relatively young and growing field of medical data mining and knowledge discovery. It was developed expressly for the purpose of making sense of large data sets. The field is inherently associated with databases. Although data mining has a great deal in common with statistics, since both strive toward discovering some structure in data, data mining also draws heavily from many other disciplines, most notably machine learning and database technology. It differs from statistics in that it must deal with heterogeneous data fields, typical for medical databases.

Data mining methods are algorithms that are used on databases for model building, or for finding patterns in data. When data mining methods are used in a process in which their outcome is evaluated, so that we can think about the product as being a new piece of information, then we speak about a knowledge discovery process. Sometimes the term knowledge discovery is used interchangeably with the term data mining; however, we understand knowledge discovery in databases as a process within which data mining methods are used.

The knowledge discovery process transforms data into knowledge. Data mining is not a one-pass undertaking. In fact, each iteration in the knowledge discovery process yields a different perspective on the data. One iteration, using one particular data mining method, reveals a different view of the data than using another preprocessing or data mining method. Various data mining methods may be equally valid or invalid. When speaking about the knowledge discovery process, we need to emphasize not only the iterative character among the data mining methods used, but also an interaction with medical professionals, who always play a crucial and indispensable role in a knowledge discovery process.

Medical data mining and knowledge discovery are not substantially different from mining in other types of databases; however, there are some characteristic features that are absent in non-medical data. The most significant is the fact that more and more medical procedures employ imaging as a preferred diagnostic tool. Thus, there is a need to develop methods for efficient mining in databases of images, which is inherently more difficult than mining in numerical databases. Other significant features are security and confidentiality concerns. Still another is the fact that the physician's interpretation of images, signals, or other clinical data, is written in unstructured English, that is very difficult to mine. This book addresses all these specific features.

The sixteen chapters of this volume, contributed by prominent researchers in the field, address many of the above-mentioned issues. The first three chapters are introductory. Chapter One summarizes the key issues of medical data mining, talks about specific features of medical data mining that are absent in mining other types of data. The second chapter explains, in layman's terms, legal policy and security issues in handling medical data. The third chapter describes medical natural language understanding as a supporting technology for data mining in healthcare. The remaining articles describe knowledge discovery processes in different types of medical databases, albeit of widely varying sizes. Chapter Four describes the development of the largest publicly accessible pathology database. The next chapter describes results of actual data mining in this database. Chapter Six uses a brain image database, and describes mining for structure-function associations in the database. Chapter Seven describes a system for an automatic diabetic retinal image screening system. Chapter Eight uses a fuzzy information theoretic approach for knowledge discovery in mortality records. Chapter Nine addresses an important problem of consistent and complete data and expert mining in medical records. Chapter Ten introduces and uses evolutionary computation for medical data mining. Chapter Eleven introduces methods of temporal data validation and abstraction in high-frequency domains. In Chapter Twelve, the authors use a data mining approach for matrix-associated regions in gene therapy. Chapter Thirteen describes the discovery of temporal patterns in course-of-disease data. Chapter Fourteen deals with the modeling of human visual perception. In Chapter Fifteen, the author uses rough sets for knowledge discovery in a bacterial test database. The final chapter discusses the use of expert knowledge for knowledge discovery in time series data.

I wish to thank the authors for their contributions and patience, and Mr. Lukasz Kurgan, a Ph.D. candidate, for formatting the chapters so that the book has a unified appearance.

Krzysztof J. Cios

Contents

1 Medical Data Mining and Knowledge Discovery: Overview of Key Issues

Krzysztof J. Cios and G. William Moore

1.1 Unique Features of Medical Data Mining 1
1.2 Defining Data Mining and Knowledge Discovery 5
1.3 Key Issues of Data Mining and Knowledge Discovery 9
1.4 Data Mining Models 11
1.5 Knowledge Discovery Process 13
1.5.1 Understanding the Medical Problem Domain 14
1.5.2 Understanding the Data 14
1.5.3 Preparation of the Data 15
1.5.4 Data Mining 15
1.5.5 Evaluation of the Discovered Knowledge 16
1.5.6 Using the Discovered Knowledge 16
1.6 Example System 17
1.7 Further Web Information 17
References 19

2 Legal Policy and Security Issues in the Handling of Medical Data

Joseph M. Saul

2.1 General Considerations 21
2.2 The United States 23
2.2.1 The Health Insurance Portability and Accountability Act (HIPAA) 23
2.2.2 The Common Rule 31
2.2.3 State Medical Records Laws 33
2.3 The European Union 33
2.3.1 The Data Protection Directive 33
2.4 Canada 36
2.4.1 The Personal Information Protection and Electronic Documents Act (Bill C-6) 36
2.4.2 The Tri-Council Code 36
2.4.3 Provincial Laws 39
References 40
United States 40
European Community 40
Canada 40

3 Medical Natural Language Understanding as a Supporting Technology for Data Mining in Healthcare

Werner Ceusters

3.1 Understanding the Problem Domain 41
3.1.1 Introduction 41
3.1.2 The Many Faces of Language Engineering 42
3.2 Understanding the Data 48
3.2.1 Types of Knowledge 48
3.2.2 Linguistic and Conceptual Knowledge 49
3.2.3 Linguistic Semantics 50
3.2.4 Conceptual and Linguistic Ontologies 51
3.3 Preparation of the Data for Subsequent Data Mining 53
3.3.1 Technologies Required 53
3.3.2 Preparing Neurosurgerical Reports for Data Mining Purposes: The MultiTale Approach 54
3.4 Data Mining 56
3.5 Evaluation 63
3.5.1 Discussion 65
3.6 Conclusion 66
References 67

4 Anatomic Pathology Data Mining

G. William Moore and Jules J. Berman

4.1 Understanding the Problem Domain 72
4.1.1 Objectives of Data Mining in Anatomic Pathology 72
4.1.2 Intended Uses for Anatomic Pathology Data Mining 72
4.1.3 Economic Issues in Anatomic Pathology Data Mining 78
4.1.4 Commercial Uses of Mined Anatomic Pathology Data 79
4.1.5 Past, Current Efforts to Standardize Pathology Data 80
4.1.6 Data Integrity Issues 81
4.1.7 Ethical and Legal Issues 82
4.2 Understanding the Data 85
4.2.1 Size of Potential Anatomic Pathology Data Domain 85
4.2.2 Description of an Anatomic Pathology Report 86
4.2.3 Converting Parts of a Report into Object Domains 89
4.3 Preparation of the Data 95
4.3.1 Data Ownership 95
4.3.2 Data Requirements 97
4.4 Data Mining Example 100
4.4.1 The Johns Hopkins Autopsy Resource 100

4.5 Conclusion 102
Appendix Internet References. 112
References 113

5 A Data Clustering and Visualization Methodology for Epidemiological Pathology Discoveries

Doron Shalvi and Nicholas DeClaris

5.1 Introduction 120
5.2 Understanding the Problem Domain 121
5.2.1 Objectives 121
5.2.2 Project Plan 121
5.3 Understanding the Data 122
5.3.1 Data Collection 122
5.3.2 Data Description 123
5.3.3 Data Quality 123
5.4 Preparation of the Data 127
5.4.1 Data Selection 127
5.4.2 Data Preprocessing 127
5.5 Data Mining 129
5.5.1 Self-Organizing Map (SOM) 130
5.5.2 Data Visualization 134
5.5.3 Adaptive Resonance Theory (ART) 143
5.6 Evaluation of the Discovered Knowledge 147
5.7 Using the Discovered Knowledge 148
5.8 Conclusions 149
References 151

6 Mining Structure-Function Associations in a Brain Image Database

Vasileios Megalooikonomou and Edward H. Herskovits

6.1 Understanding the Problem Domain 153
6.2 Understanding the Data 154
6.3 Preparation of the Data 156
6.4 Data Mining 156
6.4.1 Atlas-Based Analysis 157
6.4.2 Voxel-Based Analysis 158
6.4.3 Results from Mining BRAID 159
6.5 Evaluation of the Discovered Knowledge 164
6.5.1 The Lesion-Deficit Simulator 165
6.5.2 Results from the Evaluation of the Mining System 169
6.6 Using the Discovered Knowledge 175

References 177

7 ADRIS: An Automatic Diabetic Retinal Image Screening System
Kheng Guan Goh, Wynne Hsu, Mong Li Lee and Huan Wang

7.1 Introduction 181
7.2 Understanding the Problem Domain 182
7.2.1 Data Mining Applications on Medical Data 183
7.3 Understanding the Data 184
7.4 Preparing the Data 187
7.4.1 Optic Disc and Cup Detection 187
7.4.2 Exudates Detection 192
7.4.3 Vessel Detection 194
7.5 Data Mining 200
7.6 Evaluation of the Discovered Knowledge 201
7.6.1 Optic Disc and Cup Detection 202
7.6.2 Optic Disc Detection 202
7.6.3 Optic Cup Detection 203
7.6.4 Exudates Detection 204
7.6.5 Vessel Processing 204
7.7 Using the Discovered Knowledge 206
7.8 Conclusion 206
References 207

8 Knowledge Discovery in Mortality Records: An Info-Fuzzy Approach
Mark Last, Oded Maimon and Abraham Kandel

8.1 Introduction 211
8.2 Understanding the Problem Domain 212
8.3 Understanding the Data 214
8.3.1 Extended Database Model 214
8.3.2 Main Data Table 215
8.3.3 Additional Data Tables 216
8.3.4 Data Quality 216
8.4 Preparation of the Data 217
8.4.1 Data Transformation and Reformatting 217
8.4.2 Treatment of Missing Values 218
8.4.3 An Automated Approach to Data Cleaning 219
8.4.4 Detecting Outliers in the Main Data Table 220
8.5 Data Mining 222
8.5.1 Information-Theoretic Approach to Data Mining 222
8.5.2 Dimensionality Reduction Procedure 223

8.5.3 Discretization of Continuous Attributes 225
8.5.4 Rule Extraction 227
8.5.5 Data Reliability 230
8.6 Evaluation of the Discovered Knowledge 232
8.7 Using the Discovered Knowledge 233
8.8 Conclusions 233
References 234

9 Consistent and Complete Data and "Expert" Mining in Medicine

Boris Kovalerchuk, Evgenii Vityaev and James F. Ruiz

9.1 Introduction 238
9.2 Understanding the Data 244
9.2.1 Collection of Initial Data: Monotone Boolean Function Approach 244
9.2.2 Preparation and Construction of the Data and Rules Using MBF 253
9.3 Preparation of the Data 259
9.3.1 Problem Outline 259
9.3.2 Hierarchical Approach 262
9.3.3 Monotonicity 264
9.3.4 Rules "Mined" from Expert 267
9.3.5 Rule Extraction through Monotone Boolean Functions 268
9.4 Data Mining 269
9.4.1 Relational Data Mining Method 269
9.4.2 Mining Diagnostic Rules from Breast Cancer Data 272
9.5 Evaluation of Discovered Knowledge 275
9.6 Discussion 278
References 278

10 A Medical Data Mining Application Based on Evolutionary Computation

Man Leung Wong, Wai Lam and Kwong Sak Leung

10.1 Introduction 282
10.2 The Problem Domain 282
10.3 Understanding the Data 283
10.4 Data Preparation 283
10.5 Data Mining 285
10.5.1 Evolutionary Computation Background 285
10.5.2 Causal Structure Analysis 297
10.5.3 Rule Learning 302
10.6 Evaluation of the Discovered Knowledge 309
10.6.1 Evaluation of Causal Structure Analysis 309
10.6.2 Evaluation of Rule Learning 310

10.7 Using the Discovered Knowledge 313
10.8 Conclusions 313
References 314
Appendix The Grammar for the Scoliosis Database 317

11 Methods of Temporal Data Validation and Abstraction in High-Frequency Domains

Silvia Miksch, Andreas Seyfang, Werner Horn, Christian Popow and Franz Paky

11.1 Introduction 320
11.2 Motivation - The Characteristics of the Data 322
11.2.1 The Need for Time-Oriented Data Validation 322
11.2.2 The Need for Deriving Temporal Abstractions 324
11.3 Preprocessing: Time-Oriented Data Validation 326
11.3.1 Time-Point-Based Validation and Repair 328
11.3.2 Time-Interval-Based Validation and Repair 330
11.3.3 Trend-Based Validation and Repair 332
11.3.4 Time-Independent Validation: Reliability Ranking 336
11.4 Data Mining - Time-Oriented Data Abstraction 337
11.4.1 State Abstraction 338
11.4.2 Grade Abstraction 343
11.4.3 Bend Abstraction 343
11.4.4 Trend Curve Fitting 347
11.4.5 Derived Status Information 349
11.5 Evaluation and Discussion 350
11.5.1 Empirical Evaluation 350
11.5.2 Discussion 352
11.5.3 Overall Benefits 352
11.6 Future Research 353
11.6.1 Utilizing Qualitative Descriptions in Treatment Planning 353
11.6.2 Repetitive Temporal Patterns 354
11.6.3 Further Evaluation 354
11.6.4 Conclusion 354
References 355

12 Data Mining the Matrix Associated Regions (MARs) for Gene Therapy

Gautam B. Singh and Stephan Krawetz

12.1 Understanding the Problem Domain 360
12.2 Understanding the Data 362
12.3 Preparation of the Data 364
12.4 Data Mining for MAR Detection 367

12.5 Evaluation of Discovered Knowledge 370
12.6 Using the Discovered Knowledge 375
12.7 Conclusion 376
References 377

13 Discovery of Temporal Patterns in Sparse Course-of-Disease Data

Jorge C. G. Ramirez, Lynn L. Peterson, Diane J. Cook and Dolores M. Peterson

13.1 Understanding the Problem Domain 380
13.1.1 Determination of Objectives 380
13.2 Understanding the Data 381
13.2.1 Description of the Data 381
13.2.2 Initial Exploration of the Data 381
13.2.3 Verification of the Quality of the Data 382
13.3 Preparation of the Data 383
13.3.1 Data Cleaning 383
13.3.2 Data Selection 384
13.3.3 Constructing and Merging the Data 386
13.4 Data Mining 390
13.4.1 Selection of the Data Mining Method 390
13.4.2 Building and Assessing the Model 393
13.5 Evaluation of the Discovered Knowledge 397
13.5.1 Assessment of the Results vs. the Objectives 397
13.5.2 Reviewing the Entire Knowledge Discovery Process 399
13.6 Using the Discovered Knowledge 400
13.6.1 Implementation and Monitoring Plans 400
13.6.2 Overview of the Entire Project for Future Use and Improvements 400
References 401

14 Data Mining-Based Modeling of Human Visual Perception

Luís Augusto Consularo, Roberto de Alencar Lotufo and Luciano da Fontoura Costa

14.1 Understanding the Problem Domain 404
14.2 Understanding the Data 407
14.3 Preparation of the Data 408
14.4 Data Mining 414
14.4.1 The Σynergos 414
14.4.2 The Approach 415
14.4.3 Generalization 416
14.4.4 The Search 420

14.5 Evaluation of the Discovered Knowledge 422
14.6 Using the Discovered Knowledge 428
References 429

15 Discovery of Clinical Knowledge in Databases Extracted from Hospital Information Systems

Shusaku Tsumoto

15.1 Introduction 433
15.2 Data Selection 435
15.3 Data Cleaning as Preprocessing 436
15.4 Data Reduction and Projection as Preprocessing 438
15.4.1 Data Projection for Bacterial Test Database 438
15.4.2 Data Reduction for Steroid Side-Effect Database 440
15.4.3 Total Time Required for Data Reduction 444
15.5 Rule Induction as Data Mining 444
15.5.1 Definition of Rules Based on Rough Sets 444
15.5.2 Algorithms for Rule Induction 446
15.5.3 Application of Rule Induction Methods 447
15.6 Interpretation of Induced Rules 449
15.6.1 Induced Rules of Bacterial Tests 449
15.6.2 Induced Results of Steroid Side-Effects 450
15.7 Discussion 451
15.7.1 Summary of Time Required for KDD Process 451
15.7.2 Summary of Data Interpretation 452
15.8 Conclusions 453
References 454

16 Knowledge Discovery in Time Series Using Expert Knowledge

Fernando Alonso, Juan P. Caraça-Valente, Ignacio López-Chavarrías and Cesar Montes

16.1 Introduction 455
16.2 Understanding the Problem Domain 457
16.2.1 Overview of the System 458
16.2.2 Evaluation of the System as a KBS 461
16.2.3 Description of the KBS 462
16.3 Understanding the Data 470
16.3.1 Data Description: The Isokinetic Test 470
16.3.2 Collection of Initial Data 470
16.4 Preparing the Data 471
16.4.1 Data Analysis and Decoding 472

16.4.2 Creation of the I4 Database 472
16.4.3 Expert Cleaning of Data 474
16.4.4 Expert Pre-Processing 475
16.5 Data Mining 475
16.5.1 Detecting Injury Patterns in Isokinetic Exercises 476
16.5.2 Creation of Reference Models for Population Groups 484
16.6 Evaluation of the Discovered Knowledge 487
16.7 Using the Discovered Knowledge 492
16.8 Conclusions 493
References 495

1 Medical Data Mining and Knowledge Discovery: Overview of Key Issues

Krzysztof J. Cios[1,2] and G. William Moore[3,4,5]
[1]University of Colorado at Denver, U.S.A.
[2]Medical College of Ohio, Toledo, U.S.A.
kcios@carbon.cudenver.edu
[3]Pathology and Laboratory Medicine Service, Veterans Affairs Maryland Health Care System, Baltimore, U.S.A.
[4]Department of Pathology, University of Maryland School of Medicine, Baltimore, U.S.A.
[5]Department of Pathology, The Johns Hopkins Medical Institutions, Baltimore, U.S.A.
webmaster@netautopsy.org

In this chapter we describe unique features of medical data mining that are absent in mining other types of data. Next, we address key issues of data mining and knowledge discovery. Then we describe models of data mining, and outline a six-step knowledge discovery process. We conclude the chapter by providing links to major data mining Internet sites that provide packets of useful information.

1.1 Unique Features of Medical Data Mining

Modern medicine generates huge amounts of data, but at the same time there is an acute and widening gap between data collection and data comprehension. Thus, there is growing pressure not only to find better methods of data analysis, but also a need for automating them to facilitate the creation of knowledge that can be used for clinical decision-making. This is where data mining and knowledge discovery tools come into play, since they can help in achieving these goals (Cios et al., 1998).

Data mining and knowledge discovery in medical databases are not substantially different from mining in other types of databases. There are some characteristic features, however, that are absent in non-medical data.

One feature is that more and more medical procedures employ imaging as a preferred diagnostic tool. Thus, there is a need to develop methods for efficient mining in databases of images, which is not only different, but also more difficult, than mining in numerical databases. As an example, imaging techniques like SPECT, MRI, PET, and collection of ECG or EEG signals, can generate gigabytes of data per day. A single cardiac SPECT procedure of one patient may contain dozens of 2D images. In addition, medical databases are always heterogeneous. For instance, an image of the patient's organ will almost always be accompanied by other clinical information, as well as the physician's interpretation (clinical impression; diagnosis). This heterogeneity requires high capacity data storage devices, as well as new tools to analyze such data. It is obviously very difficult for an unaided human to process gigabytes of records, although dealing with images is relatively easier for humans, who are able to recognized patterns, grasp basic trends in data, and form rational decisions. The information becomes less useful as we are faced with difficulties of retrieving it, and making it available in an easily comprehensible format. Visualization techniques will play an increasing role in this setting, since images are the easiest for humans to comprehend, and they can provide a great deal of information in a single visualization of the results.

A second feature is that the physician's interpretation of images, signals, or any other clinical data, is written in unstructured free-text English that is very difficult to standardize and thus difficult to mine. Even specialists from the same discipline cannot agree on unambiguous terms to be used in describing a patient's condition. Not only do they use different names (synonyms) to describe the same disease, but they render the task even more daunting by using different grammatical constructions to describe relationships among medical entities.

A third unique feature of medical data mining is the question of data ownership. The corpus of medical data potentially available for mining is enormous. Some thousands of terabytes (quadrillions of bytes) are now generated annually in North America and Europe. However, these data are buried in heterogeneous databases, and scattered throughout the medical care establishment, without any common format or principles of organization. The question of ownership of patient information is unsettled, and the object of recurrent, highly-publicized lawsuits and congressional inquiries. Do individual patients own data collected on themselves? Do their physicians own the data? Do their insurance providers own the data? Some HMOs now refuse to pay for patient participation in clinical treatment protocols that are deemed experimental. If insurance providers do not own their insurees' data, can they refuse to pay for the collection and storage of the data? Some might argue that the ownership of human data, and therefore the ability to process and sell such data, is unseemly. If so, then how should the data managers, who organize and mine the data, be compensated? Or should this incredibly rich resource for the potential betterment of humankind be left unmined?

A fourth unique feature of medical data mining is a fear of lawsuits directed against physicians and other medical providers. Medical care in the U.S.A., for those who can afford it, is the best in the world. However, U. S. medical care is some 30% more expensive than that elsewhere in North America and Europe, where quality is comparable; and U. S. medicine also has the most litigious malpractice climate in the world. Some have argued that the 30% surcharge on U. S. medical care, about one thousand dollars per capita annually, is mostly medicolegal: either direct legal costs, or else the overhead of "defensive medicine", i.e., unnecessary tests ordered by physicians to cover themselves in potential future lawsuits. In this tense climate, physicians and other medical data-producers are understandably reluctant to hand over their data to data miners. Data miners could browse these data for untoward events. Apparent anomalies in the medical history of an individual patient might trigger an investigation. In many cases, the appearance of malpractice might be a data-omission or data-transcription error; and not all bad outcomes in medicine are necessarily the result of negligent provider behavior. However, an investigation inevitably consumes the time and emotional energy of medical providers. For exposing themselves to this risk, what reward do the providers receive in return?

A fifth feature is privacy and security concerns. For instance, pending U. S. Federal rules suggest that there should be unrestricted usage of medical data of patients deceased for at least two years; but for live patients, all data must be encrypted, so that it is impossible to identify a person, or to go back and decrypt the data. At stake is not only a potential breach of patient confidentiality, with the possibility of ensuing legal action; but also erosion of the physician-patient-relationship, in which the patient is extraordinarily candid with the physician in the expectation that such private information will never be made public. Thus, the encryption of data must be irreversible. A related privacy issue may apply if, for example, crucial diagnostic information were to be discovered on live-patient data, and that a patient could be treated if we could only go back and inform the patient about the diagnosis and possible cure. According to the Health Insurance Portability and Accountability Act of 1996 (HIPAA) legislation, this is unfortunately not possible. Another issue is data security in data handling, and particularly in data transfer. Before the data are encrypted, only authorized persons should have access to the data. Since transferring the data electronically via the Internet is insecure, the data must be carefully encrypted even for transfers within one medical institution from one unit to another.

A sixth unique feature of medical data mining is that the underlying data structures of medicine are poorly characterized mathematically, as compared to many areas of the physical sciences. Physical scientists collect data which they can substitute into formulas, equations, and models that reasonably reflect the relationships among their data. On the other hand, the conceptual structure of medicine consists of word-descriptions and pictures, with very few formal constraints on the vocabulary, the composition of images, or the allowable relationships among basic concepts. The fundamental entities of medicine, such as inflammation, ischemia, or neoplasia, are just as real to a physician as entities such as mass, length, or force are to a physical scientist; but medicine has no comparable formal structure into which a data miner can organize information, such as might be modeled by clustering, regression models, or sequence analysis. In its defense, medicine must contend with hundreds of distinct anatomic locations and thousands of diseases. Until now, the sheer magnitude of this concept space was insurmountable. Furthermore, there is some suggestion that the logic of medicine may be fundamentally different from the logic of the physical sciences (Moore et al, 1979; Moore et al, 1979; Moore and Hutchins, 1980, 1981a, b). However, it may now happen that fast computers and the newer tools of data mining and knowledge discovery may overcome this prior obstacle.

Finally, human medicine is primarily a patient-care activity, and only secondarily a research resource. Generally the only justification for collecting data in medicine, or refusal to collect certain data, is to benefit the individual patient. Some patients might consent to be involved in research projects that do not benefit them directly, but such data collection is typically very small-scale, narrowly focused, and highly regulated by legal and ethical considerations. On the other hand, humans are the most closely-studied species in the world, and enormous quantities of data are generated as an incidental byproduct of patient care. In Europe and North America, much of this information is now primarily generated on electronic media. These data include observations that cannot be gained from animal studies, such as visual and auditory sensations, the perception of pain, and recollection of possibly relevant prior traumas and exposures. By contrast, most animal studies are short-term, and therefore cannot track long-term disease processes of medical interest, such as preneoplasia or atherosclerosis. Furthermore, most animal studies are small-scale, and thus cannot detect or follow rare disease processes. And, there is no issue of having to extrapolate animal observations to the human species.

In summary, medical data are heavily image-based and text-based; the datasets are heterogeneous, replete with missing values; medicine lacks a formal, mathematical structure for organizing data; and there are significant issues of ownership, fairness, and privacy. Yet for all this, the unique promise of medical data mining is enormous and rich; and its potential for use in human betterment is unequalled. It is our hope that the methods and perspectives of data mining and knowledge discovery can help to exploit this emerging resource.

1.2 Defining Data Mining and Knowledge Discovery

What is data mining and knowledge discovery anyhow? We will define both, and describe the main issues associated with them. The chapter is partially based on earlier publications by Cios et al. (1999; 2000). We start by defining the two terms, and then elaborate on the issues involved.

The field of data mining and knowledge discovery is only about a decade old, and is inherently associated with databases. In this sense, knowledge discovery significantly augments databases by making them more user-friendly, and thus helping people to manage vast amounts of data. It is very important that both the inputs and outputs of a knowledge discovery system must be simple to understand and convenient to use. Thus there is a great need for visualization techniques, so that a complex output can be visualized for easy comprehension. Another issue is the realization that users do not need and, moreover, do not want to be concerned with the inner working of data mining algorithms, such as setting thresholds and various parameters. Even data mining practitioners welcome data mining tools that are easy to use, so that they can quickly turn to solving a particular problem at hand. The most significant problem, however, is the scalability problem. Many data mining algorithms may work well with medium-sized databases, but have difficulty with high-dimensional data, both in terms of the number of attributes and number of objects, encountered in large databases. In short, data mining is about reducing the dimensionality of the data and building models.

Although data mining has a great deal in common with statistics, since both strive toward discovering some structure in data, data mining also draws heavily from many other disciplines, most notably machine learning and database technology (Elder and Pregibon, 1995). Data mining, on the other hand, differs from statistics in that it must deal with heterogeneous data fields, not just heterogeneous numbers, as is the case in statistics (Friedman, 1997). The best example is medical data that may contain images, signals like ECG, clinical information like temperature, cholesterol levels, urinalysis data, etc., as well as the physician's interpretation written in unstructured English. In fact, more success stories in data mining are due to advancements in database technology than to advancements in data mining algorithms (Matheus et al., 1993). It is only after a subset of data is selected from a large database that most data mining algorithms can actually manage this reduced data set (Agrawal et al. 1993; Zembowicz and Zytkow, 1996; Ramakrishnan et al., 1998). There is simply no data mining algorithm that can handle, for example, the approximately 200 million telephone calls routed daily by AT&T.

Data mining methods can be divided roughly into those that build models and those that detect patterns. Examples of model building include rule-generation by machine learning algorithms, neural networks, and regression. Examples of the latter include methods that detect deviations from, say, "normal" ECG waveform, from shopping and travel patterns, etc.

More formal definitions of data mining and knowledge discovery follow. Data mining methods are algorithms that are used on databases, after initial data preparation, for model building, or for finding patterns / trends in the data. When data mining methods are used in a process in which their outcome is evaluated, so that we can think about the product as being a new package of information, then we speak about a knowledge discovery process. The term itself was defined by Frawley et al. (1991): "Knowledge discovery in databases is the nontrivial process of identifying valid, novel, potentially useful, and ultimately understandable patterns in data."

Data mining is not a one-pass undertaking. In fact, each iteration in the knowledge discovery process yields a different perspective on the data. One iteration, using one particular data mining method, reveals a different view of the data than using another preprocessing or data mining method. The data mining methods may be equally valid or invalid: there always exists the possibility of discovering either a golden nugget or trash. Only after deploying the discovered knowledge can the end user determine which of the two outcomes was achieved. One obviously hopes for the nugget.

The knowledge discovery process is made difficult by the fact that dozens of data mining methods can be used on any given data, and so far no theory exists for how to go about discovering new and ultimately useful knowledge. However, the general six-step knowledge discovery process (Cios et al., 2000) can help in undertaking this task. These steps are employed throughout this book, and are summarized below for the benefit of the reader.

Sometimes the term knowledge discovery is used interchangeably with the term data mining; however, we shall understand knowledge discovery in databases as a process within which data mining methods are used. The knowledge discovery process transforms data into knowledge. Data mining methods are used to build models or to find patterns in data.

When speaking about the knowledge discovery process, we need to emphasize not only the iterative character among the data mining methods used, but also an interaction with medical professionals, who always play a crucial and indispensable role in a knowledge discovery process.

There is a great need for knowledge discovery tools, or software, that concentrates not just on the preprocessing and the data mining steps, but also on a tight integration with database systems. Otherwise, a great deal of time and effort is squandered in bringing data in and out of a database.

The knowledge discovery process is still in its infancy, being rather an art than a well-understood process, which hinders its applications. Benefits of the knowledge discovery process can be measured in terms of development time, reliability, efficiency, and overall cost. In addition, the knowledge discovery process should pay attention to:

- Medical concerns, which are equally as important as data mining and knowledge discovery concerns

- Guidelines for reusing the experience gained previously on new projects

On a very high level, we distinguish three types of mining in data:

- Directed mining

  For instance, the physician is interested in acquiring some particular information, such as, "find regions of the left ventricle that were mainly affected by severe obstruction in the circumflex artery". Most medical applications probably fall into this category.

- Hypothesis testing and refinement

  The user provides some working hypotheses and expects the system to validate them, or to modify them and suggest other, more refined hypotheses.

- Undirected or pure mining

  This is the most general scenario, in which there are no constraints on the system, and at the same time no prior expectations of what the user will discover, or what type of discovery might be of interest. It is also the most difficult one to perform. Little has been done in this area.

While the field of knowledge discovery is at a relatively early stage in its development, its key features may be summarized as follows (Cios et al., 1998):

- Knowledge discovery relies on a human - system interaction. It is difficult to envision a fully automated process of knowledge discovery, since it would require the system to possess all domain knowledge, and be capable of recognizing the intentions of the user

- Knowledge discovery deals with large databases, and requires efficient ways of handling large files, by providing facilities necessary for their access and processing

- Knowledge discovery depends upon multidisciplinary research, and calls upon a number of complementary information technologies. This multidisciplinary character makes knowledge discovery very different from individual tools like statistics, machine learning, regression analysis, etc.

1.3 Key Issues of Data Mining and Knowledge Discovery

Below we enumerate fundamental issues in data mining and knowledge discovery which arise from the very nature of databases (Cios et al. 1998):

- Huge volume of data

  Because of the sheer size of databases, it is unlikely that any of the data mining methods will succeed with raw data. Data mining methods may require extracting a sample from the database, in the hope that results obtained in this manner are representative for the entire database. Dimensionality reduction can be achieved in two ways:

  - sampling in the data space, where some records are selected, often randomly, and used afterwards for data mining

- sampling in the feature space, where only some features of each data record are selected. Again, for a large number of features, the selection can be performed in a random manner.

- Dynamic nature of data

  Databases are constantly updated, either by adding, say, new SPECT images (for the same or a new patient), or by replacement of the existing ones (say, a SPECT had to be repeated because of technical problems). This requires methods that are able to incrementally update the knowledge learned so far.

- Incomplete or imprecise data

  The information collected in a database can be either incomplete or imprecise. Fuzzy sets (Zadeh, 1979) and rough sets (Pawlak, 1984) were developed explicitly for the purpose of addressing this problem.

- Noisy data

  It is very difficult for any data collection technique to entirely eliminate noise. This implies that data mining methods should be made less sensitive to noise, or care should be taken that the amount of noise in data to be collected in the future will be approximately the same as that in the current data.

- Missing attribute values

  A missing value may have been accidentally not entered, or may represent an unknown value. Missing values create a problem for most data mining methods, since most methods require a fixed dimension (number of features) for each data object. One approach to remedy this problem is to substitute missing values with most likely values; another approach is to replace the unknown value with all possible values for that attribute. The missing value problem is widely encountered in medical databases, since most medical data are collected as a byproduct of patient care activities, rather than for organized research protocols, where exhaustive data collection can be enforced. In a large medical database, almost every patient is lacking values for some feature, and almost every feature is lacking values for some patient (Moore et al, 1979, Moore and Hutchins, 1980).

- Redundant, insignificant data, or inconsistent data

  The data set may contain redundant, insignificant, or inconsistent data objects and/or attributes. We speak about inconsistent data when the same data item is categorized as belonging to more than one category.

1.4 Data Mining Models

Data mining and knowledge discovery are supported by several models that capture the characteristics of data. Below we elaborate on several of them (Cios et al. 1998, 2000).

- Summarization

  The goal is to characterize the data in terms of a small number of features/attributes in an aggregated form.

- Clustering or Segmentation

  The key objective is to find natural groupings (clusters) in large dimensional data. Objects are clustered together if they are similar to one another (according to some measure), and at the same time are dissimilar from objects in other clusters. The key concern in clustering is how to incorporate domain knowledge into the mechanisms of clustering. Without that focus and at least partial human supervision, one can easily end up with clustering problems that are computationally infeasible.

- Regression Models

  These models originate from regression analysis, and its applied field, known as system identification. Regression is the analysis of dependencies of attribute values on the values of other attributes in the same object, and generation of a model that can predict attribute values for new objects.

- Classification

  This term has its origins in pattern recognition. The task is to build a classifier, which, given a set of classes, would determine class membership for a new object. The classifiers can be regarded as a special case of regression models.

- Concept Description

  The goal is to create understandable descriptions of concepts, or categories. Machine learning, conceptual clustering, genetic algorithms, and fuzzy sets are the principal methods used for achieving this goal (Cios et al. 1995; 1997).

- Dependency Analysis

  This analysis is concerned with the determination of relationships (dependencies) among fields in a database.

- Link Analysis, or Associations

  The task is to discover associations between attributes and objects, such that the presence of one pattern would imply presence of another pattern. These associations can involve attributes of the same object, or attributes of different objects. If it is performed over time, it is called sequence analysis (see next).

- Sequence Analysis

  This analysis is geared toward problems of modeling sequential data. Methods include time series analysis, time series models, and temporal neural networks.

- Prediction

  The task, given the prediction model and a new data object, is to predict a specific value for an attribute of the object. Prediction can be used in hypotheses testing.

- Exploratory Data Analysis

Graphical models are often used to perform exploratory data analysis, i.e., to harness human visual recognition power to gain some insight into the data, such as discovering new patterns.

- Visualization

  Visualization is very important for making the discovered knowledge comprehensible for humans; although it is least developed, there is a growing demand for visualization techniques (Crevier and Lepage, 1997).

Human comprehension of numerical and other types of data is very limited. Thus we are interested in building more abstract, higher-level concepts of, say, high values in some region of the image and low in the other. Thus, when we examine data in an effort to reveal certain patterns, we examine them from a certain conceptual distance formed by packages of knowledge of a certain granularity. By information granularity, we mean a form of encapsulation of data into a single conceptual entity. For that purpose, windows of discovery were defined (Hirota and Pedrycz, 1999), which exhibit different levels of granularity. For instance, a single number has the highest level of granularity; the interval exhibits a lower granularity level, which is followed by a fuzzy set, and a rough set representation. The lowest level of granularity would occur for a set covering the entire space.

1.5 Knowledge Discovery Process

Before outlining a knowledge discovery process, we say that the outcome of a knowledge discovery process may be presented in two ways: either "blindly" or by providing some insight into the "why" question, e.g., why the patient was classified as ischemic.

Methods providing blind descriptions, also called black box methods, include artificial neural networks that, given training data, e.g., the SPECT image data and the corresponding diagnosis, can obtain a correlation between the two. Neural networks have often been used in medicine for classification purposes.

The second approach is to use a knowledge discovery process, in such a way that its outcome provides some understanding of the "why" question, say, why the data correlate to certain diseases. The methods that can be used for this purpose include machine learning, fuzzy logic, and genetic algorithms. All these methods can generate production rules in the if...then format as their output. This is in striking contrast to a trained neural network, in which only weights, associated with edges interconnecting the neurons, are provided to the user (Cios and Liu, 1992). The knowledge discovery approach is particularly important in situations where heuristic features are selected, as they make sense to the user, as opposed to some artificial features, generated by the transformed space. To illustrate the point, in our previous work, 15 new diagnostic rules were discovered, using a machine learning algorithm applied to nuclear medicine data, as compared to 68 cardiologist-specified rules, to diagnose obstructions in major coronary arteries. These rules, that subsequently made sense to cardiologists, were not previously known to them, and were obtained directly from analysis of heart images (Cios et al., 1991). Below we describe the six-step knowledge discovery process (Cios et al. 1998, 2000; Chapman et al. 1999).

1.5.1 Understanding the Medical Problem Domain

In this step, one works closely with medical professionals, to define the problem, determine medical objectives, identify key people, and learn about current solutions to the problem. This step might include high-level description of the problem, its requirements and restrictions, and determination of success criteria from the medical point of view. After understanding the availability of human expertise and the database, a specific terminology must be acquired. A key sub-goal here is translating medical goals into data mining goals. Data mining success criteria also must be defined. Finally, one prepares the project plan, identifying all critical steps.

1.5.2 Understanding the Data

Understanding medical data includes the collection of initial data, for instance a sample of existing data, and preparing plans as to which data will be used, and which additional information will be needed. An important issue is to obtain approval from the Institutional Review Board, and then to encrypt all the patient data, so that even the data miner cannot decrypt the data. This step would certainly include, say, in addition to SPECT images, also clinical patient information, as well as the physician's interpretation, and might also involve ranking of data attributes. The database must be described, including its format, size, etc. The initial data exploration may answer some of the data mining goals, confirm initial hypotheses, or demand refinement of attributes. Finally, verification of data should answer questions about data completeness (all cases should be covered), redundancy, identification of erroneous data, missing attributes, checking plausibility of values of each attribute, etc.

1.5.3 Preparation of the Data

Preparation of the data is the key step upon which the success of the knowledge discovery process, and thus of the entire project, depends. It usually consumes at least half the entire project effort, and is a major contributor to its cost. In this step, we need to decide which data from a database will be used as input for data mining methods. The rationale for inclusion or exclusion of some data records needs to be justified. Significance and correlation tests will be performed, as well as sampling of the database. Next, the selected data are cleaned. This will include correcting, removing or ignoring noise, deciding how to deal with special values, missing values, etc. Construction of the data includes production of new data, for instance derivation of new attributes, discretization, and transformation of some attributes. Integration of the data involves creating new records from the constructed data, and aggregation of information (information granularization). Reformatting the data is performed to meet requirements of the specific data mining methods. This step may involve rearranging attributes and records. For example, in a study of embryonic human central nervous system development, the authors employed data mining methods to rearrange anatomic features into their apparent chronologic order of appearance in the embryo (O'Rahilly et al, 1984).

1.5.4 Data Mining

Data mining is another key step in the knowledge discovery process. Although it is the data mining methods that actually reveal new information, this step usually takes less time than preparation of the data. The data mining step involves selection of data modeling techniques, deciding on training and test procedures, building the model, and assessing its quality.

Data mining methods include many types of algorithms, such as rough sets, fuzzy sets, Bayesian methods, evolutionary computing, machine learning, neural networks, clustering, many preprocessing methods, etc. Rough sets and fuzzy sets emphasize the representation of data at the non-numeric level. Rough sets concentrate on an enriched set theoretic apparatus, while fuzzy sets are concerned with capturing the notion of a continuous transition between complete membership and complete non-membership. Both deliver some level of summarization (granularization) of data, with the intent to place all activities of data mining within the scope implied by hints from the user. Bayesian methods are based upon the assumption that a classification problem can be expressed in probabilistic terms. Evolutionary computing can be regarded as an optimization method driven by the biological principle of survival of the fittest. Machine learning is aimed at revealing the relationships in data. The result of such summarization is provided in the form of decision trees or production rules. Neural networks are geared toward processing numeric data and building nonlinear relationships between inputs and outputs. Clustering is a key unsupervised learning technique revealing natural groupings in the data. Finally, the goal of broadly understood preprocessing is to reduce the dimensionality of data. Thorough descriptions of all these methods, within the framework of the knowledge discovery process, can be found in a book by Cios et al. (1998).

1.5.5 Evaluation of the Discovered Knowledge

Evaluation of the discovered knowledge includes understanding the results, checking whether the new information is novel and interesting, medical interpretation of the results, and checking their impact on the medical goal. Approved models (results of different data mining methods) are retained. The entire knowledge discovery process will be analyzed to identify failures, misleading steps, and alternative actions that could have been taken. Determination of possible actions will include: ranking the actions, selection of the best ones, and documenting reasons for their choice.

1.5.6 Using the Discovered Knowledge

Using discovered knowledge is basically in the hands of the owner of the database. It should include a plan for medical implementation of the results, and identification of problems associated with implementation. A plan is prepared for monitoring the implementation. A final report is written to summarize the project outcome, and the project is reviewed for future applications.

1.6 Example System

Let us finally examine one example of a knowledge discovery system, Health-KEFIR (Key Findings Reporter). It is a domain dependent system, that is, it works only for this particular domain, which is used in healthcare as an early warning system (Fayyad et al., 1996). The system concentrates on ranking deviations according to measures of how interesting these events are to the user. It focuses on discovering and explaining key findings in large and dynamic databases. The system performs an automatic drill-down through data along multiple dimensions, in order to determine the most interesting deviations of specific quantitative measures relative to their previous and expected values. Deviations are a tool used in KEFIR to identify interesting patterns in the data. They are then ranked using a measure of "interestingness", such as looking at the actions that can be taken in response to the relevant deviation. KEFIR then generates explanations for the most interesting deviations, and may even generate recommendations for corresponding actions. KEFIR presents its findings in a hypertext report, using natural language and business graphics.

1.7 Further Web Information

In this section we provide several links to web sites, which provide even more links to a wealth of data mining and knowledge discovery information. Unfortunately there is no site devoted entirely to medical data mining. The list is intentionally short. By the time this book is printed some may be defunct, and many more will appear. Not to worry - if a site is any good you will find links to it via the links listed below. These sites differ widely in nature. Some are concerned with specific data mining methods, some provide you with data, one is the largest publicly accessible source of pathology data, some are very general, while others compare existing data mining and knowledge discovery tools. Happy surfing!

Battelle,

www.emsl.pnl.gov:2080/proj/neuron/neural/systems/shareware.html

CALD,

www.cs.cmu.edu/~cald/

CRISP-DM,

www.crisp-dm.org/

CWI,

dbs.cwi.nl:8080/cwwwi/owa/cwwwi.print_themes?ID=3

Data Mine,

www.cs.bham.ac.uk/~anp/TheDataMine.html

GMDH,

come.to/GMDH

IBM,

www.almaden.ibm.com/cs/quest/

Johns Hopkins Autopsy Resource,

www.netautopsy.org

KDD Results,

www.lri.fr/~lf/results/

Kluwer,

www.wkap.nl/journalhome.htm/1384-5810

Knowledge Discovery Mine,

www.kdnuggets.com

Los Alamos,

www.acl.lanl.gov/viz/

NASA COSMIC,

www.cosmic.uga.edu/maincat.html#45

Pisa KDD Lab,

www-kdd.di.unipi.it/

STATLOG Esprit Project,

www.ncc.up.pt/liacc/ML/statlog/

Text Mining Group,

textmining.krdl.org.sg/

UCI Machine Learning,

www.ics.uci.edu/AI/ML/Machine-Learning.html

References

Agrawal, R., Imielinski, T. and Swami, A. 1993. Database mining: A performance perspective. IEEE Trans. Knowledge and Data Eng., 5: 914-924

Chapman P., Clinton J., Khobaza T.T., Reinartz T. and Wirth R. 1999. The CRISP-DM process model: Discussion paper. CRISP-DM Consortium

Cios K.J., Shin I. and Goodenday L.S. 1991. Using fuzzy sets to diagnose coronary artery stenosis. IEEE Computer Magazine (special issue on Biomedical Engineering), 24(3):57-63

Cios K.J. and Liu N. 1992. Machine learning in generation of a neural network architecture: a Continuous ID3 approach. IEEE Trans. on Neural Networks, 3(2):280-291

Cios K.J. and Liu N. 1995. An algorithm which learns multiple covers via integer linear programming, Part I - the CLILP2 algorithm. Kybernetes 24(2):29-50, www.mcb.co.uk/literati/outst97.htm#k

Cios K.J., Wedding D.K. and Liu N. 1997. CLIP3: cover learning using integer programming. Kybernetes 26(4-5): 513-536

Cios, K.J., Pedrycz, W. and Swiniarski, R. 1998. Data Mining Methods for Knowledge Discovery. Kluwer, www.wkap.nl/book.htm/0-7923-8252-8

Cios K.J., Teresinska A., Konieczna S., Potocka J., Sharma S. 2000. Diagnosing Myocardial Perfusion from SPECT Bull's-eye Maps - A Knowledge Discovery Approach. IEEE Engineering in Medicine and Biology Magazine, Special issue on Medical Data Mining and Knowledge Discovery, July

Crevier D. and Lepage R. 1997. Knowledge-Based Image Understanding Systems: A Survey. Computer Vision and Image Understanding 67, 2 (August): 161-185

Elder-IV, J. F. and Pregibon, D. 1995. A statistical perspective on KDD.In: Proc. of the 1st Int. Conference on Knowledge Discovery and Data Mining, Montreal, 87-93

Fayyad, U.M., Piatetsky-Shapiro, G., Smyth, P. and Uthurusamy, R. (eds). 1996. Advances in Knowledge Discovery and Data Mining. MIT Press

Frawley, W. J., Piatetsky-Shapiro, G. and Matheus, C.J. 1991. Knowledge discovery in databases: an overview. In: Piatetsky-Shapiro, G. and Frawley, W.J. (eds.) Knowledge Discovery in Databases, AAAI/MIT Press, 1-27.

Fayyad, U.M. and Irani, K.B. 1992. On the handling of continuous-valued attributes in decision tree generation. Machine Learning, 8:87-102

Friedman J.H. 1997. "On bias, variance, 0/1 - loss, and the curse-of-dimensionality". Data Mining and Knowledge Discovery, 1(1): 55-77

Hirota, K. Pedrycz, W. 1999. Fuzzy sets in data mining. Proc. of the IEEE, September: 1575-1600

Matheus, C.J., Chan, P.K.and Piatetsky-Shapiro, G. 1993. Systems for knowledge discovery in databases. IEEE Trans. on Knowledge and Data Engineering, 5: 903-912

Moore G.W., Hutchins G.M. and Bulkley B.H. 1979. Certainty levels in the nullity method of symbolic logic: application to the pathogenesis of congenital heart malformations. J Theor Biol, 76:53-81.

Moore G.W. and Hutchins G.M. 1980. Effort and demand logic in medical decision making. Metamedicine. 1:277-304.

Moore G.W. and Hutchins G.M. 1981a. A Hintikka possible worlds model for certainty levels in medical decision making. Synthese. 48:87-119.

Moore G.W. and Hutchins G.M. 1981b. Three paradoxes of medical diagnosis. Metamedicine, 2:197-215.

Moore G.W., Hutchins G.M. and Miller R.E. 1986. Token swap test of significance for serial medical data bases. Am J Med, 80:182-190.

O'Rahilly R., Müller F., Hutchins G.M. and Moore G.W. 1984. Computer ranking of the sequence of appearance of 100 features of the brain and related structures in staged human embryos during the first 5 weeks of development. Am J Anat, 171:243-257.

Pawlak, Z. 1984. Rough classification. Int. J. of Man-Machine Studies, 20: 469-483

Ramakrishnan, R. et al.. 1998. Database Management Systems, Mc-Graw Hill

Zadeh, L.A. 1979. Fuzzy sets and information granularity, In: Gupta M. M. et al. (eds) Advances in Fuzzy Set Theory and Applications North Holland, 3-18

Zembowicz, R. and Zytkow, J.M. 1996. From contingency tables to various forms of knowledge in databases. In: Fayyad U., Piatetsky-Shapiro G., Smyth P. and Uthurusamy (eds.), Advances in Knowledge Discovery and Data Mining, AAAI Press, 329-349

2 Legal Policy and Security Issues in the Handling of Medical Data

Joseph M. Saul
Communications Technology Consultancy
Ann Arbor, Michigan, 48103, U.S.A.
jmsaul@ctconsultancy.com

Handling of data that can be identified with a specific person always requires an awareness of privacy and confidentiality issues, but where medical data is involved care is especially important. Researchers who use such data in academic research need to be aware of applicable laws and standards in their jurisdiction. In the United States, federal standards for security and privacy of individually identifiable health information have been released in draft form as part of the Health Insurance Portability and Accountability Act of 1996 (HIPAA), and many states already have laws restricting disclosure of such information. In the European Union, the EU Data Protection Directive, while it does not specify security standards, sets out strict handling practices for any kind of individually identifiable information. Canada has federal research guidelines, and several provinces have passed or are passing laws of their own on the topic. In this chapter, we summarize the applicable laws and discuss their implications for researchers using health data.

2.1 General Considerations

Public concern about privacy has increased drastically within the last few years as people have become aware that current technology permits the processing of massive amounts of data quickly, thus enabling those with access to the data to distribute it faster and make connections between pieces of information that could not be related to each other before. Nowhere is this concern more pointed, or more valid, than in the area of medical data. As a result, any researcher making use of medical data should be especially careful about security and privacy issues, and especially aware of the sensitivity of the data itself. Researchers should also be prepared to allay public concerns by demonstrating that they are using proper procedures and taking reasonable precautions in handling the data and making use of their results. Here are some general concepts:

Obtain Legal Advice—This chapter is not a substitute for legal advice from a practitioner familiar with the laws of the country and region where the research is taking place, as well as with the specific ways in which the data are to be used. Before undertaking a project involving medical data, researchers should consult their institution's legal counsel. The issues and rules discussed in this chapter are complex, and can pose a significant risk of liability, not only to the institution where the research takes place, but in some cases also to the researcher personally.

Use Anonymized Data If Possible—Wherever possible, researchers should use data which has had all information that can be used to identify a specific person removed before the researcher sees it. Doing so will take the researcher out of the reach of some laws, as well as making it far easier (and in many cases unnecessary) to get research approval from an institutional review board or equivalent. It will also minimize risks in case of a security breach. Be aware, however, that even information such as zip or postal codes and diagnoses can be used to identify a person if the medical condition is rare or the area is lightly populated.

Have Personnel Sign Security and Confidentiality Agreements—Any and all researchers and staff with access to individually identifiable health information should sign agreements stating that they understand the confidentiality and security practices to be followed and that they agree to follow them. (This is another area where the institution's legal counsel can be helpful.) This helps to educate them about appropriate practices. It also provides a certain amount of protection from liability as it demonstrates that they have been made aware of the rules, so any breaches are not a result of the institution or investigator's failure to inform the staff of their responsibilities.

Watch for Further Developments—Given the level of public concern about privacy, especially where medical records are involved, it is likely that more privacy-related legislation will be passed at a variety of governmental levels. In the United States, further federal legislation is possible pertaining to specific types of medical data (e.g. genetic testing results) and uses of the data. Also, HIPAA permits states to create security and privacy standards of their own, provided they are at least as stringent as HIPAA's. In Europe, the EU Privacy Directive allows member nations to impose more stringent standards as well. In Canada, not only is there uncertainty about the applicability of pending federal law, but new provincial laws are likely in the near future. This is a volatile area, and researchers working with medical data should make an effort to stay up to date with developments in their locality.

2.2 The United States

Researchers working in the United States need to be aware not only of federal law and human research guidelines, but also of any state laws that may exist about the handling of medical data. The guidelines based upon the Health Insurance Portability and Accountability Act (HIPAA) will not supersede stricter state laws.

2.2.1 The Health Insurance Portability and Accountability Act (HIPAA)

The Health Insurance Portability and Accountability Act of 1996, HIPAA (Public Law 104-191) is a federal law covering a wide range of issues related to health care. It is best known for its provisions on maintaining health coverage during job transfers, pre-existing conditions, and similar issues. HIPAA also has a section discussing electronic transfers of health information, however, and two provisions of the Act are especially relevant to researchers working with medical data. The first authorizes the Federal Department of Health and Human Services (DHHS) to lay out standards for security precautions that must be taken when handling individually-identifiable medical information. These standards, Security and Electronic Signature Standards (45 CFR §142), were released in draft form in August 1998. The second ordered DHHS to produce standards on the privacy of individually-identifiable medical information if Congress did not pass legislation in that area by August 1999. Congress failed to do so, and DHHS has produced a draft set of standards, Standards for Privacy of Individually Identifiable Health Information, (45 CFR §160-164). The Act also sets criminal penalties for "wrongful disclosure or knowing misuse" of individually identifiable health information.

2.2.1.1 Status of the HIPAA Standards

At this writing, only draft versions of both sets of standards exist, but final versions are expected within the year. Once final standards are released, there is a sixty-day period before they take effect; most institutions will then have two years after that date to comply (small institutions have three years) or face possible penalties. Researchers may well have to comply earlier, however — not only are many institutions already attempting to bring their policies into compliance, but it is expected that accreditation organizations (such as JCAHO, which reviews hospitals) will modify their requirements to harmonize them with the HIPAA provisions.

2.2.1.2 Applicability of the HIPAA Standards

Exemption of Anonymized Data—Both sets of standards, Security and Privacy, cover "individually identifiable health information," so truly anonymized data is exempt. The Privacy standard includes an extensive list of the pieces of information that have to be removed for data to be considered de-identified: name; address (including street address, city, county, zip code, and equivalent geocodes); names of relatives; name of employers; birth date; telephone and fax numbers; electronic mail addresses; social security number; medical record number; health plan beneficiary number; account number; certificate/license number; any vehicle or other device serial number; Web Universal Resource Locator (URL); Internet Protocol (IP) address number; finger or voice prints; photographic images; and any other unique identifying number, characteristic, or code that the covered entity has reason to believe may be available to an anticipated recipient of the information. If the receiving organization could put the remaining data together with other information available to it and identify individuals, the data will not be considered de-identified.

Form of Data—The standards only apply to information in electronic form or, in the case of the Privacy standards, to information that has been in electronic form at some point (the final Security standards might be extended to cover such information as well).

Type of Organization—They directly apply only to organizations involved in the provision of health care services (health plans, health care clearinghouses, and health care providers). Researchers working for a hospital, health center, or health plan/HMO will be directly subject to the standards. Anyone who receives data from such an organization, however, will likely be required to comply with the standards via contract. Both sets of standards include a provision requiring covered entities to make recipients of data from them sign a contract agreeing to protect it. The Privacy standard even gives details of what must be in that contract, including a provision requiring the recipient to make its records pertaining to the use of the information available to DHHS on request.

Criminal Provisions—The criminal penalties for wrongful disclosure or knowing misuse apply to anyone who commits the prohibited acts, regardless of how they obtained the information.

2.2.1.3 Enforcement of the HIPAA Standards

The standards are enforced solely by DHHS; private individuals cannot sue over violations of the Security or Privacy standards. DHHS can impose fines of up to $25,000 per person for violations of each standard within a single year ($100 per person per instance), and may in addition be able to get an injunction forcing the organization to stop engaging in the activity in question.

In addition, the Act provides criminal penalties for knowing misuse of individually identifiable health information: normally up to $50,000 and/or a year in prison; up to $100,000 and/or five years if done under false pretenses; and up to $250,000 and/or ten years if for commercial advantage, personal gain, or malicious harm. These latter penalties will probably not be triggered by simple failure to impose appropriate security, but as they have not yet been tested in court, it is impossible to say with certainty.

2.2.1.4 The HIPAA Security Standards

The Security Standards (45 CFR §142) are intended to ensure that individually identifiable health information in electronic form is appropriately protected, both in transit and in storage. They cover a broad range of issues, from administrative policies for personnel discipline, to control of access to systems and networks, to protection of data centers. They are divided into four categories: Administrative Procedures, Physical Safeguards, Technical Security Services, and Technical Security Mechanisms. Within each category are a set of requirements, many with specific features that must be part of the implementation. In most cases, it is not enough to simply put the measures into practice; they must be backed up by "formal, documented" policies. While the standards do list specific features that must be present, they avoid specifying particular technologies, and the drafters make it clear that different organizations can implement the standards in different ways.

This section provides a summary of the requirements and implementation details (if any) in each category. Space does not permit a detailed explanation of each requirement, but the summary should give an idea of the scope of the standards and their relevance to a given organization. Required implementation features are generally quoted directly from the regulations. Obviously, some of these requirements are institution-wide; actually implementing some of the requirements would be outside the scope of most researchers' authority or responsibility.

Administrative Procedures—this category includes administrative policies and procedures; technical implementation comes in the later sections. Requirements in this category are:

- Certification (policies to evaluate and certify that appropriate security measures are in place)
- Chain of Trust Partner Agreements (contracts between the organization and any outside parties given access to individually identifiable health information, requiring the outside parties to protect the data)
- Contingency Plans (for response to emergencies; must include applications and data criticality analysis, a data backup plan, a disaster recovery plan, an emergency mode operation plan, and testing and revision procedures)
- Formal Mechanism for Processing Records (to limit risks due to processing issues)
- Information Access Control (must include policies for the authorization, establishment, and modification of access privileges)
- Internal Audit (an ongoing review of access records, etc., to identify possible security violations)
- Personnel Security (the organization must ensure supervision of personnel performing technical systems maintenance activities by

authorized, knowledgeable persons; maintain access authorization records; ensure that operating, and in some cases, maintenance personnel have proper access; employ personnel clearance procedures; employ personnel security policy/procedures; and ensure that system users, including technical maintenance personnel, are trained in system security)

- Security Configuration Management (coordinated and integrated procedures for system security; must include documentation, hardware/software installation and maintenance review and testing for security features, inventory procedures, security testing, and virus checking)
- Security Incident Procedures (must include both reporting and response procedures)
- Security Management Process (must include risk analysis, risk management, a sanction policy, and a security policy)
- Termination Procedures (to be performed when an employee leaves or loses access to the data; must include changing combination locks, removal from access lists, removal of user account(s), and turning in of keys, tokens, or cards that allow access)
- Training (security training for all staff; must include awareness training for all personnel, including management, periodic security reminders, user education concerning virus protection, user education in importance of monitoring login success/failure, and how to report discrepancies, and user education in password management)

Physical Safeguards—this category includes requirements to control and monitor physical access to systems and storage devices. Requirements in this category are:

- Assigned Security Responsibility (responsibility for security measures and personnel conduct regarding security has to be assigned to a specific person or organization)

- Media Controls (procedures covering the transport of data and software into and out of a facility; must include controls on access to media, accountability, data backup, data storage, and disposal)
- Physical Access Controls (procedures for preventing unauthorized physical access to a facility while ensuring access for those who should have it; must include disaster recovery, emergency mode operation, equipment control, a facility security plan, procedures for verifying access authorizations prior to physical access, maintenance records, need-to-know procedures for personnel access, sign-in for visitors and escort if appropriate, and testing and revision)
- Policy/Guideline on Workstation Use (how to use workstations so as to maximize security of information, e.g. log off after use)
- Secure Workstation Location (placement of workstations so as to minimize the risk of unauthorized access to information)
- Security Awareness Training (for all personnel, including contractors and the like)

Technical Security Services—this category includes requirements for technical features to control access to information and permit auditing of access. Requirements in this category are:

- Access Control (must include a procedure for emergency access, plus either context-based, role-based, or user-based control of access; encryption is optional)
- Audit Controls (recording and examination of system activity)
- Authorization Control (for obtaining consent to access information; must use either role-based or user-based control)
- Data Authentication (the ability to confirm that data has not been changed or deleted; possible methods include checksums or digital signatures, etc.)
- Entity Authentication (the ability to confirm that a person or organization accessing data is who or what they claim to be; must include automatic log off and unique user identification, as well as at least one of the following implementation features: a biometric identification system, a password system, a personal identification number, telephone callback, or a token system which uses a physical device for user identification)

Technical Security Mechanisms—protecting information as it travels over internal or external networks. There is only one requirement in this category:

- Communications/Network Controls (must include integrity controls and message authentication, plus either access controls or encryption; if data travels over a network, implementation must also include alarms, audit trails, entity authentication, and event reporting)

While the Security standards are fairly detailed, and unusual in that government has not made a practice of specifying mandatory standards for information security practices in the past, they are generally in line with current thinking on good security practices, and allow a fair amount of flexibility in their implementation.

2.2.1.5 The HIPAA Privacy Standards

The Privacy standards (45 CFR §164) are intended to ensure that individually identifiable health information is only provided to those who should have it, while ensuring that those who need to have it can get access to it. They are generally directed towards those who maintain and collect medical data as part of their core business, i.e. potential suppliers, rather than pure users, of data. As a result, most of the privacy regulations are not of direct relevance to researchers, who are accustomed to anonymizing data before publication and do not generally pass raw data on to others. They will, however, affect what data researchers can obtain from health care organizations, and may lead such organizations to be more reluctant to supply data sets because they will have to make the effort to anonymize them first.

Permission—In general, one must obtain permission from the individuals involved to use individually identifiable health information. There are, however, exemptions. One that may be relevant to researchers is for public health authorities or government agencies conducting or those acting at their direction. There is also an exemption for research use, but the request for the data must be reviewed either by an Institutional Review Board (established in accordance with the federal regulations for such boards) or a Privacy Board (for which the standards establish criteria) before the organization with the data is permitted to disclose it. In order to get approval to use identifiable health information without informed consent from all subjects, the researcher will have to show that:

(1) The use or disclosure of protected health information involves no more than minimal risk to the subjects;

(2) The waiver will not adversely affect the rights and welfare of the subjects;

(3) The research could not practicably be conducted without the waiver;

(4) Whenever appropriate, the subjects will be provided with additional pertinent information after participation;

(5) The research could not practicably be conducted without access to and use of the protected health information;

(6) The research is of sufficient importance so as to outweigh the intrusion of the privacy of the individual whose information is subject to the disclosure;

(7) There is an adequate plan to protect the identifiers from improper use and disclosure; and

(8) There is an adequate plan to destroy the identifiers at the earliest opportunity consistent with conduct of the research, unless there is a health or research justification for retaining the identifiers. (45 CFR §164.510[j])

Need for Protected Information—If the data do not have to be individually identifiable in order to perform the research, the holder of the data (assuming the holder is an organization subject to the standards) must anonymize it before the researcher gets it. This is true whether consent is obtained or not; covered organizations are required to avoid divulging any more than is actually necessary to accomplish the intended purpose.

This is actually beneficial to researchers in that, if they don't have individually-identifiable health information in their possession, they don't have to worry about the Security standards. Researchers should carefully weigh the perceived need for information such as zip codes (which could be necessary for epidemiological studies, for example), which could be regarded as making the data non-anonymized in combination with other information.

Disclosure—Researchers do not ordinarily provide raw data including personal identifiers to other organizations; it is not, therefore, worthwhile to detail the extensive regulations on disclosure here. Researchers who are part of organizations to which HIPAA directly applies should be aware that the Privacy standards place a number of restrictions on disclosure. Transfers of identifiable health data to colleagues at other institutions will be possible only with approval from their institution's Privacy Officer (a position mandated by the standards), only if certain criteria are met, and the other institution will have to sign an agreement to protect the data's confidentiality. Research organizations that are not directly governed by HIPAA, but receive data from organizations that are, will likely have to sign agreements barring them from making such disclosures.

2.2.2 The Common Rule

The "Common Rule" (the DHHS version is at 45 CFR §46) is intended to protect human subjects of federally-funded research. It lays out guidelines for what research must be approved by an Institutional Review Board (IRB), and the guidelines the IRB must follow in determining the approval and required procedures. Since individuals whose personal information is used for research are considered to be research subjects, the Common Rule can apply to medical data mining.

2.2.2.1 Status of the Common Rule

The Common Rule is currently in force; the most recent revision was in 1991.

2.2.2.2 Applicability of the Common Rule

At present, it applies to all federally-funded research involving human subjects, with some exceptions. (The most relevant to researchers performing data mining of medical data is one for the use of data that has already been collected, provided the researcher records it in such a manner that subjects cannot be identified. Under the HIPAA Privacy standards, researchers themselves would not be allowed to see identifiable data unless it was necessary for the research and they received approval, so this exemption will effectively cease to exist.) The HIPAA Privacy standards will place other research under the authority of Institutional Review Boards as well. An increasing number of institutions which receive some federal funding are now requiring that all research involving human subjects, except that which qualifies for an exemption, must be conducted subject to the policy.

Researchers using solely anonymized data should be able to receive an exemption from their IRB, as the use of anonymized data does not put subjects at risk.

2.2.2.3 Enforcement of the Common Rule

The federal government may terminate funding for any project that is not in compliance. Of late, several institutions have had all federal research funding suspended or terminated based on violations that did not necessarily involve all projects at the institution.

2.2.2.4 Common Rule Provisions

All research subject to the regulation must be approved by the institution's Institutional Review Board. The IRB will approve it only if the following criteria are met:

> (1) Risks to subjects are minimized...
>
> (2) Risks to subjects are reasonable in relation to anticipated benefits, if any, to subjects, and the importance of the knowledge that may reasonably be expected to result...
>
> (3) Selection of subjects is equitable...
>
> (4) Informed consent will be sought from each prospective subject or the subject's legally authorized representative...
>
> (5) Informed consent will be appropriately documented...
>
> (6) When appropriate, the research plan makes adequate provision for monitoring the data collected to ensure the safety of subjects.
>
> (7) When appropriate, there are adequate provisions to protect the privacy of subjects and to maintain the confidentiality of data. (45 CFR §46.111[a])

The IRB also has the ability to terminate covered research it feels is violating the guidelines. Rules where children are involved are more restrictive.

2.2.3 State Medical Records Laws

Many individual states have laws regulating the disclosure and use of medical information, though they generally apply only to insurance companies (e.g. barring the use of genetic testing information in decisions about whether to provide coverage to an individual) or employers. It is not practical to attempt to discuss all of them here. Some types of data—examples being HIV status, sexually-transmitted disease information, information on drug abuse, psychiatric records, and records of children—are more likely to have additional restrictions imposed upon their disclosure, or permit patients to withhold those portions of the record.

As yet, no state requires specific security practices for the handling of individually identifiable health information. HIPAA, however, does permit states to pass their own regulations on privacy and security of medical data, providing those regulations are at least as restrictive as the HIPAA ones are. It is certainly possible that states will do so in the future.

2.3 The European Union

The standard for laws on the privacy of personal information for member states of the European Union was set by the European Union Data Protection Directive (Directive 95/46/EC). Laws of member states must be at least as protective of privacy as is spelled out in the Directive. The Data Protection Directive lays out only very general requirements for system security, but has strong and far-reaching provisions to protect individual privacy.

2.3.1 The Data Protection Directive

2.3.1.1 Status of the Data Protection Directive

The Data Protection Directive came into force in October 1998. It is currently in force, though some governments have not yet implemented it. The European Union filed suits against a number of European governments in January 2000 for failing to comply with the Directive.

2.3.1.2 Applicability of the Data Protection Directive

National Application—As a European Union regulation, the Data Protection Directive only directly applies to EU member countries. Researchers in other nations should, however, be aware that it has a provision forbidding the transfer of personal data from a member country to any nation without sufficient privacy protections—although individual organizations in such nations can get clearance to receive data by demonstrating that the organization is in compliance. It can, as a number of financial services companies have found, wind up being relevant to organizations even outside the EU. Negotiations are currently in progress between the United States and the European Union on the transfer of personal data.

Activities Covered—The Directive applies to all automated processing, or use in even a non-automated filing system, of "personal data," i.e. all data that relates to an identifiable person. It does not, therefore, apply to anonymized data.

2.3.1.3 Enforcement of the Data Protection Directive

Member nations are required to provide a judicial remedy for violations of their privacy laws, and permit individuals who have been harmed by a disclosure to recover damages for that disclosure. Harmed individuals in nations that have not yet passed privacy laws consistent with the Directive can sue in the EU courts.

2.3.1.4 Data Protection Directive Provisions

Health Data—Processing of personal data relating to the health of an individual is prohibited unless:

- The individual gives explicit consent, or
- The processing is necessary as part of the individual's medical care, and is performed by a health care professional or someone subject to an equivalent "obligation of secrecy."

Individual nations may establish other exemptions for reasons of "important public interest," but the most relevant ones for researchers seeking to use health data are the two listed.

Notification of Subjects—If the data are collected directly from the subjects, the collector must tell them who is collecting the data, why it is being collected, and who else will be getting the data, as well as the fact that subjects have the right to correct inaccurate data about them. If the data are obtained from a third party, that third party may have an obligation to notify the subjects as above. This obligation is waived for scientific research or statistical purposes if "the provision of information proves impossible or involves a disproportionate effort" or if the member state already has specific laws regarding recording or disclosure in that context.

Notification of the Government—Those wishing to process data must notify whatever supervisory authority their nation has established for dealing with data privacy issues before beginning automated processing of personal data for a given purpose. (At academic institutions, this will probably be part of the research approval procedure.)

Security—The security provision is more general than the United States' HIPAA security standards, requiring the controller of the data to implement technical and organizational measures that "ensure a level of security appropriate to the risks represented by the processing and the nature of the data to be protected." The data must be protected against destruction, modification, or access, as well as against "unlawful forms of processing." The provision states that security measures are particularly important when the data is traveling over a network.

If the controller of a set of data needs to transfer it to a third party for processing, they must execute a contract requiring the processor to follow the same regulations that apply to the controller of the data. It is the controller's responsibility to make sure that the processor has adequate security measures in place.

While the Data Protection Directive does not give specific direction on security measures, individual member states may do so. One possible model for such standards may be British Standard 7799, which lays out a set of appropriate security practices and procedures. The lack of specific standards is actually more dangerous to those handling protected data than a set of standards would be. It is impossible to know what a court would consider "appropriate" until the laws have been tested.

2.4 Canada

Canadian researchers primarily need to be concerned with the Tri-Council Code (promulgated by the federal councils that fund research, but applied by institutions that receive any such funding even to research that is not funded by one of the councils) and the laws of the province within which they operate. Canadian federal laws on information privacy, including the proposed Bill C-6, will probably not affect academic research but should be watched closely over the next few years.

2.4.1 The Personal Information Protection and Electronic Documents Act (Bill C-6)

Though Bill C-6 is wide-reaching and high-profile, it will not apply to most academic research uses of data. First, there is some question about the applicability of a federal law to activities that occur solely within a single province. Second, Bill C-6 is limited to for-profit activity. It governs inter-provincial data transfers "for consideration," but it is uncertain whether the providing of data for research in exchange for printed credit or the opportunity to benefit from publicly-printed research results would be covered. Issues relating to provision of data in exchange for "finders' fees," and research funded by commercial organizations, are as yet unresolved. As a result, we will not discuss the provisions of Bill C-6 here.

In any event, the provisions of the Act will not apply to transactions of personal health information across provincial lines until 1 January 2002, or to activities within a province until 1 January 2004.

2.4.2 The Tri-Council Code

The Tri-Council Code is a set of guidelines for research involving human subjects. It was developed by representatives of the Medical Research Council of Canada, the Natural Sciences and Engineering Research Council of Canada, and the Social Sciences and Humanities Research Council of Canada.

2.4.2.1 Status of the Tri-Council Code

The Tri-Council Code is currently in force.

2.4.2.2 Applicability of the Tri-Council Code

Funding Source — The Tri-Council Code most directly applies to research funded by one of the councils. Its provisions, however, require that it be applied to all research involving human subjects regardless of funding source. The Code, therefore, applies in practice to all research involving human subjects that is conducted at an institution receiving any funding from one or more of the councils.

Covered Data — The Code applies to all research involving human subjects. Research involving the use of any non-public data about human subjects is considered to involve human subjects, even if the data has been anonymized. Research using purely information in the public domain, including archival documents, is not considered to involve human subjects.

2.4.2.3 Enforcement of the Tri-Council Code

The councils can refuse to fund or withdraw funding from projects that fail to adhere to the Code. Institutions are expected to refuse to approve non-complying projects.

2.4.2.4 Tri-Council Code Provisions

All research involving human subjects must be reviewed for compliance with the Code by the institution's Research Ethics Board (REB). The REB has the power to disallow research that does not comply. Requirements include:

Informed Choice —Subjects must be competent to consent, must be informed well enough to understand the risks of participation, and must not be coerced into participating. Researchers have to tell participants about:

a) conditions under which identifying information will be released to third parties and the identification of those third parties;

b) any modes of observation (e.g., photographs or videos) or access to information (e.g., sound recordings) in the research that allows identification of particular participants;

c) any anticipated secondary uses of data from the research;

d) any anticipated linkage of data gathered in the research with other data about participants, whether that data are contained in public or private records; and

e) provisions for confidentiality in publications resulting from the research. (Tri-Council Code, Article 3.2.)

Confidentiality — "Adequate provision" must be made for keeping data confidential. Researchers who want access to identifiable information must demonstrate that:

a) identifying information is essential to the research; and

b) they have taken appropriate measures to protect the privacy of the individuals, to ensure the confidentiality of the data, and to minimize harms to participants. (Tri-Council Code, Article 3.3.)

While the Code does not mandate specific security measures, this provision can be read as requiring measures to secure the data that are commensurate with its sensitivity.

Secondary Use of Data — Secondary use is the use of preexisting information, instead of collecting information specifically for the project. If identifiable data is involved, such use must be approved by the REB. Approval is not required for secondary use of non-identifiable data.

Secondary use complicates the issue of consent. If the risks of use of the data are low, the REB may simply require that researchers meet the confidentiality regulations but waive consent. At the other end of the spectrum, they may require full informed consent as described above, or may at least require that the participants be informed. Where it is extremely difficult to locate the participants, one possible alternative is to consult with representative members of the affected group (the example cited is consulting an AIDS advocacy group where data from AIDS patients is involved) or polling a representative sample of the participant pool.

If researchers need to contact the subjects of the data, e.g. to obtain additional information, they may be required to do so through the party that originally collected the data.

Data Linkage — linkage of multiple databases that may result in identification of research participants must be approved by the REB, and as few people as possible should be involved in the linking process.

Anonymized Data — Research using anonymized data is still subject to REB review. If the REB finds that the data is actually anonymized, they should permit access. In making their decision, however, they are instructed to consider the possibility that the data in question could be linked with other available data to identify individuals.

2.4.3 Provincial Laws

Several provinces — among them Alberta, British Columbia, and Quebec — have legislation proposed or in force on the topic of information privacy. Others are likely to follow, given the provision in Bill C-6 allowing "comparable" provincial laws to trump the federal legislation. For activities conducted solely within a province, these laws will be the most relevant. Unfortunately, they differ from province to province, and it is not feasible to outline them in detail here. Researchers should stay aware of developments in information privacy within their province, as this is a volatile area.

Acknowledgements

Thanks to Tom Fitzpatrick and Melanie Millar of the Office of the Privacy Commissioner of Canada, and Michael Yeo of the Canadian Medical Association, for answering questions on Canadian law.

References

References are organized by nation (or supranational organization, in the case of the European Community) and follow US legal citation standards.

United States

The Health Insurance Portability and Accountability Act of 1996, Public Law 104-191.

Security and Electronic Signature Standards, 63 Federal Register 43,242 (1998) (to be codified at 45 C.F.R. §142) (proposed Aug. 12, 1998).

Standards for Privacy of Individually Identifiable Health Information, 64 Federal Register 59,918 (1999) (to be codified at 45 C.F.R. §160-164) (proposed Nov. 3, 1999).

Protection of Human Subjects ("The Common Rule"), 45 C.F.R. §46 (1999).

European Community

Council Directive 95/46/EC of 24 October 1995 On The Protection Of Individuals With Regard To The Processing Of Personal Data And On The Free Movement Of Such Data, 1995 O.J. (L 281) 31.

Canada

Tri-Council, Tri-Council Policy Statement: Ethical Conduct for Research Involving Humans (July 1997).

Personal Information Protection and Electronic Documents Act, Bill C-6, 2nd Ses., 36th Parl., 48 Elizabeth II, 1999.

3 Medical Natural Language Understanding as a Supporting Technology for Data Mining in Healthcare.

Werner Ceusters
Language and Computing
B9520 - Zonnegem, Belgium
www.landc.be

In this chapter, we describe the role of language engineering techniques in text mining, a discipline focusing on information extraction from free texts. Indeed, text mining expands the idea of data mining in structured databases towards information discovering in natural language documents. After an introduction of the various tools and techniques that are available for text mining from the linguistic engineering point of view, we concentrate on a specific application in the domain of medicine.

3.1 Understanding the Problem Domain

3.1.1 Introduction

Medicine is one of these complex domains where new knowledge is accumulated at a daily basis, and at an exponential rate. Most of this knowledge resides in textbooks and papers, a big portion of them resulting from studies conducted on data and information accumulated in patient records. Despite the growing tendency to make this information available in electronic format, turning the information into knowledge is not an easy task. Indeed, faithful recording of patient data can only be achieved by using natural language. This was already stated in the early eighties by Wiederhold who claimed that *the description of biological variability requires the flexibility of natural language and it is generally desirable not to interfere with the traditional manner of medical recording* (Wiederhold 1980). At the other hand, it is evenly true that without proper mechanisms in place, free natural language registrations are impossible to be understood by machines, if not to say, quite often also by colleagues. Very often, medical statements are written down in a context that is obvious at the time of registration, but that is difficult to reconstruct later on by third parties, or even by the original source. Also, in order to allow a computer to process healthcare data further such as for data mining purposes, the data must be available in a coded and structured format. Making that happen in a transparent way for healthcare specialists, is the ultimate goal, if not even the "raison d'être" of natural language understanding applications in healthcare. A necessary condition is however that systems could be built that transform sentences into a meaning representation that is independent of the subtleties of linguistic structure that nevertheless underlie the way language works (Bateman et al. 1995).

Natural language processing systems are already looked at since the sixties, though mostly only in academic environments. Now it is recognised by major technology consultants in the healthcare domain as an emerging technology with great prospects for the near future. Real applications start to become available, and once the current problems related to continuous speech recognition will be solved, a massive penetration of natural language understanding applications will undoubtedly occur.

In this paper, we give an overview of the many faces of language engineering applications, focusing on their impact on data mining in healthcare. It is not the idea to give a detailed course in theoretical computational linguistics. In line with the new ideas on successful management in business, we prefer to pay attention to solutions, while not loosing time by focusing too much on the problems (Drucker et al. 1997).

3.1.2 The Many Faces of Language Engineering

3.1.2.1 Definitions

The development of a machine that understands a human being has been a great dream ever since the beginning of computers. Proof of that are the numerous science-fiction stories in which a computer is addressed in ordinary human speech, i.e. natural language, upon which the machine promptly answers with a metallic sounding voice. The obstacles between that dream and today's reality are still enormous, but the light is beginning to shine in certain specialised domains.

Natural language processing applications come in many flavours. At the heart of the technology is a specific discipline of science called *computational linguistics*, aiming to develop computational models of language that explain how language works in human beings, and how this insight can be used to allow computers to work with language. If the focus is more on the development of practical applications rather than on theoretical studies, the term *linguistic engineering* is preferred.

As with many disciplines, sub-branches of linguistic engineering emerged very quickly. A first major division is to be recognised between *language processing* and *speech processing*. The basic aim of *speech processing* or *speech recognition* is to turn the sound wave generated by a speaking human being into a digitally represented text, f.i. by using the ASCI set of characters. Speech recognition is not be confused with *voice recognition* which aims to identify or authenticate individual people based on some physical characteristics of their voice.

The result of a speech recognition application can be used in word processors or printed on paper. The computer processing the speech signal has however no understanding of the meaning of what has been said, nor is the resulting text by any means a representation that is immediately understood by the machine. *Language processing* at the other hand starts with the verbal representation of - say - an ASCI text, and uses this format to do some further useful processing.

A second major subdivision that cuts orthogonally through the previous one, is whether or not understanding of speech or language is at stake. It is possible to do many tricks with language - and even to build very useful applications by doing so - without a need for true understanding of spoken or written texts. Many information retrieval packages operate in this way by doing string searches, some basic stemming procedures - such as transforming conjugated verbs or plurals to their base form - and counting words, with fairly adequate success. Also the *command & control* paradigm where a computer user can dictate commands to a computer instead of using a mouse, belongs to this class. For this kind of applications, the general terms *natural language processing*, versus *speech processing* apply, whereas if true understanding is achieved, the term *natural language understanding* is preferred.

A third division has to do with the direction of processing. While generally with natural language understanding, *natural language analysis* is understood (going from a text to its meaning), the opposite (going from a meaning representation to a text) is called *natural language generation*. For speech applications, the terms *speech-to-text* or *text-to-speech* are often used. Be aware that also here the understanding issue cuts orthogonally through the applications. It is perfectly possible to have text-to-speech applications that do not understand what is being said. Also specific paradigms of *machine translation* work quite well without deep understanding of the texts that must be translated.

Natural Language Understanding is being considered as one of the most complex problems in artificial intelligence. Up to now, a computer is not yet capable of really understanding the true meaning of ordinary human language. The necessary background knowledge is so extensive and complex that even today's description-possibilities are unable to describe everything. Food for thought is the idea that a human child needs at least six years to adopt a language and that even today's supercomputers don't posses even a fraction of the comprehension capabilities of the human brain.

However ! Under certain specific circumstances it is possible to have a computer understand natural language. Medical language, as a sub-language of ordinary human language, is a field that complies in an excellent way with the 'specific circumstances' required: a closed world with restricted domains and disciplines easily separated from each other, a relatively uniform terminology, and the availability of numerous descriptions (textbooks, classifications, ...). Because the principles of understanding natural language in the world of medicine could have immediate and huge advantages, the conception of systems to make a machine understand medical language has been a field of research for nearly 20 years. The results of this research are now becoming available as *medical natural language understanding*.

3.1.2.2 Natural Language Understanding Applications for Healthcare Telematics

There are numerous applications for which medical language technology may pay off. Quite a bit of those have an immediate added value in the present and future clinical-care organisations, most often as enabling tools in the field of traditional telematics. Medical Language Technology is the new engine that will provide the power to stimulate the next generation of medical software applications. Table 1 summarises the possibilities. Some are discussed more deeply in the following paragraphs.

3.1.2.2.1 Automatic Encoding

To overcome the problems related to the use of natural language in communication and clinical registration, coding and classification systems have been introduced as interlingua. Systems such as ICD, Snomed International, ICPC, CPT and many others are now widely used to register medical findings, diagnoses or procedures. Similarly, terminological systems such as NIC, NANDA, ICNP and others are proposed to be used as interlingua in a nursing environment.

- semi- and full-automatic ICD-registration and coding based on full-text-reports.
- medical terminology-management on all levels (departmental, hospital, HMO, National)
- natural-language data-entry-facilities for EPR-systems
- tools for building, selection and evaluation of clinical guidelines on all levels (departmental, hospital, HMO, national)
- automatic translation of medical files into a multiple range of languages (for telematic or telemedicine-purposes)
- automatic conversion of medical files into different classifications and mapping between classifications (ICD9, ICD10, Snomed, CPT4, UMLS, Mesh, Read, ICPC, ICNP, CISP, ...)
- tools for medical-data-cleaning and uniformisation for datawarehouses
- tools for full-text-retrieval and semantic searches
- access tools for internal and external knowledge-bases

Table 1. Use of NLU in the healthcare domain.

Coding patient data means that a physician (or professional encoder) has to describe the patient data by means of codes that are a kind of placeholders for the concepts available in systems such as ICD. The requirements to be met in order to perform the coding task adequately are (Ceusters et al. 1996) : 1) a perfect understanding of the meaning of the patient data (the source concepts), 2) a perfect understanding of the meaning of the concepts available in the concept system (the target concepts), 3) at least a certain level of similarity and coherence between the source concepts and target concepts, 4) facilities to search the concept system for the target concept(s) that match(es) a given source concept as closely as possible.

It is common knowledge that coding performed by humans is of rather low quality, both in terms of recall/precision, inter-rater variability, and even reproducibility by the same team. Natural language understanding tools can improve coding quality dramatically.

3.1.2.2.2 Medical Terminology Management

Coded data are the most convenient way for computers to turn data into information. This is the main reason for the success of coding and classification systems. Hélas, the one omni-potent classification system that fulfils the needs of all doctors, nurses, hospital managers, governments, librarians and international organisations, has yet to be developed. We are even quite convinced it never will be built ! There always will be a need for local variations, for additional dimensions, for greater detail, etc. And as long as a variety of systems continues to be available, the need for integration, mappings and translations will also continue to exist.

That is why people working in the domain of medical natural language processing invest in the development of tools that allow them to work with various classifications, without however becoming too much dependent on them. Assisted by such language analysis tools, mappings can be created from local systems to any other, while guaranteeing that they will remain compatible with future and previous versions. By doing so, users can be sure that their precious data don't become worthless once a new version of an official classification system becomes available.

3.1.2.2.3 Natural Language Data Entry

Continuous speech recognition software will soon become available at a level of quality that is acceptable to be used in routine medical practice. Discontinuous speech applications are on the market since many years but cannot be said to be a big success. Speaking discontinuously, i.e. pausing after each word or word cluster, is not really practical. Also "command and control" speech applications where - if we may say so - not just the keyboard is replaced by a microphone, but also the mouse movements are to be guided by the voice ("go to medication", "enter 3 tablets of Aspirin", "go back", ...) are only useful in some uncommon situations where it is impossible to use the hands to operate a mouse, light pen, keyboard, or whatever other "conventional" input device.

The availability of continuous speech recognition software will have as consequence that the structured data entry of today will disappear gradually, probably even completely in a not so far future. This requires for powerful full text understanding systems that can capture the true semantics of what is said by the user. For specific domains (radiology, pneumology, ...), such "text-to-meaning" applications are already available, and this in various languages. Interest in such systems is constantly growing thanks to XML, a format that is perfectly suited to capture the recursively embedded meaning-representations resulting from free text analysis.

3.1.2.2.4 Clinical Trials and Practice Guidelines

Language understanding services are needed when free text entries (whether being full text or short phrases) entered in a certain context, are to be used for other purposes. A typical example is matching patient selection criteria for clinical trials. It is not easy for a physician seeing patients on a routinely basis to bear in mind constantly what clinical trials are running in his department, and what criteria must be met by a patient to enter a trial. It is not feasible to run over the inclusion criteria for each single patient during an encounter. It is more sensible to have a software "watchdog" that constantly monitors the data entered by a physician, and that produces an alert when specific criteria are met. If data are entered in free text, this means that such a watchdog must have enough language understanding power to identify "numbness in left lower leg since last week" as satisfying an inclusion criterion such as "sensory disorders of the limbs lasting for more than 24 hours".

The same goes for checking whether or not practice guidelines are followed when registering patient data, or to generate other alerts upon specific criteria.

3.1.2.2.5 Intelligent Querying, Information Retrieval

Many electronic patient record systems keep collections of text documents (discharge summaries, referral letters, surgery reports, ...) related to individual patients. Documents in these "result servers" are only accessible through general indicators such as the original source, the kind of document or the creation data. Searching documents on the basis of their content is seldom possible, or only by means of string search or some crude pattern matching mechanisms with jokers. Natural language understanding techniques can add a lot of functionalities to these primitive mechanisms.

Searches could be improved by using a thesaurus. A basic problem is however where to get one that is suitable for your needs. For medical bibliographic retrieval, one could use the well known MESH thesaurus from the National Library of Medicine. But this thesaurus is largely insufficient to be used in clinical practice. With the proper natural language processing tools, special purpose thesauri that respond to local demands can be built.

Having a thesaurus is not enough. The next step is to attach thesaurus entries to the documents. This is the problem of indexing. Traditionally, indexing is done manually. Professional indexers read a document, and assign the relevant thesaurus entries to it. Natural language understanding software is able to automate this process partly or even completely. The result is an electronic index that gives you fast access to documents on the basis of their "conceptual content" and not limited to the occurrence of specific words.

However, this is not the end of the story. Using a thesaurus to index properly a collection of documents, guarantees that you will find all (and not more) the documents that you need, provided that you know perfectly the terminology used in the thesaurus. To overcome this restriction, "query enhancement" techniques can be used to match a user's query to one or more relevant thesaurus entries. This requires the use of a semantic network.

3.1.2.2.6 Text Mining

Together with the recent interest in data mining, also *text mining* has been introduced as a new discipline. Text mining applications support knowledge workers who must extract meaning and relevance from large amounts of information available in textual format. Both text and data mining have much in common with archeology, because underlying each is the assumption that knowledge lies buried in a scattered mass of information.

Typical text mining applications cluster documents in sets that have a common semantic basis. The semantic basis can be queried beforehand by the user, or discovered automatically by the software using statistical techniques. Other text mining applications try to summarize documents, or pinpoint the user to parts of documents that contain information that the user probably did not see before.

3.2 Understanding the Data

3.2.1 Types of Knowledge

The different forms of knowledge that traditionally are claimed to be required for proper written text understanding are: *morphology*, *syntax*, *semantics*, *pragmatics* and *discourse* or *world knowledge* (Allen 1987). It is obvious that these forms of knowledge do not stand on their own, but that they are tightly related. At morphological level, inflection may be seen as a pure syntactic phenomenon, whereas compounding is merely guided by semantic principles. The actual form of a sentence depends amongst others on the situation under which a meaning is to be conveyed. As such pragmatics and discourse have an influence on syntax. Some authors even deny or reduce the distinction between some of these kinds of knowledge. Quine for instance showed that semantic knowledge and world knowledge cannot sharply be delineated (Quine, 1953).

When dealing with terminology rich domains and with automated knowledge acquisition from written text understanding as a primary goal, it is possible to simplify the picture and to adopt a rather reductionist view. First, we can abstract away from the discourse level. Authors of medical textbooks, developers of terminologies or physicians writing patient reports, merely want to convey facts, and not to invoke emotions or to initiate actions by the reader. As such, we can limit our analysis to what in the speech-act literature is known as *constative inscriptions*, sentences uttered in a descriptive context (Searle et al. 1980), however without being too narrow as is the case in the traditional formal linguistic semantics scene where sentence-meaning is viewed as being exhausted by propositional content and is truth-conditionally explicable (Bach 1989).

We also can abstract away from pragmatics - although not ignore its existence - as it is not our aim to provide theories on how context changes the surface forms of the expressions we are looking at. When looking to terminological phrases, we can certainly abstract away from indexical information. Terminological phrases by definition have to be self-explaining and do not refer to entities that are outside the domain covered.

In a monolingual environment, we could also ignore morphology, but as multilinguality is one of the main objectives in large scale text understanding, this would be too big a sacrifice. However, for the sake of simplicity and quietly assuming that the principles that govern word-formation are similar to the principles that govern syntax, we will not further deal with morphology in this chapter.

3.2.2 Linguistic and Conceptual Knowledge

In our reductionist view, we can see a medical text as the product of a process in which words or word groups that refer to concepts, are put together following linguistic rules to form larger word groups that refer to new concepts that have a certain relationship with the original concepts.

Since the early activities of CEN/TC251, the Technical Committee of the European Standardisation Centre that deal with healthcare informatics, references to *conceptual* models, *concept* systems and *conceptual* semantics are dominating the medical informatics literature (Rossi-Mori 1994). For the purpose of this book, we mean by *conceptual knowledge* that knowledge that exclusively deals with concepts and the organisation of these concepts in a structure that is independent of any language. This is not a fortiori the same as what in the linguistic literature is known as *conceptual semantics*, which is a particular theory on *meaning as conceptual structure* (Jackendoff, 1988; Lakoff, 1988). Central in this theory is that semantic structures (what we denote) and conceptual structures (what we mean) converge, or even are the same. However, this probably is the case in a terminology rich domain such as medicine. Hence the *semantics* (i.e. the linguistic meaning) of a medical expression can be said to be equal to the concept that is referred to.

In the light of our data mining objective starting from written text understanding, we mean by *linguistic knowledge* that knowledge that specifies the rules of how valid expressions in a particular language are formed. This kind of knowledge comes in different flavours, two of which in our reductionist view are of importance. First there is the pure grammatical or syntactic knowledge that f.i. dictates phrase constituent order. Typical examples are the adjective - noun order in English, and the noun - adjective order in French. Gender agreement between nouns and adjectives in French is another example.

A second kind of linguistic knowledge is the one that is influenced by meaning. It is this kind of knowledge that tells us that actions usually are denoted by verbs, and entities by nouns. It is also this kind of linguistic knowledge that dictates us that adjectives denoting colour must appear just in front of nouns, and after other adjectives. This knowledge is extremely interesting for our purposes, as it holds the key of the door that leads from denotation to meaning. The particular branch of semantics that deals with this issue is *linguistic semantics*: *the study of literal meanings that are grammaticalised in a language* (Frawley 1992).

3.2.3 Linguistic Semantics

A first principle of linguistic semantics is that one looks only at the *literal*, i.e. *decontextualised* meaning of an expression. From the standpoint of literal meaning, the expression

(E-1) *removal of cardiac pacemaker from epicardium or myocardium.*

represents a state of affairs that involves an event of *removing* and certain entities namely a *cardiac pacemaker*, an *epicardium* and a *myocardium.* There is no discussion about that. If we know that this expression is the rubric-term for SNOMED-code *P1-315C4*, then we know also that the implicational, i.e. contextualised meaning of this expression is that if on a patient a cardiac pacemaker is removed from one of the two specified places, this may be registered in his medical record as *P1-315C4* if there is an agreement in the institution where the procedure is carried out that such interventions are coded in SNOMED. The notions *patient*, *institution*, *agreement*, etc, are required to understand the full semantics of the expression, but it is obvious that these notions are not encoded in the sentence itself. Hence they are not part of the linguistic semantics, or the *grammatical meaning* of the sentence.

At the other hand, the entities pacemaker, epicardium and myocardium appear in sentence (E-1) as structural categories, in casu nouns, that are essential to the formation of English sentences. From expression (E-1), we know also that it is the pacemaker that is the entity on which the event of removing acts, and not the epi- or myocardium. We are sure about that just because of the form of the expression in English, and not because we have to infer it from other information, e.g. because this expression is a rubric in SNOMED. It is the preposition *of* that marks the object that is removed, and the preposition *from* that encodes the source from which the removal is carried out.

3.2.4 Conceptual and Linguistic Ontologies

All knowledge based approaches rely on an *ontology*, a more or less formal representation - to be used in computer systems - of what concepts exist in the world, and how they relate to one another. Ontologies are often viewed as strictly language independent models of the world, especially in the medical informatics community (Rector et al. 1996), though the need for an ontology in natural language processing applications is generally well accepted (Bateman 1993). This is not to say that knowledge structuring based on a linguistic approach leads to the same result as when opting for a conceptual approach. A typical example is the ontological distinction between *nominal* and *natural kinds* (Kripke 1972), that in no language is grammaticalised just because the difference is pure definitional (Welsh 1988).

Situated ontologies - i.e. ontologies that are developed for solving particular problems in knowledge based applications (Mahesh and Nirenburg, 1995) - that have to operate in natural language processing applications, are better suited to assist language understanding when the concepts and relationships they are built upon, are linguistically motivated (Deville and Ceusters, 1994).

In the perspective of re-usability, two dimensions have however to be explored: (relative) independence from particular languages and (relative) independence from particular domains.

Linguistic semantics based analyses allow us to separate f.i. entities from events and property concepts, a rather crude distinction being the fact that in most languages these concepts are respectively grammaticalised by means of nouns, verbs and adjectives. Linguists are concerned on how these concepts give overt form to language, while from a computational point of view, these concepts also have to be "anchored" in an ontology.

A relative new notion related to ontologies is that of the *interface ontology*, standing between conceptual (or domain) and linguistic ontologies. Approaches based on interface ontologies differ in the "distance" between the interface ontology and the domain ontologies at the one hand, and the linguistic ontologies at the other hand. In the MikroKosmos initiative, an interface ontology is developed for machine translation purposes in the domain of commercial merges and acquisitions of companies (Mahesh 1996). Hence, it is more close to a given conceptual domain, although general concepts are included as well as unrestricted texts are envisaged to be processed. The KOMET project resulted in the "Generalised Upper Model 2.0", where a closer contact with linguistic realisations is maintained: *if there is no specifiable lexicogrammatical consequences for a 'concept', than it does not belong in the Generalised Upper Model* (Bateman et al. 1995 : p5). As a linguistically oriented ontology, the GUM is fundamentally different in design from domain- or world-knowledge oriented ontologies in that it captures those distinctions which have influences for grammatical expressions in distinct languages without committing to just what the grammatical distinctions of any particular language are. This therefore provides a powerful point of language localisation that maintains theoretical independence from particular linguistic theories and language engineering techniques.

A relatively similar, though more simple approach is used in EuroWordNet (Vossen et al. 1997). In this project, semantic databases like WordNet1.5 (Miller et al. 1990) for several languages are combined via a so-called inter-lingual-index (ILI). This allows language-independent data to be shared over the languages, while language-specific properties are maintained as well in each individual database. The only organisation provided to the ILI is via two separate ontologies. The first one is the top-concept ontology which is a hierarchy of language-independent concepts, reflecting explicit opposition relations. The second is a hierarchy of domain labels. Both the top-concepts and the domain labels can be transferred via the equivalence relations of the ILI to the language-specific meanings and, next, via the language-internal relations to any other meaning in the individual database of a specific language.

3.3 Preparation of the Data for Subsequent Data Mining

The application of natural language understanding that will interest most the readers of this textbook, is to prepare textual documents in such a way that the information they contain can be used for traditional data mining. This requires applications that can re-arrange the unstructured information that resides in texts, into a structured format.

In the remaining part of this chapter, we will first describe the prinicples and technologies that underly natural language understanding applications in the context of information discovery in healthcare. Then we'll describe a system that has achieved these objectives.

Various technologies are indispensable in the process of representing medical natural language in a format understandable by machines. Some of these technologies are used "off line", i.e. they assist in the development of resources that are needed to drive the "on-line" technologies such as syntactic-semantic taggers and parsers. We refer to these resources and technologies together as "lingware" because contrary to traditional informatics tools, they are specifically designed for linguistic processing, and software and knowledge bases are tightly interconnected.

3.3.1 Technologies Required

3.3.1.1 Machine Readable Multilingual Medical Lexicons

Dictionaries are usually large books intended to be used by humans to look up the meaning of unknown words. Most electronic dictionaries currently available differ only from paper dictionaries in their being published on a digital medium. The major advantage is that they can be used from within the most popular word processors without the need for retyping. But their audience consist still of human readers...

For medical natural language understanding purposes, dictionaries have to be fundamentally different in nature: they are primarily intended to be used by machines ! Such dictionaries can be used by some of the knowledge extraction software to represent the meaning of full text documents. But they also can be integrated in third party systems for information retrieval, spell checking, automatic translation, etc.

3.3.1.2 Automatic Term Extractors

Linguistic engineering is a very labour intensive activity. Hence there is a need for tools that can be used to automatically extract new words and terms from text documents. Whether they are in English, Dutch, French or whatever other European language, the vast majority of typical expressions contained in documents pertaining to a specific domain should be extracted on the fly. In addition, semantic relationships between the content words of the documents (i.e. those words pertaining to the domain) are to be made explicit.

3.3.1.3 Taggers and Parsers

These tools are linguistic analysers that are able to make the implicit knowledge available in texts more or less explicit.

Taggers are pieces of software that take as input a text, and that "decorate" these texts with syntactic and/or semantic descriptions pertaining to the sentence constituents identified.

Parsers provide a complete structural analysis of sentences. Here also, analysis can be limited to syntactic structure, or complemented by semantic decorations.

3.3.2 Preparing Neurosurgerical Reports for Data Mining Purposes: The MultiTale Approach

3.3.2.1 Rationale

For data-collection in healthcare, two major issues are generally well recognised. Firstly, coherent models for the representation of data, information and knowledge are urgently needed. Indeed, only when such models are available, data coming from different sources may be compared and used for various purposes. Secondly, despite the increasing use of healthcare information systems in which data are registered in a structured and standardised way, the clinical narrative remains an important source of information when delivering optimal care to patients. However, the format in which this information is expressed, cannot readily be used for automatic data-processing, and is inefficient in terms of computer assisted medical management, data transfer between different information systems, quality assurance and surveillance.

The Multi-TALE syntactic-semantic tagger has been developed as a tool for factual information retrieval from neuro-surgical procedure reports, hence making this information suitable for further processing (Ceusters et al. 1998). In the remaining part of this chapter, we describe the underlying semantic model and the overall technical architecture of the prototype, sketch the results of two validations, and compare the results with those of similar systems.

3.3.2.2 The CEN/TC251 ENV on Surgical Procedures

A project Team (PT002S) of CEN/TC251 (Technical Committee 251 on Medical Informatics of CEN (Comité Européen de Normalisation) was given the task to develop a structure for classification and coding of surgical procedures. The purpose of this standard is to *identify the concepts within the text of surgical procedure notes and to structure them to represent the concepts and their internal relations* (CEN ENV 1828:1995).

According to this standard, a surgical procedure is conceptually composed of a *surgical deed* (deed that can be done by the operator to the patient's body during the surgical procedure) which is semantically linked to the concept fields *human anatomy*, *pathology* and *interventional equipment*. Potential semantic links are *direct object* (referring to that on which the surgical deed is carried out), the *indirect object* (referring to the site of the surgical deed) and the *means* (referring to the means with which the deed is carried out).

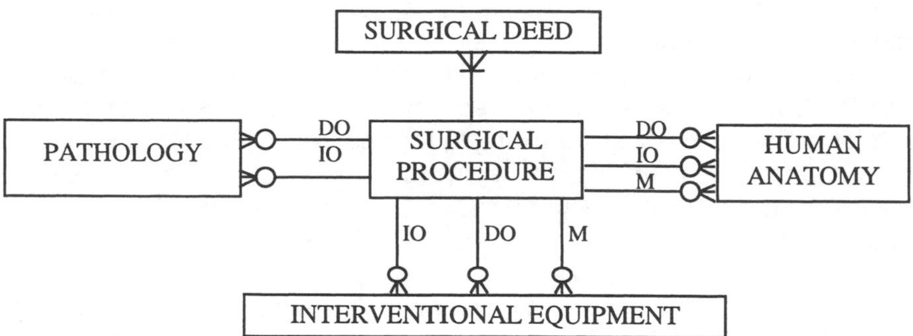

Although the standard was developed for the description of elementary surgical procedure expressions as they can be found in classification and coding systems, one of the hypotheses of the Multi-TALE project was that the same structure could be used to represent the particular tasks described in full text reports. To test this hypothesis, a functional approach to the medical language was adopted, recognising that the language structure is not to be separated from language use. The functional dimension of natural language has been convincingly introduced by Dik in theoretical linguistics (Dik 1989), and successfully applied and adapted by Deville for the modelisation of administrative language (Deville 1989). By using the same approach, we could semantically model surgical procedure expressions as structures that consist of a predicate (surgical deed) with an adequate number of terms, specified by means of a semantic function or case, and functioning as arguments of that predicate. We identified the concept field *surgical deed* as predicate primitive and the semantic links *direct object, indirect object and means* as the expression of semantic functions labelled case roles that can be ascribed to the arguments of a predicate (i.e. concept of surgical deed). We also redefined the notion of combinatorial rule as a specification at surgical deed level, constraining on semantic grounds the case roles that are prototypical of a given surgical deed. We finally defined 12 classes of surgical deeds by appealing to the notion of predicate primitive. To each class of surgical deed corresponds a cluster of arguments with specific semantic constraints.

3.4 Data Mining

The function of an automatic *tagger* is mainly to perform the first and essential pre-processing for any natural language processing application: labelling words in sentences with their grammatical (sub-)categories, only taking into account a limited context. The output of an automatic tagger is a list of the words of a text with the appropriate labels. This output can be used for further processing, for example by a parser. With *parsing* is meant here performing a complete syntactic analysis of a sentence, distinguishing syntagms (noun phrase, verb phrase, etc.) with their syntactic functions (subject, direct object, main verb, etc.). In addition to this syntactic tagging, the Multi-TALE prototype also provides semantic tags to the texts. More specifically, semantic decoration is provided on the basis of the CEN\TC251model for Surgical Procedures as explained above.

The existing DILEMMA-1 tagger-lemmatizer for English general language was used as a starting-point for the analysis (Paulussen and Martin, 1992). Its output, a list of lemmatised words with their basic syntactic categories (adj, noun, verb, ...) was then processed by the semantic tagger. This tagger uses a rule-set to combine in a bottom-up approach words and word groups in the sentences to be analysed, to more complex elements, up to the level of a predicate, or one of its arguments. Each rule contains information regarding the syntactic and semantic conditions to be fulfilled by the word or word group in focus, and its left and right neighbours within in a specified distance.

Other resources used by the Multi-TALE prototype are a small syntactic lexicon to correct the systematic mistakes of DILEMMA-1 (Mommaerts et al. 1994), and a semantic lexicon of 2000 words (base-forms) with additional information on case-assignment and usage of prepositions.

Finally, a heuristic scoring procedure is used to select the best solution when more than one analysis for a given sentence is possible.

For example: the sentence "After insertion of the ventricular catheter, removal of cerebral fluid was performed.", is analysed by Multi-TALE as:

Semantic link	Semantic type	Syntactic tag	Rule	Syntagm	Meaning (Snomed-code)
		prep		**After**	**G-4004**
Action	**install**	**sg**		**insertion**	**P1-05500**
		prep		**of**	
Do	**inte**	**detnoun**	**4**	**the ventricular catheter**	**(T-A1600,A-26800)**
		comm		**,**	
Action	**remove**	**sg**	**bac**	**removal was performed**	**P1-03000**
		prep		**of**	
Do	**anat**	**adjnoun**	**2**	**cerebral fluid**	**(T-A0110,fluid)**

Table 2. Typical output of Multi-TALE.

3.4.1.1 The Multi-TALE Reference Lexicon

3.4.1.1.1 Macro-Structural Entities

A macro-structural entity of the MULTI-TALE augmented reference lexicon is defined here as a lexical entry as it is coded in the lingware of the application. This macro-structural entity can be of three basic types: bounded morphemes, words, and word groups. We will discuss these three types on the basis of linguistic and operational criteria. The examples illustrating this section are taken from the corpora of English and Dutch corpora of neurosurgical procedures that were used in the development of the system.

a) Sublanguage bounded morphemes

The first type of macro-structural entities consists of sublanguage bounded morphemes. These morphemes are :

• each word stem under its different variation patterns, provided that these variations are unpredictable. In the following examples, the stems 'skull' and 'crani' are encoded as two different lexical entries (the alphanumeric string preceding the expressions are identification tags of corpus extracted expressions):

SDY_E_88_011.2 *The resultant craniectomy was then extended as a 2 cm strip a long fused metopic suture down to the skull base in the region of the crista galli.*

• the predictable orthographic variants of a given word. In the following example, the term 'haemostasis' can also be written as 'hemostasis'. In that case two different lexical entries are foreseen:

SDY_88_E_010.7. *Haemostasis was achieved without difficulty and without use of Surgicel.*

Unpredictable orthographic variants (i.e. spelling errors) can only be taken into account by means of a matching algorithm that would check the user's input before processing it, and are not part of the lexicon.

b) Single words

The second type of macro-structure consists of the sublanguage's single words in their lemmatised version.

c) Word groups

The third type of macro-structure consists of word groups (in their lemmatised form) that are considered as one single conceptual entity. Note that the structure of these word groups cannot be computed. Examples of such compounds are respectively "spinous process(es)" and 'Infant delta Shunt' in the two following report abstracts :

SDY_88_E_055.1. *Under general orotracheal anaesthesia, in the prone position, through a midline incision, the muscles were separated from the spinous processes and laminae of L2 to the sacrum and levels identified by reference to the sacrum.*

SDY_88_E_037.5 *Peritoneum exposed through an epigastric incision and an Infant Delta Shunt, Performance Level I was tunnelled between the two incisions.*

3.4.1.1.2 Micro-Structure of Lexical Entries

Each entry in the lexicon has the following structure, consisting of a set of 5 fields with syntactic semantic information.

```
<lemma>
  Meaning: <snomed-code>
  Superconcept: <supertype>
  Superord. Concept: <subtype>
  Main Syntactic Cat: <syntactic category>
 [ Roles:
                <role_desc 1>
                <role_desc 2>
                ...
                <role_desc n>
   Preps:
          <prep_desc 1>
          <prep_desc 2>
          ...
          <prep_desc n> ]
```

Table 3. Micro-structure of entries in the Multi-TALE lexicon.

The <snomed-code>-field contains the SNOMED-code of the entry when available.

The <supertype> fields specifies the main semantic type to which the entry belongs. Potential values are the central semantic types as defined in ENV1828:1995.

The <subtype>-field refers mainly to the occurrences of concept types for surgical deeds such as *install*, *remove*, *inspect*, etc.

The <syntactic category> field specifies the syntactic categorial (and subcategorial) information regarding the lemma. Examples of such categories are Noun, Adjective, Verb, Adverb. In case of surgical deeds, potential entries for this field are “verb” and “noun”. The syntactic category does not of course influence the semantics of a lemma, but depending on whether a surgical deed syntactically is realised by means of a verb or a noun, specific prepositions may be used or not.

The <role>- field (only applicable for surgical deeds) indicates for the surgical deeds the prototypical case structure that is in relation with the deed in question, together with some semantic constraints -expressed in terms of other supertypes or specific concepts- on each of the cases. Theses cases are DO (direct object), IO (indirect object), and MEANS (manner/means).

The <prep>-field indicates the case markers (prepositions, or prepositional locutions) that univoquely mark the term they refer to with a given case. Note that one lemma can have more that one case marker, as the example of the surgical deed "removal" that combines with the preposition 'from' (marking an IO -indirect object-) and 'of' (marking a DO -direct object).

3.4.1.2 The Syntactic-Semantic Grammar

A separate linguistic knowledge base attached to the system contains the Multi-TALE syntactic-semantic grammar for English neurosurgery procedure reports. The purpose of this grammar is to combine in a bottom-up approach syntactic elements in the sentences[1] to be analysed, to more complex elements, up to the level of a "clause".

A sentence is considered to have the following structure:

<sentence>	::=	{ <segment> }* [<segmentor> { <segment> }*]
<segment>	::=	{ <clause> }*
<clause>	::=	{ <intercon> }*
<intercon>	::=	{ <token> }*

E.g.: The sentence "*A big fatty tumour was removed rapidly from the brain and the hole filled with pieces of artificial tissue*", is composed of the segments "*A big fatty tumour was removed rapidly from the brain*" and "*the hole filled with pieces of artificial tissue*". The two segments are connected by the segmentor "and". The first segment contains the clauses "*a big fatty tumour*", "*was removed*", "*rapidly*", and, "*from the brain*", while the second segment is composed of the clauses "*the hole*", "*filled*", "*with pieces of artificial tissue*".

This aggregation process is shown in the file MULTITAL.BRS of the developers version of Multi-TALE, as outlined in the next table.

---

[1] The "decision" on what parts of a full-text are to be considered sentences, is taken earlier in the process.

```
SENTENCE 001, SOLUTION 001, SEGMENT 001: remove
do      path     detnoun 4      A big fatty tumour
 -        -      art     -        A
 -      path     adjnoun 2        big fatty tumour
 -        -      adj     -            big
 -      path     adjnoun 2            fatty tumour
 -        -      adj     -                fatty
 -      path     sg      -                tumour
action  remove   papa    11a    was removed
 -        -      past    -        was
action  remove   papa    -        removed
 -      velocity adv     -      rapidly
 -        -      prep    -      from
io      anat     detnoun 4      the brain 1
 -        -      art     -        the
 -      anat     sg      -        brain


SENTENCE 001, SOLUTION 001, SEGMENT 002: fill
do      mcr      detnoun 4      the hole
 -        -      art     -        the
 -      mcr      sg      -        hole
action  install  past    -      filled
 -        -      prep    -      with
m       anat     adjnoun 16mcrOf pieces of artificial tissue
 -      mcr      pl      -        pieces
 -        -      prep    -        of
 -      anat     adjnoun 2        artificial tissue
 -        -      adj     -            artificial
 -      anat     sg      -            tissue
```

Table 4. Bottom-up syntactic-semantic tagging in Multi-TALE.

Each grammar rule has the following general format:

<u>**IF**</u> you find in the sentence to analyse a <token> or <intercon> (further called *left-element*) with a syntactic category occurring in the list <leftsyn>, and a semantic type featuring in the list <leftsem>,

ANDIF (optionally) this <token> or <intercon> is followed by a <token> or <intercon> (further called *mid-element*) with a syntactic category occurring in the list

[1] In this version of MULTITAL.BRS, clauses starting with a preposition are displayed over two lines.

	<midsyn>, and a semantic type featuring in the list <midsem>,
ANDIF	you find also after that a right <token> or <intercon> (further called *right-element*) for which applies respectively <rightsyn> and <rightsem>,
ANDIF	before *left-element* there is (optionally) within a given <distance> a <token> or <intercon> with a syntactic category occurring in the list <left-context>,
ANDIF	after *right-element*, described by <rightsyn> and <rightsem>, there is (optionally) within a given <distance> a <token> or <intercon> > with a syntactic category occurring in the list <right-context>,
THEN	take the *left-element*, *mid-element* and *right-element* together as indicated by the <demon> of <midsyn>,
AND	give the resulting <intercon> as syntactic category what is expressed in <syntactic_result>
AND	finally assign the resulting <intercon> the semantic type as specified in <semantic_result>.

When an action can be performed on consecutive elements within a sentence, three <demon>s can be applied:

"join":	take the elements together as they occur in the sentence
"reloc":	join *left-element* and *right-element*, and put *mid-element* at the right of it
"break":	insert a <segmentor> before *mid-element*

For instance, the rule:

```
sc("16start","@1",
  [scope("break","",1),scope("segm","",2)],
  ["pred","detnoun","noun","ind","sg","pl"],
  join(["prep"]),
  ["sg","pl","detnoun","noun","adjnoun","pers","prop","adjprop"],
  [], ["nil","anat","path","inte","mcr"], [], [], "@1").
```

specifies that at the beginning of a sentence, or when occurring 1 or 2 places after a <segmentor>, noun-phrases separated by a preposition, may be grouped together to form one constituent that receives the syntactic and semantic features of the left-element. This rule will cause in the sentence "*the catheter in the third ventricle was withdrawn*" the combination of "*the catheter*", "*in*" and "*the third ventricle*", while in the sentence, "*I inserted the catheter in the third ventricle*", this combination will not be allowed as the rule would not fire.

All the rules are thoroughly documented following a rigorous schema. As a consequence, updates to the grammar can be implemented without mayor difficulties. The following documentation tags are provided:

- **RULE_ID :** the original identification label (digital or alphanumeric code) that has been used in the development of the grammar itself. As the rule set has evolved in the course of development, this label does not systematically indicate any sequential or logical order of the rules.
- **RULE_SHORTHAND :** as the RULE_ID gives few indications on the type and content of the rule, we identified each rule with an transparent shorthand (string of characters) on type and role content. This shorthand can appear in the multi-tale output in order to easily trace and check the rules that have fired.
- **RULE_FORMAT :** the rule as expressed under its original format
- **RULE_DESCRIPTION :** the rule as interpreted in a condition action structure
- **EXAMPLE_REF :** indicates the reference of the example
- **EXAMPLE_TXT :** indicate the example taken from the English and Dutch Representative Base-Corpora of Neurosurgical Procedure Reports.
- **EXAMPLE_OUTPUT:** indicates the example in its Multi-Tale output format
- **COMMENTS :** motivates the rule both in a functional and linguistic perspective.

3.5 Evaluation

Two types of validation have been carried out: one to test the intermediate performance of the system with fine-tuning as primary objective, and a second one to assess the results of the final modifications. Ten surgical reports (138 sentences) from the corpus, five having been used for the development of the syntactic-semantic rule-base (training sample), and five for which this is not the case (testing sample), have been manually validated. Two human experts (physicians) were used as gold standard. Recall (number of entities retrieved and relevant over number of relevant entities in the report) and precision (number of entities retrieved and relevant over number of entities retrieved (only for second validation)) were calculated separately for testing and training sample. Calculations were based on the correct recognition of syntactic entities such as sentences, segments (surface form of the predicates), clauses (surface form of predicate arguments), simple and complex noun phrases and verb phrases, as well as on semantic information (types and semantic links correctly identified). In total 2139 syntactic units (to be mapped into 6 categories) and 857 semantic-contextual entities (to be mapped into 8 categories) were to be retrieved.

The next table shows the results for both validations (* indicates test not performed). The first validation revealed an acceptable performance for syntactic tagging (except for complex noun phrases) and semantic type recognition, with only very modest results for case assignment. In addition, recall in the training sample appeared to be much higher than in the test sample. Fine-tuning of the system turned out to be very effective, and led to syntactic recall for the test sample of 95.7% (precision being 95.7% also) and 89.3% for semantic recall with a precision of 94.8%. Semantic labelling still appeared to be more successful than case-assignment (recall 93.4% versus 77.4%, 60.0% and 77.8%, $p < 0,01$).

	First Evaluation		Second Evaluation			
	Known	Unknown	Known		Unknown	
	Recall	Recall	Recall	Precision	Recall	Precision
Sentences	100	99	100	100	98.7	100
Segments	88	86	98.0	88.3	98.5	92.3
Clauses	91	80	91.9	92.6	95.2	93.3
Simple NP's	93	85	92.8	100	94.3	100
Complex NP's	79	56	88.6	93.9	86.7	100
VP's	93	85	92.6	98.9	95.2	100
Tot. Syntax	91	82	93.3	94.4	95.7	95.7
Deeds	*	*	96.5	94.3	98.1	97.1
Anatomy	*	*	93.9	95.8	98.4	98.4
Pathology	*	*	100	88.6	94.7	100
Instrument	*	*	87.5	97.2	71.1	96.4
Tot. Sem. Types	90	71	94.6	94.2	93.4	97.8
Action	97	82	96.5	90.1	97.1	93.5
Direct Object	84	69	83.3	88.7	77.4	92.9
Indirect Object	78	61	75.0	80.0	60.0	70.6
Means	68	50	70.6	100	77.8	93.3
Tot. Semantics	83	71	91.3	92.0	89.3	94.8

Table 5. Validation results of the Multi-TALE syntactic-semantic tagger.

3.5.1 Discussion

Some existing systems can be compared with Multi-TALE from a functional and implementational viewpoint. The LSP system was originally designed to extract factual information from medical reports (Sager et al. 1987). The medical sublanguage is viewed by this system as consisting of 6 information formats onto which a total of 54 semantic classes (represented in the lexicon) can be mapped. The system uses a parser that can deal with incomplete analyses. When it was used to find 13 important details of asthma management in a total number of 31 discharge summaries (testing set), recall appeared to be 82.1% (92.5% counting only omissions instead of errors) and precision 82.5% (98.6%) (Sager et al. 1994). Haug et al. report recall and precision rates of 87% and 95% for detecting clinical findings in 839 chest x-ray reports by using SPRUS (Ranum 1988), and rates of 95% and 94% respectively for the detection of diagnoses (Haug et al. 1990). SPRUS is mainly semantically driven, and is not able to exploit syntactic information. Hence complex noun-phrases and whole sentences cannot be processed. The CAPIS system was able to recall 92% of the relevant physical findings (156 in total in 20 reports on patients with gastro-intestinal bleeding), with a precision of 96% (Lin et al. 1991). CAPIS uses a finite-state machine parser that is specifically designed for the more structured parts in medical narrative such as the clinical findings section.

The main conclusion from this work was that tagging, as a more simple procedure compared to parsing, may be an effective strategy to extract factual information from clinical narrative. The main advantage is that a complete parse of a sentence is not needed to map the semantic contents of a sentence onto a predefined classification or conceptual model. But at the same time, the approach has its limits. Full natural language understanding cannot be realised by a semantic tagger alone. It is our believe that when full understanding of a sentence is required, semantic taggers are however useful as they can enhance the performance of a parser used subsequently by rapidely eliminating alternatives that only after a long processing time would turn out not to lead to an acceptable solution.

Another conclusion was that the CEN/TC251/PT002S standard for surgical procedure classifications can be used for syntactic-semantic tagging of neurosurgical procedures provided that the concept type *surgical deed* is thought of as predicate primitive and the semantic links *direct object, indirect object and means* as the expression of semantic functions labelled case roles that can be ascribed to the arguments of a predicate (i.e. concept of surgical deed). In this context, Multi-TALE is in line with the

World Health Organisation's view in that *the challenge is now to clarify how we can pass from traditional encoding of medical data to automatic encoding of natural language, and how the universally accepted classifications with their advantages and disadvantages can be used in this context* (Jardel 1989).

3.6 Conclusion

Medical information systems are sufficiently large and varied such that no one vendor can expect to provide all of the systems needed in even a single hospital, let alone for the health service as a whole. Many of these varied systems would benefit from natural language interfaces and some, such as automatic linkage to abstracts of the literature, are even impractical without it. Generic multilingual solutions are required if the range of services to be built is to meet the demand. Furthermore, it is essential that the natural language processing components share the underlying concept structure used by the various applications.

Electronic patient record systems are no exception to this. A wealth of knowledge is needed to enter information in those systems consistently and to use the information afterwards for various purposes. Provided that a highly acceptable system can be designed in a specific environment, then developers surely will want to make it available to other users. Whilst much re-use of system components is feasible within a given market segment, there are significant costs associated with the 'localisation' of systems to the needs of other markets. Perhaps the most important of these costs is the localisation to the linguistic needs of each national market in Europe.

Medicine is a descriptive, language intensive activity, and the costs of developing, and perhaps more importantly maintaining, the linguistic resources needed to localise clinical systems are clearly high. Any practical approach to the management and exploitation of linguistic resources in large scale clinical information systems must be based on common methods and internal representations for linguistic information. This information must be reusable across a wide range of systems and local variants of those systems, and the cost of maintaining that information must be separable from those of maintaining the rest of the system.

Data mining is also one of these new disciplines that can benefit from natural language understanding applications. Numerical data are hard to get in domains such as medicine where most data are only available in textual format. Preprocessing textual information through natural language analysers will be one of the solutions to resolve the knowledge acquisition bottle neck.

References

Allen J. 1987. Natural Language Understanding. Menlo Park: The Benjamin/Cummings Publishing Company Inc.

Bach E. 1989. *Informal lectures on formal semantics.* Albany, NY: Suny Press.

Bateman J, R. Henschel and F. Rinaldi. 1995. Generalised Upper Model 2.0: documentation, GMD/Institute for integrated publication and information systems Technical Report, Darmstadt, Germany.

Bateman JA. 1993. Ontology construction and natural language. *In Proc. International Workshop on Formal Ontology.* Padua, Italy, 83-93.

CEN ENV 1828:1995. Medical Informatics - Structure for classification and coding of surgical procedures.

Ceusters W, Lovis C, Rector A, Baud R. 1996. Natural language processing tools for the computerised patient record: present and future. In P. Waegemann (ed.) *Toward an Electronic Health Record Europe '96 Proceedings*, 294-300.

Ceusters W, Spyns P, De Moor G, Martin W (eds.) 1998. Syntactic-Semantic Tagging of Medical Texts: the Multi-TALE Project. Studies in Health Technologies and Informatics, IOS Press Amsterdam.

Deville G. 1989. Modelisation of Task-Oriented Utterances in Man-Machine Dialogue System. Ph.D. Thesis, University of Antwerp.

Deville G, Ceusters W. 1994. A multi-dimensional view on natural language modelling in medicine: identifying key-features for successful applications. Supplementary paper in *Proceedings of the Third International Working Conference of IMIA WG6*, Geneva.

Dik S. 1989. A Theory of Functional Grammar, Foris, Dordrecht.

Drucker P, Dryson E, Handy Ch, Saffo P, Senge P. 1997. Looking ahead: Implications of the present. In: Harvard Business Review, sept-oct 1997.

Frawley W. 1992. Linguistic Semantics. Hilsdale, Hove and London: Lawrence Erlbaum Associates.

Haug PJ, Ranum DL, Frederick PR. 1990. Computerized extraction of coded findings from free-text radiologic reports. Radiology, 174, 543 - 548.

Jackendoff R. 1988. Conceptual semantics. In Eco U et al. (eds.) *Meaning and mental representation.* Bloomington: Indiana University Press, 81-97.

Jardel JP. 1989. Opening address for the International Working Conference on Natural Language Processing of the International Medical Informatics Association. In: Scherrer JR, Côté RA, Mandil SH (eds.) Computerized Natural Language Processing for Knowledge Engineering. Elsevier Science Publishers, p 1.

Kripke S. 1972. Naming and Necessity. In Davidson D & Harman G (eds.) *Semantics of natural language*. Dordrecht: Reidel, 253-355.

Lakoff G. 1988. Cogintive semantics. In Eco U et al. (eds.) *Meaning and mental representation*. Bloomington: Indiana University Press, 119-154.

Lin R, Lenert L, Middleton B, Shiffman S. 1991. A free-text processing system to capture physical findings: Canonical Phrase Identification System (CAPIS). Proc-Annu-Symp-Comput-Appl-Med-Care, 843-7.

Mahesh K. 1996. *Ontology Development for Machine Translation: ideology and methodology.* Technical Report MCCS-96-292, Computing Research Laboratory, New Mexico State University, Las Cruces, NM.

Mahesh K and Nirenburg S. 1995. A situated ontology for practical NLP. In *Proceedings of the Workshop on Basic Ontological Issues in Knowledge Sharing, IJCAI-95*. Montreal, Canada.

Miller GA, R. Beckwidth, C. Fellbaum, D. Gross, and K.J. Miller. 1990. Introduction to WordNet: An On-line Lexical Database, International Journal of Lexicography ¾, 235-244.

Mommaerts JL, Ceusters W, Deville G. 1994. Are taggers for general language useful for medical sublanguage ? A case-study with DILEMMA (Dutch). In: Beckers WPA, ten Hoopen AJ (eds) Proceedings of MIC'94, Velthoven, The Netherlands, 25-26/11/94, 283-290.

Paulussen, Hans & Willy Martin. 1992. *DILEMMA-2: a lemmatizer-tagger for medical abstracts*, in Proceedings of the Third Conference on Applied Natural Language Processing (ACL), Trento, 141-146.

Quine W. 1953. Two Dogma's of Empiricism. In Quine W (ed.) *From a logical point of view*, New York.

Ranum DL. 1988. Knowledge based understanding of radiology text. Proceedings of the 12th Annual Symposium on Computer Applications in Medical Care, Washington, DC, 141 - 145.

Rector AL, Rogers JE, Pole P. 1996. The GALEN High Level Ontology. In Brender J, Christensen JP, Scherrer J-R, McNair P (eds.) *MIE 96 Proceedings*. Amsterdam: IOS Press, 174-178.

Rossi-Mori A. 1994. Towards a new generation of terminologies and coding systems. In Barahona P & Christensen JP (eds.) *Knowledge and decisions in health telematics*. Amsterdam: IOS Press, 208-212.

Sager N, Friedman C, Lyman MS. 1987. Medcial Language Processing: Computer Management of Narrative Data. Reading, MA: Addison - Wesley.

Sager N, Lyman MS, Bucknall C, Nhan N, Tick LJ. 1994. Natural language processing and the representation of clinical data. J. Am Med Infomatics Assoc, 1, 142-160.

Searle JR, Kiefer F, Bierwisch M (eds.) 1980. *Speech Act Theory and Pragmatics*. Dordrecht: Reidel.

Vossen P, P. Diez-Orzas, and W. Peters. 1997. The Multilingual Design of the EuroWordNet Database. in: Proceedings of the IJCAI-97 workshop on Multilingual Ontologies for NLP Applications, Nagoya, August 23.

Welsh C. 1988. *On the non-existence of natural kind terms as a linguistically relevant category.* Paper presented at the Liguistic Society of America, New Orleans, LA.

Wiederhold G. 1980. Databases in healthcare. Stanford University, Computer Science Department, Report No. STAN-CS-80-790.

4 Anatomic Pathology Data Mining

G. William Moore [1,2,3] **and Jules J. Berman** [3,4]

[1]Pathology and Laboratory Medicine Service, Veterans Affairs Maryland Health Care System, Baltimore, Maryland, U.S.A.

[2]Department of Pathology, University of Maryland School of Medicine, Baltimore, Maryland, U.S.A.

[3]Department of Pathology, The Johns Hopkins Medical Institutions, Baltimore, Maryland, U.S.A.

[4]Resource Development Branch, National Cancer Institute, National Institutes of Health, Rockville, Maryland, U.S.A.

G. William Moore: webmaster@netautopsy.org

Pathology is the study of disease. Anatomic pathology is that area of pathology that studies the gross anatomy and microanatomy (histology) of diseased organs, in order to render specific diagnoses, and to acquire new knowledge related to disease biology. One of the chief functions of the anatomic pathologist is to issue diagnostic reports on tissue samples (biopsies) taken from suspected lesions. Pathology reports are needed to guide treatment of the individual patient. The aggregate collection of free-text reports contains a wealth of information related to almost every serious human disease. The goal of data mining in anatomic pathology is to extract research value from collections of pathology reports. Intended uses for anatomic pathology data mining include: epidemiology; human tissue resources linked to clinical data; trial and outcomes analysis; and monitoring the quality of patient care. Issues facing anatomic pathology data mining include: security and patient confidentiality; data integrity; and standards for pathology reports. In the future, with improved data mining technology, we can anticipate wide use of anatomic pathology reports in support of medical research.

4.1 Understanding the Problem Domain

4.1.1 Objectives of Data Mining in Anatomic Pathology

In the course of providing patient care, anatomic pathologists issue diagnoses in the form of *free-text pathology reports.* Almost every new diagnosis of cancer, and many diagnoses of non-neoplastic diseases, results in a pathology report, issued from a hospital or an independent pathology laboratory. The main, and until now essentially the only, purpose of most of these reports has been to provide a correct and timely diagnosis for the individual patient. The goal of *data mining* in anatomic pathology is to extract additional value from these reports, beyond their initial, designated purpose.

Over the past decade, with the growth of computers and word processors, nearly every anatomic pathology report exists for a period of time as a computer-readable document. Approximately 40 million pathology reports are issued each year in the United States (American Board of Medical Specialists, Appendix; Smith et al, 1989; Anderson et al, 1991). If even a small percentage of these reports could be analyzed with modern data analysis techniques, the benefits to society could be enormous. Currently this potential data-source is essentially untapped, due to technical, legal, and social obstacles, none of which is insurmountable. The principal areas for potential application of anatomic pathology data mining include: epidemiologic studies; as a link to archival tissue specimens for research use; for monitoring and improving patient treatments; and for the development of new diagnostic tests.

4.1.2 Intended Uses for Anatomic Pathology Data Mining

4.1.2.1 Epidemiology

Epidemiology is the study of the distribution and determination of disease in specified populations, and the application of this knowledge to the control of health problems (Lilienfeld and Stolley, 1994). Almost every new diagnosis of cancer, issued in the USA or in other technically advanced medical environments, results in a pathology report being generated, and an accompanying tissue sample being processed and stored. Thus, in the field of cancer epidemiology, anatomic pathology reports represent an enormous, but at this time largely untapped resource, for determining the epidemiologic distribution of cancer diagnoses, by sex, by age, by geographic location, and by a variety of environmental and occupational risk factors.

Currently, 48 U. S. states have a reporting requirement for cancer diagnoses. That is, each physician or medical institution that renders a report containing the patient's original cancer diagnosis (i.e., the biopsy upon which the patient and physician initially document the patient's cancer) has a legal obligation to report the diagnosis to state authorities. State agencies then submit this information to the *Centers for Disease Control and Prevention (CDCP)* (1995). In addition, many cancer diagnoses are collected by other agencies, including *Surveillance, Epidemiology, and End-Results (SEER)* (Lilienfeld and Stolley, 1994; U. S. Centers for Disease Control and Prevention, 1995; Nelson et al, 1999; Moulton, 1999; Surveillance, Epidemiology, and End-Results, Appendix), and the American College of Surgeons (Appendix), which maintains the National Cancer Database.

Once collected, the information is evaluated by a team of experts in medicine, public health, and statistics, who do not necessarily foresee the needs of all possible end-recipients who might eventually use the information. For example, SEER excludes non-melanoma skin cancer cases. Non-melanoma skin cancer (represented primarily by squamous carcinoma and basal cell carcinoma) account for well over one million cases per year in the USA, the same order of magnitude as the sum of cancer incidences from all other organ sites combined. In addition, the SEER data do not include precancerous lesions, including adenomas of colon, dysplasias of cervix, esophagus, bronchus, oral mucosa, liver, etc. SEER also excludes atypical nevi, a precursor lesion for malignant melanoma. The *U. S. National Cancer Institute* has recognized the importance of studying the precursor lesions that precede invasive cancer (Klausner, 1999). However, there is no national database that collects the pathology reports for all newly-occurring pathologic lesions in the USA. At present, all pathology databases and registries are designed to fulfill a specific objective, and are not publicly available for data mining projects. It would seem that for many potentially important cancer studies, national databases are inadequate, and data mining efforts with pre-existing archives residing in large medical institutions and clinical service laboratories may become the most practical way of supporting exploratory data mining efforts.

From time immemorial, it has been commonplace for privileged experts, who have access to biomedical data, to claim that the mechanics of releasing these data into a public venue are impractical and expensive.

With the rise of the Internet, large biomedical databases have been made available, at no cost, to the general public (e.g., the U. S. National Library of Medicine's PubMed (Appendix), the Human Genome Research Institute's GenBank and Cancer Genome Anatomy Projects (Appendix), and summary SEER data (Surveillance, Epidemiology, and End-Results, Appendix)).

The most important obstacles against using laboratory-based collections of pathology reports for data mining projects are:

Inadequate and inconsistent data-representation. Reports often have missing information, and contain errors in grammar and spelling. Further, there is currently no standard format for pathology reports, so that data collected from different institutions cannot be consistently merged.

Pathology data are always highly sensitive for the individuals involved, and the confidentiality of these data are protected by law.

Although data miners may have strong incentives to acquire pathology data, there are at present no incentives for the data-holders to dispense data to researchers. On the contrary, there are numerous disincentives to sharing pathology data, including a bewildering array of still-unresolved legal, ethical and administrative issues (U. S. Code of Federal Regulations, 1995; U. S. Health Insurance Portability and Accountability Act, 1996; U. S. Code of Federal Regulations, 1999; U. S. Office of Protection from Research Risks, Appendix; U. S. National Bioethics Advisory Commission, Appendix; Berman et al, 1996).

If these issues were addressed and settled acceptably, researchers could, in principle, have access to every record of every pathology diagnosis rendered. This information would have enormous benefit to medical researchers, epidemiologists, public health policy experts, and, ultimately, all patients.

4.1.2.2 Data Mining for Human Tissue Resources

Pathology informatics is inseparable from the field of *tissue banking* (U. S. National Cancer Institute, NCI Cooperative Human Tissue Network, and NCI Cooperative Breast Cancer Tissue Resource, Appendix; Naber et al, 1992;Grizzle et al, 1998). This relationship is exemplified by the pathology report's specimen accession number, which is used to identify the tissue specimen, the microscope slides prepared from the tissue specimen, and the pathology report. One unique number immutably links tissue to data. Data linked to tissue samples is one of the most important resources in the area of biomedical research that deals with translating basic research discoveries into clinical practice.

Furthermore, tissue banking can reduce the need for animals in clinical research. Research using human tissues can sometimes spare researchers the time and costs involved in developing and validating animal models for human disease. In addition, retrospective studies using existing collections of pathology data and human tissue specimens may sometimes obviate the need for costly prospective clinical studies, and reduce the time required to convert laboratory discoveries into actual patient benefits.

Pathology informatics provides a mechanism whereby researchers can test new markers and reagents on a wide variety of human tissues, collected from large archives maintained by pathology departments. Since the specimens are human tissues obtained from live patients and archived for future use, the tests performed are directly applicable to patients (i.e., do not require extrapolation from an animal model). Since each specimen is associated with a diagnosis as well as clinical and demographic information, researchers can answer questions pertaining to specific clinical conditions and outcomes. The task of the pathology informatician, more often than not, includes the identification and retrieval of archived tissue, selected for specified criteria related to diagnosis, stage of disease, patient demographics, treatment status, and clinical history.

Tissue microarrays are a new tool that will have a wide range of uses, including validation studies, as well as development of new prognostic markers and new diagnostic tests (Moch et al, 1999; Bubendorf et al, 1999; Kononen et al, 1998). A tissue microarray is a composite tissue-block, containing as many as one thousand small sections of tissue. Each microscope slide cut from this block can be stained in a single procedure. The advantage of a tissue microarray is that it permits a scientist to perform the equivalent of hundreds of experiments at once, on a single slide, using only a small amount of reagent. Since one tissue microarray block can be used to produce up to several hundred near-identical glass slides, different laboratories can compare their results obtained from slides all obtained from the same tissue-block (i.e., from the same set of tissues). For instance, a researcher might have a small amount of monoclonal antibody raised against a putative marker for prostate cancer of low malignant potential (i.e., a prognostically favorable variant of prostate cancer). To test the value of the new marker, she performs an immunostain procedure on a tissue microarray that contains prostate cancer sections selected from hundreds of patients. For each tissue on the microarray, she measures the immunostaining intensity of the marker. In order to validate the stain, she will need pathologic and clinical information for each patient. At this point, the tissue microarray serves as a pathology database, consisting of a patient-record for each tissue specimen, that contains staining information, staging and Gleason scores for the tissue, clinical course of the patient, recurrence data, treatment data, demographics, etc. The results at different laboratories can be compared using a set of tissue microarray glass slides all prepared from the same tissue-block.

Each tissue microarray requires an informatics effort, in which large archives of pathology data are mined. The desired result will be the creation of an array of tissues and associated data, all tailored to the goals of the researcher. Once the microarray is complete and stained, a second informatics phase begins, involving the association of images and measured data derived from each of the sampled tissues included in the microarray. In the case of microarray blocks that have several hundred slides parceled to multiple investigators, all the test result data collected from each investigator will ideally be merged into a large database that includes clinical data and test data for each of the thousand samples included in each tissue microarray. This second informatics phase will require methodology to store and access terabytes of image and other data associated with a single microarray block. The third informatics phase is the data analysis phase, in which conclusions and new hypotheses are generated from the collected tissue microarray database. This will spawn a major data mining effort involving the development of novel informatics methodology to evaluate image data with data linked to textual and conceptual biologic and medical information.

The *Cancer Genome Anatomy Project* (U. S. National Cancer Institute, Appendix; Clark et al, 1993; Schmitt et al, 1999) of the U. S. National Institutes of Health consists of a an ever-growing wealth of genetic information related to human tumors. Data include *Expressed Sequence Tag* (EST) databases (Clark et al, 1993; Schmitt et al, 1999; Choi et al, 1999; Hawkins et al, 1999), gene microarray data, and data related to oncogenes and tumor suppressors found in human tumors.

Data miners are welcomed at this important public resource. It is now possible to link together data mined from pathology reports, and associated clinical data, with publicly available CGAP data. This data ensemble, in turn, can be linked to genetic data held in laboratory databases, where genetic studies were performed on clinical specimens. Trends and associations found by data mining databases that contain clinical, pathologic, and genetic data from related specimens, have enormous potential value. As a hypothetical example, suppose a laboratory with access to clinical specimens and related data has found a mutated gene present in a morphologic and clinical variant of a lung carcinoma. A search through the CGAP database might indicate the presence of the same mutation sequence in a specific set of tumors. This finding might initiate further studies, leading to the identification of a cancer gene, and also to new clinical approaches in the treatment of these cancers.

4.1.2.3 Trial and Outcome Analysis

Much of medical practice has developed as an empiric art. Treatment protocols are often accepted as standard of care, with no objective evidence. Radical mastectomies for breast cancer, hiatal hernia repairs, laser endarterectomes for advanced atherosclerotic disease, bone marrow transplants for advanced breast carcinoma, and tonsillectomies for throat infections, are all examples of medical procedures whose uses have been reduced or eliminated as the result of well-designed clinical studies showing general ineffectiveness, or effectiveness restricted to a small subset of the diseased populations.

The medical community and the public are demanding that the practice of medicine be evidence-based (Bubley, 1999; Junor et al, 1999; Connell et al, 1999; Compton, 1999; Mapp et al, 1999). This means that the validity of a treatment or test must be based on well-designed studies yielding statistically signficant results. Unfortunately, such studies are extremely expensive and time-consuming. Considering the enormous number of old, new, and developing medical tests and procedures, it would be impossible to implement expensive prospective studies in every case.

However, retrospective studies using collections of pathology data, linked to clinical data and specimens, may sometimes yield evidence related to the value of medical procedures, treatments, and tests. Data and specimens can be analyzed in large numbers, especially when variables such as gender, age, ethnicity, and clinical presentation, treatment and outcome are known.

4.1.2.4 Monitoring and Improving Patient Care

There is an enormous potential for monitoring and improving individual patient care with mined anatomic pathology data. Currently the only universal purpose for issuing an anatomic pathology report is to provide a correct and timely diagnosis for the individual patient. However, as aggregate data, anatomic pathology reports can identify potential risks to the individual patient, as well as managerial and administrative problems in medical institutions.

This fact is recognized by national regulatory bodies, such as the *College of American Pathologists* (CAP) and the *Joint Commission for the Accreditation of Healthcare Organizations* (JCAHO) (Appendix), who currently inspect most of the pathology laboratories in the USA. For example, a new anatomic pathology diagnosis, such as malignant melanoma of the skin with a positive surgical margin (indicating that not all of the malignancy was removed by the procedure), should trigger two consequences, documented in the records of the pathology laboratory. First, there should be evidence that the clinician caring for the patient has been notified of an urgent diagnosis in a timely manner. In principle, every clinician should read his/her own pathology reports on a periodic basis, and should pursue delinquent reports. However, for very serious diagnoses, there is a recognized value in having a back-up notification mechanism. Second, the original urgent diagnosis of malignant melanoma should eventually be followed by a second specimen, documented in pathology laboratory records, namely, the definitive excision specimen. The absence of such a specimen in laboratory records after a predetermined period of time, should trigger a documented attempt to verify that the patient has:

- undergone the appropriate procedure at another institution;
- undergone another, acceptable treatment;
- refused treatment;
- been considered too ill to receive the usual treatment.

While the CAP and JCAHO require that each accredited institution should have such policies in place, every physician who has been in practice for a few years knows of an occasional instance where these policies have failed for the individual patient. Data mining procedures could automatically generate lists of problem cases that might require additional medical attention. Through an automated process, pathology departments could alert clinicians to potential problem cases.

4.1.3 Economic Issues in Anatomic Pathology Data Mining

Pathology departments offering new services, such as informatics and specimen-related support, should be compensated for providing those services. As an example, one major reason for the long and dramatic decline in autopsy rates has been the inability of most pathology departments to find mechanisms for adequate monetary compensation for autopsies.

In addition to specimen-handling costs, the preparation of reports in a manner that supports informatics initiatives will also require incentives. Third parties might pay a bonus for reports that are well-coded using standard terminologies that permit more accurate billing, better data analysis, improved outcome studies, etc. Advocacy groups might be motivated to seek support for efforts to standardize pathology reports when they come to understand the potential value of pathology data mining. It has also been suggested that laboratory information system vendors might invest in informatics initiatives that are likely to add value to their services. It is a commonly held perception that pathology informatics could add significant value to pathology reports, as well as facilitate better research support. Some examples of improved reporting include: posting images on reports; coding data to make reports more useful to third parties; using *The Bethesda System* and other reporting standards in a more consistent manner (Hutchins, 1990; Hutchins et al, 1999; Rosai and Ackerman,1996; Hruban et al, 1996; Association of Directors of Anatomic and Surgical Pathology, 1997; Kurman et al, 1991); and permanently and securely associating tissue specimens with pathology data.

4.1.4 Commercial Uses of Mined Anatomic Pathology Data

Pathology data and archived tissues have enormous potential value to commercial entities. Imagine the case of an ambitious genomics company that has just cloned a gene found in an EST (expressed sequence tag) gene library obtained from a prostate cancer cell line, and which was not found in EST libraries derived from normal cells or from other types of cancer cells. The company knows that if a prostate-specific gene can be isolated, it might potentially be useful as a diagnostic test for prostate cancer. The gene may even be exploitable for prostate cancer treatment, if an antisense version of the gene could be produced that interferes with production of the normal gene *in vivo*. The company would need information and tissues related to prostate cancer patients, in order to locate prostate cancer cases representing the spectrum of human disease, including precancerous lesions and lesions of varying clinical stage and prognosis. The company would use the tissues to help develop a gene assay and to test for the presence of the gene in a large number of prostate specimens, as well as in specimens from normal tissues and cancer tissues from other organs. Since bioinformatics companies do not have their own pathology departments, they would need to obtain contractual services from a pathology laboratory. The laboratories would need to be large, with high-quality pathology and clinical data, and with well-characterized, retrievable tissues. The laboratory would need to provide its service in such a way that ethical and legal standards of operation are maintained. The company would need to compensate the laboratory to an extent commensurate with the market value of the service.

The pharmaceutical industry, genomics companies, privately supported laboratories, and federally supported research and development laboratories, all have a growing need for data and tissues. Even academic researchers in need of pathology data and tissues must compete with commercial laboratories in producing a satisfactory incentive for pathology laboratories to provide them with data and tissues.

4.1.5 Past, Current Efforts to Standardize Pathology Data

Efforts to standardize anatomic pathology data have proceeded on three fronts: standardized coding; standard formatting of anatomic pathology reports; and standards for publishing collections of reports. The three dominant coding systems in anatomic pathology are: SNOMED, Read, and UMLS. *The Systematized Nomenclature of Human and Veterinary Medicine* (SNOMED International, or SNOMED III) (Appendix, Cote et al, 1993, Moore and Berman, 1994) is a copyrighted product of the *College of American Pathologists* (Appendix), and one of the recognized standard nomenclatures in medicine. SNOMED is used in most pathology laboratories that employ standardized coding systems. The *Read Classification* is employed by the National Health Service in Great Britain (Read and Benson, 1986; Payne, 1995), and is owned by the the British crown. SNOMED, Read, MeSH, and over fifty other classifications are subsumed within the *Unified Medical Language System (UMLS) Metathesaurus* of the *U. S. National Library of Medicine* (Appendix).

The UMLS is by far the largest of all medical concept systems (Hahn et al, 1999), and is the best tool for research studies in controlled medical vocabularies. UMLS serves as an indexing tool for PubMed (Appendix), a collection of over nine million medical citations available on the Internet to the general public. It has been estimated that only 1-3% of medical concepts in general medical text are not present in UMLS (Humphries, Appendix; Kao and Moore, 2000). UMLS provides a uniform, integrated distribution format from over fifty biomedical vocabularies and classifications. The 1999 UMLS Metathesaurus contains 625,530 biomedical concepts and 1,362,823 different concept-names. Each *Concept Unique Identifier* (CUI) consists of C followed by seven decimal digits, with an accompanying *synonym-name*. Different synonym-names have the same CUI. UMLS is updated annually and made available to registered users, with a complete listing of CUIs and synonym-names. Since the UMLS is available cost-free to researchers worldwide for research projects, it makes the most sense to develop pathology data mining applications in UMLS.

One of the major limitations in coding systems for anatomic pathology today is that there is no agreed-upon syntax for an anatomic pathology report, and no agreed-upon method for translating an anatomic pathology report written in plain English into a given coding system for publication. It is our perception that no two hospital systems encode their reports with the same set of coding rules. Consequently, there are no examples of different hospital systems merging their encoded pathology datasets into an aggregate database.

4.1.6 Data Integrity Issues

Currently nearly every anatomic pathology report exists for at least a while as an electronic file; but beyond this, there are few standards. Patient identification, provider identification, date/time conventions, name of tissue source, name of diagnosis, and even word processor formatting conventions, are all idiosyncratic to the pathology laboratory that issues the report. Even the presence or absence of certain pieces of information is not guaranteed.

The most unstructured part of the pathology report, and perhaps the part in greatest need of accurate data mining, is the *microscopic diagnosis* (Moore and Berman, 1994). At a minimum, this field should contain the *disease name* and *bodysite* for each anatomic diagnosis. Almost equally important, the sentences must be appropriately separated from one another. At this time, there is virtually no control on data-integrity in the microscopic diagnosis, beyond the fastidiousness of the pathologist and the competence of the typist. Sentences may not contain complete information. Sentences may be written with convoluted grammatical constructions, including run-on sentences and vaguely placed negations. There may be spelling errors, idiosyncratic abbreviations, or ambiguous terms. The following examples are potentially ambiguous sentences. In most cases, the meaning is more-or-less apparent to a trained health professional, but might easily be misinterpreted by a data mining program.

Squamous cell carcinoma. *(Which bodysite?)*

Liver showing metastatic adenocarcinoma, portal lymph node showing reactive hyperplasia. *(Run-on sentence.)*

Liver showing metastatic adenocarcinoma No tumor present in portal lymph node. *(Ambiguous negation.)*

Skin with sqamous cell carcinoma. *(Spelling error.)*

Skin with BCC. *(Idiosyncratic abbreviation: BCC=basal cell carcinoma.)*

Cervical soft tissue with metastatic adenocarcinoma. *(Neck? Uterine cervix?).*

RLL. *(Right lobe of lung? Right lower lung? Right lower lobe of lung? Right lower lid of eye?)*

4.1.7 Ethical and Legal Issues

Current U. S. federal regulations governing the protection of human subjects are contained in *Title 45 of the Code of Regulations, Part 46* (also known as *Common Rule*, or *45CFR46)* (Appendix). Although different U. S. states have passed their own laws that restrict the uses of medical information, 45CFR46 is the most general and comprehensive document on this subject, detailing the functions and operations *of Institutional Review Boards (IRBs),* and applicable to all research funded by or regulated by any U. S. Federal Department or Agency. *The National Bioethics Advisory Commission (NBAC)* (Appendix) has recently expressed their views in a document that provides researchers, IRB members, and federal agencies with the NBAC's interpretation of 45CFR46 (Appendix).

Several provisions of 45CFR46 directly relate to pathology informatics initiatives. Under 45CFR46, a subject must be living in order to be a human subject protected under Common Rule. Consequently, autopsy data and tissues may be used freely by the research community.

In addition, records and tissues that have have irreversibly unlinked from patient identifiers are specifically exempted from 45CFR46 restrictions (so-called Exemption 4). Research involving anonymous tissue and data can proceed without IRB review, but this exemption only applies to data and tissues that can never be traced back to the patient, either by the pathologist who contributes materials to the researcher, or by the researcher who generates new data based on evaluation of the provided material (e.g., data mining), or through laboratory examinations of the tissue.

The practice of removing all links between a patient's data and the patient's identity is called *anonymization*. The anonymization process relieves the researcher from the regulatory burdens and the IRB review process required by 45CFR46. It has been our experience that many researchers believe that anonymizing data is a foolproof method for protecting the interests of both patient and researcher. It would seem reasonable that in an anonymized study, the patient would certainly be no worse off than if the study had not been performed at all.

Nonetheless, ethicists have made some cogent arguments against research using anonymized tissues or data. In our view, the most compelling argument against research using anonymized tissues arises in the instance in which life-saving information is discovered during the course of the research. Imagine the researcher's predicament when a treatable disease is diagnosed on an anonymized tissue sample. By definition, anonymized tissue samples have had all identifying links to the patient removed. There would be no way of identifying the patient who should be notified of research findings.

From the researcher's perspective, anonymized tissues and data make it impossible to validate research results. When the unique linkage between tissue (or data) and the patient is removed, there is no way of verifying data. In an anonymized database, one cannot be certain that the data haven't been biased by multiple submissions on a single patient. If one suspects that a particular laboratory may have contaminated its contributions to the archive, there is no way of identifying those samples. Suppose that particular data-records are incomplete. Anonymized data do not permit the researcher to identify and contact a subject, in order to verify or complete a data-record. In the absence of any mechanism to verify data-records, how can one accept the conclusions drawn from the data?

Drafted NBAC recommendations consider a mechanism whereby certain types of studies might be approved by the IRB without meeting Exemption 4. Under opinions emerging under NBAC, IRBs may categorize research proposals by the risks they impose on human subjects. In general, research that utilizes in-place data and tissues (i.e., materials collected in the regular course of patient treatment and not collected as part of a research protocol), would be considered *minimal risk research projects.* The only risk to the patient would be the loss of confidentiality of medical record data. In these cases, the IRB may examine the proposal to determine whether the researchers have a plan that assures that patient confidentiality will be well-protected. The IRB, at that point, might address the question of whether the potential value to society of the proposed research outweighs the minimal risk to the patient for whom confidentiality might be breached. If the research meets these requirements, then the IRB may grant approval for the research without requiring data anonymization or obtaining informed consent (in the case of retrospective data and tissues).

How can patient confidentiality be protected when the data are not anonymized? The authors have previously demonstrated the use of a doubly-encrypted brokered tissue database (Berman et al, 1996). In this model, providers of pathology data encrypt patient identifiers and send their data to a database administrator. The database administrator then performs a second encryption on the identifiers, before releasing the data to the scientific community. Data miners could freely use the data in such a pathology database, without access to the identity of the patients included in the database. Suppose, for some reason, a data miner needs to collect additional data on certain patient records (e.g., survival or treatment data). The researcher would send a request for additional information to the database administrator, along with the relevant records, each containing doubly-encrypted patient identifiers. The database administrator would perform a single decryption of the patient identifiers, and forward the request to the institution that contributed the data-record. The provider IRB then reviews the request, and determines whether it would be legal and ethical to perform the final decryption step linking the data-record with the patient. This decision might involve obtaining patient consent. If the final decryption is approved, then the patient is identified. The additional information is returned to the database administrator, after tagging the data-record with the re-encrypted identifier. The database administrator then sends the records to the researcher, after tagging the data with the doubly-encrypted identifier. Throughout the process, the database administrator and the researcher never learn the identity of the patient. It is interesting that the field of cryptography provides the solution (double-encryption) to the greatest legal and ethical obstacle against progress in the field of pathology informatics.

Of some interest is the fact that 45CFR46 applies to all federally funded research involving human subjects. However, research conducted with absolutely no federal tie-in is not covered by 45CFR46 regulations. Today, medical insurers and health maintenance organizations freely use data collected on patients for a variety of data mining activities, that may eventually impact negatively on certain groups of patients. Consider the medical insurer who employs data mining techniques to identify persons at high risk for cancer or other chronic diseases, for the purpose of removing those patients from insurance enrollment. Is this an ethical use of data mining?

4.2 Understanding the Data

4.2.1 Size of Potential Anatomic Pathology Data Domain

On August 1, 1998, there were 17,974 board-certified pathologists in the USA (American Board of Medical Specialists, Appendix), who spend an estimated 42.5% of their time in the practice of diagnostic surgical pathology (Smith et al, 1989; Anderson et al, 1991). Other activities that occupy a pathologist include: teaching, research, administration, diagnostic cytopathology, autopsy pathology, and clinical pathology (laboratory medicine). A fulltime surgical pathologist, who does nothing but practice diagnostic surgical pathology, is expected to issue approximately 5,300 surgical pathology reports per year. Autopsies account for only a tiny percentage of anatomic pathology reports. Cytopathology reports are predominantly screening procedures, and usually do not contain the final diagnoses required for data mining investigations.

Hence, the pathology establishment in the USA issues approximately

$$17{,}974 \times 5{,}300 \times 42.5\% = 40 \text{ million}$$

surgical pathology reports annually, or about one surgical pathology report per year for each six persons in the USA.

In general, large medical centers and large health-care networks, such as the Veterans Affairs medical centers and Kaiser Permanente, maintain archival computerized surgical pathology reports indefinitely. However, many community hospitals maintain computerized reports for two years (as required by pathology laboratory regulatory bodies), and then transfer surgical pathology reports to an inactive storage medium, such as microfiche, in which reports are essentially unrecoverable for data mining purposes. This downloading policy made economic sense about a decade ago when computer storage was relatively expensive. The persistence of this policy in this modern era of cheap computer storage represents administrative inertia, and the absence of financial and social incentives to convert laboratories toward more computerized medical record management.

Each surgical pathology report is approximately one kilobyte in size, i.e., one double-spaced typewritten page, of which approximately 100 bytes form the *free-text microscopic diagnosis*. The other 900 bytes consist of accession numbers, patient identifiers, date/time stamps, and the gross description text. Thus each year, an estimated 40,000,000,000 bytes (40

Gigabytes, 40 GB) of surgical pathology reports are issued in the USA, an amount of data small enough to fit on a single hard-disk drive.

Academic medical centers and Veterans Affairs medical centers generate an estimated 30% of all reports (Anderson et al, 1991), with a decade of legacy data, for a total of 12 GB of surgical pathology report information. Community hospitals generate 70% of all reports, with two years of legacy data, for a total of 5.6 GB of surgical pathology report information. Thus we estimate that there is a total of 17.6 GB of legacy surgical pathology report information potentially available for data mining in the USA, with 4 GB of new information generated annually.

Clinical pathology (laboratory medicine) involves medical laboratory tests on fluids taken from the patient's body (blood, urine, etc.). Each byte of anatomic pathology data corresponds to approximately 150 bytes of clinical pathology data. Thus each year, six terabytes (six trillion bytes) of clinical pathology data are generated in U. S. medical centers. While most of these data are numerical in character, the data often require non-numerical contextual information about the patient in order to be meaningfully interpreted in data mining investigations.

4.2.2 Description of an Anatomic Pathology Report

Every pathology report begins as pieces of human tissue, submitted to a pathology laboratory with accompanying paperwork. In the simplest case, there is one piece of tissue, obtained from one surgical procedure, arriving in one container, from one appropriately identified patient, with one accompanying page of paper that contains matching identifiers, and a relevant medical history in plain English, with correct spelling and grammar. Roughly half the specimens received in a typical pathology department conform to this description. Furthermore, this model can serve as the basis for understanding the more complex situations, in which an accessioned case arrives in the pathology laboratory with multiple specimens from one or more procedures performed on the patient.

When the specimen and paperwork arrives in the laboratory, an *accession clerk* verifies the paperwork, and assigns a unique *accession number* to the specimen-and-paperwork ensemble, known as an *accession*. A sample surgical pathology report is illustrated in Table 1. The format for this pathology report is United States Government Tissue Examination Form, Standard Form 515. All U. S. Government installations use the same form, and academic and community hospital tissue examination forms contain essentially the same information, although details differ. Different institutions enforce the completion of these forms with different degrees of strictness. For example, at our institution, a form with a patient-name not recognized in the hospital database, a form without a physician-name or unsigned by a physician, or a form without a patient-history, are not accepted, and an effort is made to resolve any problems with the submitting physician. These procedures are minimum requirements set by the College of American Pathologists (Appendix).

There are four general classes of data in an anatomic pathology report:

- Assigned numbers (accession number, procedure number, etc.).
- Date/time stamps (date obtained, date received, date released).
- Person (patient, submitting physician, pathologist).
- Clinicopathologic information (brief clinical history, gross description, microscopic diagnosis).

Accession numbers are assigned by the pathology laboratory, and are used to keep track of what specimens arrived in the laboratory. This accession number assignment is ideally carried out in one physical location, using a computerized *Laboratory Information System (LIS)* with a parallel offline accessioning system (*logbook*). The LIS assigns the accession number, which should be sequential and non-duplicated. If specimens are accepted and accession numbers are assigned at more than one physical location, then great care must be taken to keep numbering assignments at all the physical locations in synchrony. This requirement is trivial as long as the LIS is always functioning everywhere, but may become very convoluted when different accession areas have dyssynchronous periods of computer downtime.

Date/time stamps include: *date obtained, date received, date released.* The LIS should not accept date/time information that is inconsistent, such as a specimen obtained at a date/time later than specimen received. On the other hand, reality is unpredictably complex, and there must be mechanisms to override apparent inconsistencies in the usual sequence-of-events in a pathology report. For example, what if the exact date of a particular event is not known? When a patient cannot recall the appearance of a particular symptom; or, for some older or immigrant patients, birthdate.

There must be a formalism for managing inexact dates. In the VISTA computer system used by Veterans Affairs Medical Centers, date/time is denoted by seven decimal digits, followed by a decimal point, followed by six decimal digits. The first digit denotes century (0=1700, 1=1800,

2=1900, etc.). Thus, U. S. Veteran George Washington (born 1732) has a century digit of 0; and U. S. Veteran George Bush (born 1924) has a century digit of 2 (DeGregorio, 1997). Digits two and three denote year; digits four and five denote month (01=January, etc.); and digits six and seven denote day. The first and second post-decimal digits denote hour (24-hour clock); the third and fourth post-decimal digits denote minute; and the fifth and sixth post-decimal digits denote second. Missing values in the date/time are denoted with zero. Thus, an event happening during an unknown month in 1999 is denoted 2990000.000000; and an event happening at an unknown time on August 27, 1908 (birthdate of U. S. President Lyndon B. Johnson (DeGregorio, 1997)) is denoted 2080827.000000. The VISTA date/time numbering system is ideally suited for managing patient confidentiality on in a public data mine resource. All events can be rounded off to year-of-occurrence, simply by replacing all digits past the third digit with zero; or to decade-of-occurrence, by replacing all digits past the second digit with zero.

Each person named on the report (*patient, submitting physician, pathologist*) must match up to a person on a list, who can be reached as necessary for purposes of notification, billing, and followup. It is critical that the paperwork reliably identifies the patient and the submitting physician, and unambiguously links the paperwork to the specimen. Correct identification is not easy to achieve, but is not an idle luxury. A misidentification could mean the failure to assign a serious diagnosis to a patient, or assigning a diagnosis to the incorrect patient. Patient injury and legal action could ensue.

Unusual names must be spelled correctly, and common names must be distinguished for different actual patients. For example, a thousand-bed U. S. hospital can expect to add one new *Mary Smith* every week to its patient identification system. The U. S. Social Security Number is *not* an acceptable method for distinguishing among all the Mary Smiths, since there is a known error rate in the social security system (about one percent), and the immediate consequence of a misidentified patient is far more serious than that of a misplaced social security payment. It is *not* acceptable to assign Mary Smith a new identification number each time her physician submits a new specimen to the pathology laboratory, because the certain knowledge of a patient's prior diagnoses is critical toward understanding each subsequent diagnosis. Finally, uncommon names with unusual spellings must be spelled consistently for each entry into the LIS, and *aliases* (i.e., different names used by the same patient) must be known and managed appropriately by the LIS.

Clinicopathologic information includes*: brief clinical history, gross description, microscopic diagnosis*, and typically appears on a pathology report as *free-text*. This free-text is the most unstructured part of the pathology report, and is difficult both to enter correctly and to recover satisfactorily in data mining investigations. Clinical histories are received from other departments, so that one makes the effort to clarify an unintelligible clinical history only if the clinical information is perceived as critical to the final diagnosis on the pathology report. In many cases, medical histories replete with misspellings, nonsequiturs, and missing information are accepted. Gross description and microscopic diagnosis are under the administrative control of the pathology laboratory, but there is typically little motivation to achieve standards of spelling and punctuation beyond those necessary for a presentable report.

The microscopic diagnosis field contains the final result of the anatomic pathology examination. The microscopic diagnosis is referred to by a number of different names, including *diagnostic impression, diagnosis, microscopic evaluation*, and even *report*. The lack of consistent terminology for common data elements poses yet another obstacle for data mining efforts using stored pathology reports. In our experience, approximately half the microscopic diagnosis fields from anatomic pathology reports must be copyedited before the reports are optimally suitable for data mining investigations. In some cases, this copyediting might consist of little more than inserting appropriate sentence terminators. In other cases, major revision might be necessary to correct misspellings, and to reconstruct sentences into a grammatically correct and unambiguous text.

4.2.3 Converting Parts of a Report into Object Domains

4.2.3.1 Pathology Report Database

In the Laboratory Information System (LIS), the report database is separated into *fields*, and certain minimum standards are enforced by the system. For example, the date/time that the specimen was removed from the patient must precede temporally the date/time that the specimen was received in the pathology laboratory; and in turn, the date/time that the specimen was received in the pathology laboratory must precede the date/time that a final report was issued by the pathology laboratory. The name of the patient must correspond to an identifier recognized by a third-party-payer (insurance carrier); the name of the submitting physician must correspond to an identifier to whom the report can be sent (in order to receive payment); and the name of the attending pathologist must correspond to an identifier who can be disciplined if the report is tardy. The advantage of such a LIS is a level of managerial control over workloads, turnaround times, and billing that a simple word processor system cannot offer. An important byproduct of this enforced structure is that such systems contain data that are usable in data mining projects. However, in the commercial setting, there is always a tradeoff between strict enforcement of standards and offending the customer, so that optimal data standards are not always achieved.

In complex cases, the submitting physician may submit multiple pieces of tissue from the same patient, taken during a single outpatient visit or inpatient encounter. For example, Table 1 describes two *containers* taken at the same encounter from the patient, and consecutively numbered by the submitting physician. The final pathology report must reproduce the numbering produced by the submitting physician. All discrepancies in the actual containers received and their descriptions on accompanying paperwork must be resolved in the final report.

There are two other natural divisions in a multi-container anatomic pathology accession: *procedure* and *bodysite*. Many multi-part pathology reports do not unambiguously reflect these divisions; and in our conversations with colleagues, we are convinced that some of our colleagues do not clearly understand these divisions. However a correct assignment of these divisions is essential for making sense of the data in any anatomic pathology data mine resource, and for many quality assurance surveys.

For example, suppose that a surgeon performs a total laryngectomy on a patient with previously diagnosed squamous cell carcinoma of the left true vocal cord. The patient has hard, palpable lymph nodes (probable metastatic cancer) on both sides of the neck, so the surgeon performs a bilateral radical neck dissection in the same operative session. The surgeon also notices two small, irregular black macules (i.e., flat skin discolorations), one over the right clavicle, the other over the left scapula, and removes them for diagnosis. The laryngectomy specimen arrives in the pathology laboratory in container #1. Ten surgical margin specimens arrive in containers #2 through #11. The right radical neck dissection arrives in container #12, and the left radical neck dissection arrives in container #13. The right clavicular skin excision arrives in container #14, and the left scapular skin excision arrives in container #15.

These fifteen containers separate logically into five surgical procedures, namely, laryngectomy, right radical neck dissection, left radical neck dissection, right clavicular skin excision, and left scapular skin excision. The laryngectomy procedure subdivides into at least sixteen bodysites; the right and left radical neck dissections subdivide into nine bodysites apiece; and each of the skin excisions and their surgical margins subdivide into five bodysites apiece (Rosai and Ackerman, 1996; Hruban et al, 1996; Association of Directors of Anatomic and Surgical Pathology,

1997). The structure of the mined database must capture these divisions and subdivisions, in order to be optimally useful to epidemiologists and tissue resource specialists.

Furthermore, the relationship between one specimen and another specimen taken from the same patient at a different time may be indeterminate. For example, for many skin cancers, a particular report may correspond to a new lesion on the patient or to the recurrence of a previously diagnosed lesion, taken either at the same hospital or at another institution. All too often, the bodysite designation provided by the submitting physician does not provide enough anatomical detail even for a human expert to make this distinction from the content of the report alone.

Multiple cancer lesions from the same patient might represent metastases or multiple independent lesions. Sometimes, the submitting physician does not include relevant clinical or radiologic information that might resolve this question.

Sometimes the submitting physician does not even accurately identify the site of origin of a specimen, omitting such details as left versus right, medial versus lateral, or superior versus inferior. Sometimes the anatomical orientation is resolved in such a convoluted manner that only an expert can reasonably understand what is intended. In any event, no commercially available LIS enforces the correct disambiguations from carelessly composed pathology reports. Ensuring that reports can be automatically parsed into data elements that accurately represent the concepts included in the free-text report is one of the greatest impediments (and challenges) to the advancement of pathology informatics.

4.2.3.2 Parsing Free-Text into Sentences

The introduction of sentence boundaries into the free-text of an anatomic pathology report is a surprisingly necessary and complicated undertaking.

For example, this text report:

Liver showing metastatic adenocarcinoma

Portal lymph node showing reactive hyperplasia.

might easily be misinterpreted by an autocoder (computer translator) as including the diagnosis: *Metastatic adenocarcinoma portal lymph node.* After all, the disease-concept, *Metastatic adenocarcinoma,* and the bodysite-concept, *Portal lymph node,* are not separated by any intervening words or punctuation.

One could insist that the pathologist punctuate the report as:

Liver showing metastatic adenocarcinoma.

Portal lymph node showing reactive hyperplasia.

This insistence is no help in processing legacy (retrospective) anatomic pathology reports. Different pathologists have different punctuation styles. Even the two authors of this chapter, who practiced pathology together for eight years, could never reach agreement on a consistent style of punctuation of their department's anatomic pathology reports. Furthermore, uniform punctuation standards may not be enforceable even in the future, unless it is demonstrated that the pathologist is rewarded, either financially or by substantially improved case management, for correctly punctuating her reports, and that this goal can be achieved with a minimum of fuss.

It should be noted that the period-character (ASCII 46) is neither an unambiguous sentence-terminator, nor is it the only possible sentence terminator. The period is also used as a decimal-point (4.2, 10.17), for honorifics (Dr., Mr., Ms.), and (often ambiguously) in abbreviations (AIDS., A.I.D.S., A. I. D. S.), all of which may occur in mid-sentence of a pathology report. For example, the abbreviation MS. may be used legitimately in a free-text medical document to denote: female-honorific, Mississippi, Microsoft®, multiple sclerosis, mitral stenosis, morphine sulphate, millisecond, microsecond. Conversely, *colon, semicolon, question-mark*, and *exclamation-point* may also serve as *de facto* sentence-terminators for some sentences appearing in a pathology report.

4.2.3.3 Discovering Terms for Translation into Coded Nomenclature

The process of *autocoding (computer-translating)* a large collection of legacy free-text reports is interactive and iterative. One begins with the entire, text-file (*source-text*), and a computerized *coding system*, such as UMLS. One concludes with a database that maps each text-sentence into either a syntactically acceptable sequence of codes recognized by the autocoder, or else into an error message. The goal of the autocoder is to minimize the number of text-sentences that generate an error-message.

Both the source-text and the coding system can be modified and enriched. The source-text may be pre-edited, with sentence boundaries corrected, and with misspellings and ambiguities resolved.

If the original source-text is relatively well-formed, then pre-editing may be targeted at those few sentences that fail a grammatical parser. One may discover additional, as yet unforeseen sentence structures that must be added to the autocoder. The coding system may be enriched to include new synonyms encountered in the source text. For example, in the UMLS Metathesaurus coding system, C0007117 is the *Concept Unique Identifier* (CUI) for *Basal Cell Carcinoma*. However, pre-editing the source-text might uncover *Basal Cell Epithelioma* or *Basalioma* as synonyms for C0007117. A very ambitious researcher might even collect a list of *false-negative concepts*, present in the source-text but absent in the coding system, and petition the administrators of the coding system to include the additional codes and synonyms in a future revision of the coding system (Kao and Moore, 2000).

Concepts within the source-text are further discoverable by the *Barrier Word Method* (Tersmette et al, 1988; Moore GW et al, 1989; Nelson et al, 1995). In the barrier word method, natural-language medical text is regarded as a sequence of medical concepts linked together with grammatical objects, or *barrier words*, which serve to delimit sentence boundaries or phrase boundaries. Barrier words include: all punctuation, all numerals, nearly all one-letter and two-letter words, articles, prepositions, and common verbs and modifiers. *Medical concepts* are one-word or multiple-word terms, consisting of medically significant component words (*keywords*).

For example, consider the source-text appearing in Table 3 (Colby et al, 1995). In this example, the *barrier words are shown in lower case*, and the *KEYWORDS ARE SHOWN IN UPPER CASE*. In general, each *SEQUENCE OF KEYWORDS uninterrupted by barrier words* should point to one or more UMLS Metathesaurus CUIs. Thus the entire message contained in this table, not including punctuation, may be translated into a sequence of CUIs, namely, C0206704, C0396473, C0225355,....

4.2.3.4 Preparing the Zipf Distribution of Phrases and Words

It is helpful to prepare a descending-order frequency distribution, or *Zipf Distribution*, of single words occurring in the source-text. *Zipf's Law* (Zipf, 1949) states that a few hundred common words (typically, barrier words) account for over half the word-occurrences in a large text-database, an observation confirmed in large text-databases in English (Fedorowicz, 1982; Moore et al, 1988), German (Giere, 1981), and Chinese (Zhang, 1981). Very high frequency words and terms have almost no recall value in a computerized indexing system, and should not be indexed. High frequency words that are not barrier words provide the data miner with a snapshot of the common concepts in the data source. Greater attention should be focused on matching these words to UMLS synonym-names, since failure to match common concepts will result in poor overall data mining performance. Many low frequency words are highly specific for indexing and data mining purposes. These words are also important to match to UMLS synonym-names, particularly if one of the goals of data mining is to identify unusual disease conditions and outcomes.

4.2.3.5 Translating Source Terms into UMLS Codes

As a first approximation, one can obtain an exact match between keyword terms in the source-text and UMLS Metathesaurus synonym-names, in order to achieve a preliminary mapping into UMLS. For example, *Large Cell Carcinoma* maps exactly into the official UMLS Metathesaurus CUI, C0206704. Next, some non-matches may be mapped as more complete forms. For example, *Nuclei* is not an official UMLS Metathesaurus synonym-name, but *Cell Nucleus* maps into the UMLS Metathesaurus CUI, C0007610. Additional non-exact matches may be mapped into obvious synonym-names. For example, *Cluster* and *Clusters* are not official UMLS Metathesaurus synonym-names, but the synonym-name, *Aggregate*, maps into the UMLS Metathesaurus CUI, C0205418.

Misspellings in the source text may be managed either by declaring a *popular misspelling* as a synonym-name, or by correcting the misspelling in the source text. For example, *abcess* is a popular misspelling for *abscess* (C0000833) in many surgical pathology reports. Some orthographic purists would shudder at the prospect of placing *abcess* in a synonym-name table, but this action may be a necessary concession to practicality. *Popular abbreviations* may be matched to UMLS codes in a comparable manner, such as C.O.L.D. for *Chronic-Obstructive-Lung-Disease* (C0024117). However, this action can eventually lead to a jungle of unresolved ambiguities, as for example: COLD for *Chronic-Obstructive-Lung-Disease* (C0024117); *Cold-Coryza* (C0009443); and *Cold-Temperature* (C0009264).

As a general rule, it is preferable for an expert copyeditor to annotate an obvious ambiguity in the source text than to relegate this step to the autocoder. Thus for example, *Adnexa* is ambiguous, but the annotations, *Skin-Adnexa* (C0221943), *Uterine-Adnexa* (C0001575), or *Ocular-Adnexa* (C0229243), are unambiguous, and would be properly translated by the autocoder.

Another compelling reason to initially disambiguate the source-text in a pre-editing step is our belief that the real goal of preparing source-text for pathology data mining should be recoding or retranslation. This is the view that the anatomic pathology report should initially be written in plain English: unambiguous, orthographically and syntactically correct, short sentences. Then, as the philosophy or goals of the autocoder evolve and improve, the entire set of anatomic pathology reports can be re-autocoded, and re-mined.

4.3 Preparation of the Data

4.3.1 Data Ownership

Pathologists, patients, and laboratories all lay claim to ownership of tissue specimens and pathology report data. When a pathologist renders a diagnosis on a microscopic slide (which contains a stained sample of tissue that the pathologist has carefully selected and described), she creates a medicolegal document that often creates a drastic change in the life of the patient from that point onward. For many patients, the notification of cancer (or absence of cancer) on a pathology report may represent one of the most important moments of their lives. The pathologist's signature appears on each report, and the pathologist must be prepared to accept the legal and social consequences of any errors or inaccuracies in her rendered diagnosis. Pathologists spend a good portion of their professional life archiving tissues and contributing their reports to the pathology database. It is no wonder that pathologists tend to think of pathology specimens and reports as their professional property. This belief, long held by pathologists, is currently under attack by patients and patient-advocates, who believe that the tissues obtained from a patient and the report rendered on the tissues belong to the patient.

Legal theory treats ownership in relation to commerce. The owner of an item is considered to be the person who has the right to sell the item. Since it is almost universally held that human tissue has special status and should not be sold or bartered, legal precedent demures from assigning ownership of human tissue. Instead, current practices provide specific rights to use human tissues to several parties. Patients have the right to know the content of pathology reports rendered on their biopsied tissues. In certain cases, such as when a patient seeks treatment at an institution different from the institution that rendered the original diagnosis, or when the patient chooses to have the pathologic material reviewed by a different laboratory or pathologist, the pathologist must transfer those materials according to the patient's request. In this instance, the original pathologist concedes that her fiduciary responsibility to the patient is more compelling than her rights to own the specimen.

Institutions rendering pathology diagnoses have certain rights and obligations regarding patient information. The *Health Insurance Portability and Accountability Act of 1996 (HIPAA, Kennedy-Kassebaum Bill, H.R. 3103 of 104th Congress* (Appendix)) requires standards to be established for the transfer of information regarding health claims. Institutions may also be required to establish registries, particularly cancer registries. This involves compiling data, including synopses of pathology data, and contributing the collected data to a centralized registry, such as the registry operated by the *Centers for Disease Control and Prevention (CDCP).* In addition, institutions may on occasion need to acquire and transfer reports and tissues, in order to comply with legal subpoenas filed in the interest of patients.

The pathologist who uses a patient's tissues and associated data in a research study, is likely to claim ownership. If she can satisfy herself that the study is designed in such a way that the patient's welfare is protected, and that the fiduciary responsibilities to the patient are satisfied, then she will most likely argue that she has the right to use her acquired specimens and data without obtaining the patient's consent.

Currently, regulations guiding the use of tissues and data for research purposes abound. A number of states have enacted laws that place special restrictions on genetic research. However, the current U. S. Federal legislation that is directly germane to the use of human tissues and associated data for research involving federally funded institutions or researchers is found in *Article 46 of 45 CFR, U. S. Code of Federal Regulations (USCFR)* (1995). These regulations are used by researchers, by Institutional Review Boards, and by the *U. S. Federal Office of Protection from Research Risks (OPRR)* (Appendix), to ensure the safety of individuals entered into research projects. Some suggestions for the ethical conduct of research and for the interpretation of 45 CFR 46, have been prepared by *the U. S. National Bioethics Advisory Commission (NBAC)* (Appendix).

In general, in research involving pathology data and tissues that are stored in pathology archives, but which were obtained in the standard course of patient treatment (i.e., that were not obtained to satisfy a research protocol), the risk to the patient is the risk that the patient's confidentiality will be breached. All physicians have a fiduciary obligation to ensure that information related to a patient's medical condition can never be used to harm the patient.

In response to the HIPAA legislation, the Department of Health and Human Services has issued proposals for Standards for Privacy of Individually Identifiable Health Information. The Proposed Rules appeared in the Federal Register, and are designated as 45 CFR Parts 160 to 164 (Appendix). In the Proposed Rule, the concept of deidentification is discussed. In 45 CFR 46 (*Common Rule*), researchers who use medical information can be excluded from regulation, if the medical data are completely stripped of all patient identifiers (*anonymization*) as well as all links to patient identifiers. Because anonymization is irreversible, discoveries, inconsistencies or errors found in anonymized data cannot be relinked back to a patient. Consequently, studies using anonymized data cannot be used to inform patients of any discovered risks to their health; cannot have data inconsistencies rectified; and cannot be checked for the accuracy of the original data included in the dataset.

De-identified data are data for which the recipient of the data cannot determine the patient's identity, but the institution that provided the data can, if needed, relink the patient's identity to the data (Appendix; Berman et al, 1996). For instance, if an institution encrypts a patient's name and gives the data to a third party, then the third party does not know the identity of the patient (i.e., the data are anonymized for the recipient). But if the third party contacts the institution and suggests that they have information that the patient may need to know, then the institution can take the encrypted patient identifier from the third party, decrypt the patient's identifier, and contact the patient. Although the mechanism for patient deidentification is unspecified in the Proposed Rule, it is clear that institutions will need to develop deidentification methods that are reasonable for their own operational circumstances, and that such methods will require approval from Institutional Review Boards before de-identified medical data can be shared with researchers.

De-identification methods may offer institutions a way of sharing encrypted, masked, or otherwise modified data for research efforts, in which the value to public health is deemed to outweigh the minimal risk to patient confidentiality.

4.3.2 Data Requirements

4.3.2.1 What Constitutes Acceptable Anatomic Pathology Data?

Every surgical pathology report is identified by a unique case accession number (usually assigned when the patient's specimen is received in the pathlogy laboratory), and a patient identifier (typically the patient's name and a unique identifying code assigned by the hospital, or the patient's social security number). Many institutions prefer the social security number, because it is presumed to be unique, and lasts for a lifetime. We have heard unverified anecdotal stories of the re-use of social security numbers from deceased patients. If this is true, then it implies that social security numbers might be unique among the set of living persons, but that some living persons may share the same social security number of persons who are deceased. In any event, it can be safely assumed that social security numbers provided by patients to hospitals may be transcribed with human data-entry errors. The most common data-entry error is associated with remembering sequences of digits, or transcribing sequences of digits is transposition of consecutive digits. For long sequences of digits, error rates can exceed 10%. It is a certainty that hospital databases contain incorrect social security numbers, and that some of these numbers are non-unique (i.e., erroneously match one individual to another individual).

Relevant demographic material might include: date of birth, gender, ethnicity, and date of death when applicable. Additional clinical information is often obtained in the form of other pathology reports for a given patient, clinical history that precedes a diagnostic report, and clinical history, including treatment, that results from a rendered pathology diagnosis. Finally, there is the pathology diagnosis itself, which may be recorded as free-text, and translated (either manually or automatically) into a standardized coding system.

For a well-formed pathology report, the laboratory information system should be able to markup the report with document tags, that serve as a roadmap for a data mining system. The *Hypertext Markup Language (HTML)* is a document formatting language that permits Internet web designers to attach markup tags to elements of text (e.g., font size, formatting information, color selection, etc.). The *Extensible Markup Language (XML)* permits document elements to be tagged with markers that that describe the actual content of data elements in the text (Simpson, 1996; Light, 1997).

Table 2 shows a valid XML file for the surgical pathology report listed in Table 1. The significant elements in the pathology report (accession number, lab identifier, time obtained, etc.) are marked by XML tags. These tags, in turn, may have certain required properties (date/time, size in cm, bodysite-name, UMLS-CUI, etc.), and may be iterated.

The open challenge for anatomic pathology data miners is to develop a structure for XML tags that is acceptable to our colleagues, and then to translate large collections of pathology reports into corresponding XML files.

4.3.2.2 Security and Confidentiality

There are two levels of security that must be addressed in any data mining project for anatomic pathology:

- Concealment of the patient's name.
- Concealment of the patient's detailed medical history.

At the first level of security, the patient's exact identifiers must never be disclosed in a public venue. These identifiers include (U. S. Code of Federal Regulations, Appendix): name; address, including street address, city, county, zip code, or equivalent geocodes; names of relatives and employers; birth date; voice telephone and fax numbers; email addresses; social security number; medical record number; health plan beneficiary number; account number; certificate/license number; any vehicle or other device serial number; web URL; Internet Protocol (IP) address; finger or voice prints; photographic images; and any other unique identifying number, characteristic, or code (whether generally available in the public realm or not) that the one has reason to believe may be available to an anticipated recipient of the information. The methods for achieving simple encryption of the patient's identifiers are well-understood, commercially available, and if used properly, are essentially unbreakable (Schneier, 1996). These include: the *one-time-pad method* and *public-private encryption methods*.

At the second level of security, one must recognize that a detailed medical record, even when purged of the patient's exact identifiers, might still contain information sufficiently detailed to identify the patient. For example, suppose that the hypothetical autopsy report in Table 4 had been deposited in a public autopsy resource. Then public knowledge regarding this U. S. President's medical history might be sufficient to identify the subject of this hypothetical autopsy report. Furthermore, there might be additional, previously private information in the report that would embarrass or otherwise harm the family. Even if it were legal to disclose this report, such wholesale disclosures of personal information would erode public confidence in the doctor-patient relationship, cause future patients to conceal parts of their medical history, and eventually damage the overall quality of medical care.

On the other hand, had the public autopsy report identified the patient's occupation solely as *Politics* (C0032382), seventh decade at death, autopsied in the 1970s, and contained no exact numeric information regarding the dates of birth and of various diagnoses, then it might represent the autopsy report of thousands of middle-aged men.

This example is further mitigated by an important qualification. Anyone who campaigns and serves on a job as public as the President of the United States must reckon with a loss of privacy, and with possible exposure of private aspects of one's life. Should a public medical resource be deemed culpable for revealing additional facts about an already-public person?

A patient's detailed medical history may be concealed by a distinction between public demographics and private demographics (Carter et al, 1981; Peery, 1978). Public demographics must include enough information to have value for epidemiologic studies, but not so much as to disclose the identity of the patient. All other demographics could be withheld from the public, and should be disclosed only under subpoena or with IRB approval.

4.4 Data Mining Example

4.4.1 The Johns Hopkins Autopsy Resource

Over the past three decades, there have been proposals in the anatomic pathology literature for inter-institutional sharing of pathology data (Carter et al, 1981; Peery, 1978; Wagner, 1996; Mullick, 1997; Moore et al, 1996). *The Johns Hopkins Autopsy Resource (JHAR)* (Appendix) is an Internet website, founded as an institutional database in 1980, and posted publicly in 1995, that lists over 50,000 autopsy facesheets, on patients born over a span of two centuries. An autopsy facesheet is the summary of final diagnoses, typically appearing as the first page in an autopsy report. The JHAR corresponds to an estimated one million tissue blocks, predominantly formalin-fixed and paraffin-embedded, which may be obtained as part of collaborative research investigations. Over 1300 publications in scholarly journals have resulted from the cases listed in the JHAR, and all citations, many with PubMed hyperlinks, are available on the website. Studies based upon data mining the JHAR include case reports (Hutchins et al, 1996), large autopsy case series (Arcidi et al, 1981; Vigorita et al, 1980; Moore and Hutchins, 1982), and even linguistic studies of medical text (Moore et al, 1988; Moore et al, 1989).

For example, in one of the autopsy studies based upon cases listed in the JHAR, the investigators sought to determine whether the severity and duration of adult-onset diabetes mellitus (AODM) is correlated with the severity of coronary atherosclerosis observed at autopsy. Clinical and autopsy findings were studied in 185 patients with AODM, who ranged in age from 37 to 91 years, and had had a clinical diagnosis of AODM established between a few days and up to 50 years before death. The JHAR was used to identify age-sex matched control subjects autopsied during a similar period. In comparison with age-sex matched controls, patients with AODM showed significantly more coronary artery disease, more diffuseness of coronary disease, more coronary collateralization, more vessels involved by atherosclerosis, and more myocardial infarcts. On the other hand, the progression of this atherosclerotic disease was unrelated to duration or severity of AODM (Vigorita et al, 1980).

The authors of that study cautioned against drawing conclusions from large datasets without a thorough understanding of the contained data (Moore and Hutchins, 1982). For example, severity of AODM was significantly correlated with short stature at autopsy. Further investigation of this initially interesting observation revealed that each patient's height at autopsy was measured from the head to the termination of the lower extremities. It turned out that many severe diabetics were double amputees!

Studies such as this one underscore the value of data mining efforts, in which valuable conclusions could be drawn quickly and inexpensively from existing patient records, radiographs, and microscope slides alone, without the expense and ethical problems inherent in designing a prospective clinicopathologic investigation.

In order to achieve patient confidentiality in the JHAR, each autopsy facesheet consists of a *demographic line*, followed by *diagnoses*. The only public demographic information provided is: age in decades, race, sex, decade of autopsy, and a *key-number*, which can be used to decrypt the patient identification, if necessary. Confidentiality is protected by the double-brokered encryption system of patient identifiers, which requires the participation of both the JHAR administrator and officials of the Department of Pathology of The Johns Hopkins Medical Institutions to re-identify the individual patients (Berman et al, 1996). As an additional security measure, the key-number may correspond to multiple patients, with the number-of-patients for a given key-number known only to the JHAR administration. Diagnoses in the original autopsy facesheet have been stripped of names of persons, locations, and institutions; and diagnoses have been autocoded into generic medical language as well as into UMLS codes in XML format. The only mechanism for obtaining additional information regarding an individual JHAR autopsy facesheet is to correspond with the database administrator, who forwards the correspondence to the appropriate official at The Johns Hopkins Medical Institutions. The Johns Hopkins Medical Institutions responds in accordance with policies set by its Institutional Review Board.

4.5 Conclusion

Data mining in anatomic pathology is an emerging field. In the past, data mining efforts consisted of small projects conducted with the existing electronic records within a given institution. Five developments over the past several years have enormously expanded the potential for anatomic pathology data mining:

1. The accumulation of millions of pathology records in electronic form. Approximately 40 million new anatomic pathology reports are created and stored each year in the USA.

2. The emergence of legislative guidelines that ensure patient confidentiality, while establishing ethical and legal paradigms by which researchers can acquire pathology data for legitimate research needs.

3. The availability of comprehensive common medical terminologies (including SNOMED, Read, and UMLS), that will support translation of diagnostic information into coded terms that can be aggregated and queried.

4. Community acceptance of standard document structures, such as XML. Electronic reports will contain data, along with information that describes the data, using community-standard data tags (metadata). Such standardized reports will remove the greatest technical impediment to sharing pathology data, namely, unclassifiable data.

5. The availability of Internet technology that allows the rapid and secure transfer of medical data. The most promising technology for data mining is the distributed network query. Through this mechanism, a client query is sent to multiple institutional databases, and a reply is created by a middleware agent that merges the responses from each of the cooperating institutions into a single database.

Access to pathology data is the rate-limiting factor to advancement in the field of pathology data mining. The next few years will be critical to the development of this new and promising field of research.

Table 1. Surgical Pathology Sample Report.

U. S. Government Standard Form 515

MEDICAL RECORD I SURGICAL PATHOLOGY

PATHOLOGY REPORT

Laboratory: BALTIMORE VAMHCS Accession No. BSP 99 8888

Submitted by: J SURGEON MD Date obtained: Jan 14, 1999

Specimen (Received Jan 15, 1999 10:32):

1. LARYNGECTOMY.

2. LEFT RADICAL NECK DISSECTION

Brief Clinical History:

SQUAMOUS CARCINOMA, LEFT TRUE CORD.

Preoperative Diagnosis:

SQUAMOUS CARCINOMA, LEFT TRUE CORD.

Operative Findings:

SAME.

Postoperative Diagnosis:

SAME.

Surgeon/physician: J SURGEON MD

Gross description:

PATIENT IDENTIFICATION AGREES WITH REQUISITON AND TWO CONTAINERS.

1. THE SPECIMEN IS RECEIVED FRESH, LABELED WITH THE PATIENT'S NAME, AND ADDITIONALLY LABELED "LARYNGECTOMY".

THE SPECIMEN CONSISTS OF A LARYNGECTOMY RESECTION, MEASURING 10.5 X 5.5 X 3.5 CM. THE LARYNX

IS EDEMATOUS. THE LARYNX IS OPENED POSTERIORLY, TO REVEAL AN IRREGULARITY OF APPARENT TUMOR, ON THE SURFACE OF THE LEFT TRUE VOCAL CORD, MEASURING 3.0 X 1.5 CM. THE TUMOR DOES NOT APPEAR TO INVOLVE THE SUBGLOTTIS, NOR THE ANTERIOR COMMISSURE. THE SUPERIOR, INFERIOR, ANTERIOR, AND POSTERIOR MARGINS ARE GROSSLY UNINVOLVED BY TUMOR REPRESENTATIVE SECTIONS OF TUMOR ARE SUBMITTED, AS WELL AS THE SURGICAL MARGINS, AS FOLLOWS:

SUMMARY OF SECTIONS:

1-1, 1 PIECE. TRACHEAL MARGIN.

1-2, 1 PIECE. BASE OF TONGUE MARGIN.

1-3, 1 PIECE. RIGHT PYRIFORM SINUS MARGIN.

1-4, 1 PIECE. LEFT PYRIFORM SINUS MARGIN.

1-5, 1 PIECE. ANTERIOR SOFT TISSUE MARGIN.

1-6, 1 PIECE. POSTERIOR SOFT TISSUE MARGIN.

1-7, 1 PIECE. LESION OF THE LEFT TRUE CORD.

1-8, 1 PIECE. LESION OF THE LEFT TRUE CORD.

1-9, 1 PIECE. LESION OF THE LEFT TRUE CORD.

1-10, 1 PIECE. EPIGLOTTIS.

2. THE SPECIMEN IS RECEIVED FRESH, LABELED WITH THE PATIENT'S NAME, AND ADDITIONALLY LABELED "LEFT RADICAL NECK DISSECTION". THE SPECIMEN CONSISTS OF A LEFT RADICAL NECK DISSECTION, MEASURING 25.0 X 15.0 X 5.0 CM.

THE SPECIMEN IS DIVIDED INTO LEVELS 1, 2, 3, 4, AND 5. IN LEVEL 1, THE SALIVARY GLAND AND ONE PROBABLE LYMPH NODE ARE SUBMITTED.

IN LEVEL 2, SIX PROBABLE LYMPH NODES ARE SUBMITTED.

IN LEVEL 3, TWO PROBABLE LYMPH NODES ARE SUBMITTED.

IN LEVEL 4, ELEVEN PROBABLE LYMPH NODES SUBMITTED.

IN LEVEL 5, FIVE PROBABLE LYMPH NODES ARE SUBMITTED.

REPRESENTATIVE SECTIONS ARE SUBMITTED, AS FOLLOWS:

SUMMARY OF SECTIONS:

1-1, 1 PIECE. LEVEL 1.

2-1, 5 PIECES. LEVEL 2.

3-1, 5 PIECES. LEVEL 2.

4-1, 4 PIECES. LEVEL 3.

5-1, 3 PIECES. LEVEL 3.

6-1, 6 PIECES. LEVEL 3.

7-1, 5 PIECES. LEVEL 4.

8-1, 5 PIECES. LEVEL 4.

9-1, 4 PIECES. LEVEL 5.

Microscopic exam/diagnosis:

1. SQUAMOUS CELL CARCINOMA OF LEFT TRUE CORD, WELL-DIFFERENTIATED, INVASIVE. SURGICAL MARGINS OF RESECTION ARE FREE OF TUMOR.
2. RADICAL NECK DISSECTION. SALIVARY GLAND WITH NOEVIDENCE OF MALIGNANCY. ELEVEN OF TWENTY-THREE LYMPH NODES WITH METASTATIC SQUAMOUS CELL CARCINOMA, AS FOLLOWS.

LEVEL I: SALIVARY GLAND AND ONE LYMPH NODE WITH NO EVIDENCE OF MALIGNANCY.

LEVEL II: THREE OF FIVE LYMPH NODES WITH METASTATIC SQUAMOUS CELL CARCINOMA.

LEVEL III: ONE OF TWO LYMPH NODES WITH METASTATIC SQUAMOUS CELL CARCINOMA.

LEVEL IV: SEVEN OF TEN LYMPH NODES WITH METASTATIC SQUAMOUS CELL CARCINOMA.

LEVEL V: FIVE LYMPH NODES WITH WITH NO EVIDENCE OF MALIGNANCY.

JOHN Q PATHOLOGIST MD xyzl Date Jan 16, 1999

VETERAN,JOHN Q. STANDARD FORM 515

ID:123-45-6789 SEX:M DOB:12/01/1940 AGE:58 LOC:ENT J SURGEON

Table 2. XML File for Surgical Pathology. Sample Report *

```
<?xml version="1.0" ?>
<!DOCTYPE path_report
[
<!ELEMENT path_report (accession)>
<!ELEMENT accession (lab_identifier, time, submission, pathologist, patient, procedure)>
<!ELEMENT lab_identifier (#PCDATA)>
<!ELEMENT time (time_obtained, time_received, time_reported, time_amended, time_supplemented)>
<!ELEMENT time_obtained (#PCDATA)>
<!ELEMENT time_received (#PCDATA)>
<!ELEMENT time_reported (#PCDATA)>
<!ELEMENT time_amended (#PCDATA)>
<!ELEMENT time_supplemented (#PCDATA)>
<!ELEMENT submission (submitting_physician, submitting_service)>
<!ELEMENT submitting_physician (#PCDATA)>
<!ELEMENT submitting_service (#PCDATA)>
<!ELEMENT pathologist (#PCDATA)>
<!ELEMENT patient (patient_name, patient_identifier, date_of_birth,
patient_gender, patient_ethnicity)>
<!ELEMENT patient_name (#PCDATA)>
<!ELEMENT patient_identifier (#PCDATA)>
<!ELEMENT date_of_birth (#PCDATA)>
<!ELEMENT patient_gender (#PCDATA)>
<!ELEMENT patient_ethnicity (#PCDATA)>
<!ELEMENT procedure (specimen)>
<!ELEMENT procedure_cui (specimen)>
```

```
<!ELEMENT specimen (unique_specimen_identifier,container)>
<!ELEMENT unique_specimen_identifier (#PCDATA)>
<!ELEMENT container (container_number,label,gross,diagnosis)>
<!ELEMENT container_number (#PCDATA)>
<!ELEMENT label (#PCDATA)>
<!ELEMENT gross (gross_description,lesion_size)>
<!ELEMENT gross_description (#PCDATA)>
<!ELEMENT lesion_size (#PCDATA)>
<!ELEMENT diagnosis (diagnosis_number, disease_concept, disease_modifiers, comment)>
<!ELEMENT diagnosis_number (#PCDATA)>
<!ELEMENT disease_concept (#PCDATA)>
<!ELEMENT disease_concept_cui (#PCDATA)>
<!ELEMENT disease_modifiers (#PCDATA)>
<!ELEMENT disease_modifiers_cui (#PCDATA)>
<!ELEMENT comment (#PCDATA)>
]>
<path_report>
 <accession> BSP 99 8888
  <lab_identifier> BALTIMORE VAMC SURGICAL PATH </lab_identifier>
  <time>
   <time_obtained> Jan 14, 1999 14:18 </time_obtained>
   <time_received> Jan 15, 1999 10:32 </time_received>
   <time_reported> Jan 18, 1999 09:18 </time_reported>
   <time_amended></time_amended>
   <time_supplemented></time_supplemented>
  </time>
  <submission>
   <submitting_physician> J SURGEON MD </submitting_physician>
   <submitting_service> SURGERY </submitting_service>
```

```
</submission>
<pathologist> JOHN Q PATHOLOGIST MD </pathologist>
<patient>
  <patient_name> VETERAN,JOHN Q. </patient_name>
  <patient_identifier> 123-45-6789 </patient_identifier>
  <date_of_birth>  12/01/1940 </date_of_birth>
  <patient_gender> M </patient_gender>
  <patient_ethnicity> WHITE </patient_ethnicity>
</patient>
<procedure> LARYNGECTOMY AND LEFT NECK DISSECTION
  <procedure_cui> C0023065, C0205091, C0034542 </procedure_cui>
  <specimen> LARYNX
    <specimen_cui> C0023078 </specimen_cui>
    <unique_specimen_identifier> 9876543 </unique_specimen_identifier>
    <container>
      <container_number> 1 </container_number>
      <label> LARYNGECTOMY </label>
      <gross>
        <gross_description> THE SPECIMEN IS RECEIVED FRESH, LABELED WITH THE PATIENT'S NAME, AND ADDITIONALLY LABELED "LARYNGECTOMY". THE SPECIMEN CONSISTS OF.... </gross_description>
        <lesion_size> 3 cm </lesion_size>
      </gross>
      <diagnosis>
        <diagnosis_number> 1 </diagnosis_number>
        <disease_concept> SQUAMOUS CELL CARCINOMA </disease_concept>
        <disease_concept_cui> C0280324, C0007137 </disease_concept_cui>
```

<disease_modifiers> WELL DIFFERENTIATED SQUAMOUS CARCINOMA OF LARYNX </disease_modifiers>

<disease_modifiers_cui> C0205615 </disease_modifiers_cui>

<diagnosis_number>2</diagnosis_number>

<disease_concept> MARGINS FREE OF TUMOR

</disease_concept>

<disease_concept_cui> C0332648 </disease_concept_cui>

<disease_modifiers></disease_modifiers>

<comment> </comment>

</diagnosis>

</container>

</specimen>

<specimen> LEFT NECK

<unique_specimen_identifier> 9876544

</unique_specimen_identifier>

<container>

<container_number> 2 </container_number>

<label> LEFT </label>

<gross>

<gross_description> THE SPECIMEN IS RECEIVED FRESH, LABELED WITH THE PATIENT'S NAME, AND ADDITIONALLY LABELED

"LEFT RADICAL NECK DISSECTION". THE SPECIMEN CONSISTS OF.... </gross_description>

</gross>

<diagnosis>

<diagnosis_number>1</diagnosis_number>

<disease_concept> METASTATIC SQUAMOUS CARCINOMA </disease_concept>

<disease_concept_cui> C0334246, C0280399

</disease_concept_cui>

<disease_modifiers></disease_modifiers>

```xml
        <disease_modifiers_cui></disease_modifiers_cui>
        <comment> METASTATIC SQUAMOUS CARCINOMA FOUND IN 11 OF 23 EXAMINED LYMPH NODES </comment>
        <diagnosis_number>2</diagnosis_number>
        <disease_concept> NO EVIDENCE OF MALIGNANCY </disease_concept>
        <disease_concept_cui> C0391857 </disease_concept_cui>
        <disease_modifiers></disease_modifiers>
        <disease_modifiers_cui></disease_modifiers_cui>
        <comment> SALIVARY GLAND </comment>
      </diagnosis>
    </container>
    </specimen>
   </procedure>
  </accession>
</path_report>
```

* This sample XML format can be expanded to associate UMLS (CUI) descriptor tags with every text-containing tag.

Table 3. Barrier Word Method, Illustrated by Sample Source Text from the Armed Forces Institute of Pathology Electronic Fascicles.

Sample Legend-Text from the Armed Forces Institute of Pathology Electronic Fascicles (Colby et al, 1995). *Barrier words are displayed in lower case*, and *KEYWORDS ARE DISPLAYED IN UPPER CASE.* Each sequence of keywords uninterrupted by barrier words, maps to one or more CUIs in the UMLS Metathesaurus.

LARGE CELL CARCINOMA . BRONCHIAL WASH CYTOLOGY SPECIMEN shows CLUSTERS of NEOPLASTIC CELLS with LARGE NUCLEI, PROMINENT NUCLEOLI , and ABUNDANT CYTOPLASM .

LARGE CELL CARCINOMA............... C0206704

BRONCHIAL WASH C0396473

CYTOLOGY SPECIMEN C0225355

shows C0332265

CLUSTERS C0205418

of C0332285

NEOPLASTIC C0027651

CELLS C0007634

with C0332287

LARGE C0205164

NUCLEI C0007610

PROMINENT C0205402

NUCLEOLI C0007609

and C0332287

ABUNDANT C0205172

CYTOPLASM C0010834

Table 4. Hypothetical Autopsy Report

Male. Caucasian. 1.91 m. 95.5 kg. (DeGregorio, 1997).

b. 8/27/1908. d. 1/22/1973.

Occupation: U. S. Congressman, U. S. Senator, U. S. President.

Status post: Appendectomy. (C0003611)

Status post: Cholecystectomy. (C0008320)

History of: Renal Calculi. (C0022650)

Myocardial Infarct, 1955. (C0027051)

Myocardial Infarct, April, 1972. (C0027051)

Myocardial Infarct, January 22, 1973. (C0027051)

Marked Generalized Atherosclerosis. (C0205082, C0205046, C0205246)

Appendix Internet References.

American Board of Medical Specialists.
http://www.abms.org/

American College of Surgeons.
http://www.facs.org/

College of American Pathologists.
http://www.cap.org/

Humphries BL. NLM/AHCPR Large Scale Vocabulary Test.
http://www.cpri.org/events/meetings/terminology/blh/sld001.htm

Johns Hopkins Autopsy Resource.
http://www.netautopsy.org/

Joint Commission for the Accreditation of Healthcare Organizations.
http://www.jcaho.org/

Surveillance, Epidemiology, and End-Results (SEER):
http://www-seer.ims.nci.nih.gov

Systematized Nomenclature of Human and Veterinary Medicine.
http://www.snomed.org/

U. S. Code of Federal Regulations, 45 CFR Parts 160 - 164.
http://aspe.hhs.gov/admnsimp/

U. S. Health Insurance Portability and Accountability Act of 1996.
http://thomas.loc.gov

U. S. Human Genome Research Institute, GenBank.
http://www.ncbi.nlm.nih.gov/Genbank

U. S. National Bioethics Advisory Commission.
http://bioethics.gov/general.html

U. S. National Cancer Institute, Cancer Genome Anatomy Project.
http://www.ncbi.nlm.nih.gov/CGAP

U. S. National Cancer Institute, Cooperative Breast Cancer Tissue Resource.
http://www-cbctr.ims.nci.nih.gov/FAQ.html

U. S. National Cancer Institute, Cooperative Human Tissue Network.
http://www-chtn.ims.nci.nih.gov/

U. S. National Library of Medicine, PubMed.
http://www.ncbi.nlm.nih.gov/PubMed/

U. S. National Library of Medicine, Unified Medical Language System.
http://www.nlm.nih.gov/research/umls/

U. S. Office of Protection from Research Risks (OPRR).
http://grants.nih.gov/grants/oprr/oprr.htm

References

Anderson, R.E., Smith, R.D. and Benson, E.S. 1991. The accelerated graying of American pathology. Hum Pathol 22:210-214.

Arcidi, J.M. jr., Moore, G.W. and Hutchins, G.M. 1981. Hepatic morphology in cardiac dysfunction. A clinicopathologic study of 1000 autopsied patients. Am J Pathol 104:159-166.

Association of Directors of Anatomic and Surgical Pathology. 1997. Recommendations for the reporting of specimens containing laryngeal neoplasms. Mod Pathol. 10:384-386.

Berman, J.J., Moore, G.W. and Hutchins, G.M. 1996. Maintaining patient confidentiality in the public domain Internet Autopsy Database (IAD). Proc AMIA Annu Fall Symp. 328-332.

Bubendorf, L., Kononen, J., Koivisto, P., Schraml, P., Moch, H., Gasser, T.C., Willi, N., Mihatsch, M.J., Sauter, G. and Kallioniemi, O.P. 1999. Survey of gene amplifications during prostate cancer progression by high-throughout fluorescence in situ hybridization on tissue microarrays. Cancer Res. 59:803-806.

Bubley, G.J., Carducci, M., Dahut, W., Dawson, N., Daliani, D., Eisenberger, M., Figg, W.D. Freidlin, B., Halabi, S., Hudes, G., Hussain, M., Kaplan, R., Myers, C., Oh, W., Petrylak, D.P., Reed, E., Roth, B., Sartor, O., Scher, H., Simons, J., Sinibaldi, V., Small, E.J., Smith, M.R.,

Trump, D.L., Vollmer, R. and Wilding, G. 1999. Eligibility and Response Guidelines for Phase II Clinical Trials in Androgen-Independent Prostate Cancer: Recommendations From the Prostate-Specific Antigen Working Group. J Clin Oncol. 1999 Nov;17(11):3461-3467.

Carter, J.R., Nash, N.P., Cechner, R.L. and Platt, R.D. 1981. Proposal for a national autopsy data bank. A potential major contribution of pathologists to the health care of the nation. Am J Clin Pathol. 76 (Suppl): 597-617, 1981.

Choi, S.S., Kang, Y.S., Kim, U.J., Lee, K.H. and Shin, H.S. 1999. Chromosomal localization of ESTs obtained from human fetal liver via BAC-mediated FISH mapping. Mol Cells. 9:403-409.

Colby, T.V., Koss, M.N. and Travis, W.D. 1995. Armed Forces Institute of Pathology Atlas of Tumor Pathology. Tumors of the Lower Respiratory Tract. Electronic Fascicle version 2.0.Armed Forces Institute of Pathology.

Compton, C.C. 1999. Pathology Report in Colon Cancer: What Is Prognostically Important? Dig Dis. 17:67-79.

Connell, P.P., Rotmensch, J., Waggoner, S.E. and Mundt, A.J. 1999. Race and clinical outcome in endometrial carcinoma. Obstet Gynecol. 94:713-720.

Cote, R.A., Rothwell, D.J., Beckett, R.S., Palotay, J.L. and Brochu, L. 1993. SNOMED International. The Systematized Nomenclature of Human and Veterinary Medicine. College of American Pathologists.

Degregorio, W.A. 1997. The Complete Book of U.S. Presidents. Fifth Edition. Barricade Books. 1997.

Fedorowicz J. 1982. A Zipfian model of an automatic bibliographic system: An application to MEDLINE. J Am Soc Info Sci 33:223-232.

Giere, W. 1981.Foundations of clinical data automation in cooperative programs. Proc 5th Ann Symp Comp Applic Med Care.1142-1148.

Grizzle, W.E., Aamodt, R., Clausen, K., LiVolsi, V., Pretlow, T.G. and Qualman, S. 1998. Providing human tissues for research: how to establish a program. Arch Pathol Lab Med 122:1065-1076.

Hahn, U., Romacker, M. and Schulz, S. 1999. How knowledge drives understanding -- matching medical ontologies with the needs of medical language processing.Artif Intell Med 15:25-51.

Hruban, R., Westra, W.H. and Phelps, T.H. 1996. Surgical Pathology Dissection. Springer Verlag.

Hutchins, G.M. 1990. Autopsy. Performance and Reporting.College of American Pathologists.

Hutchins, G.M., Meuli, M., Meuli-Simmen, C., Jordan, M.A., Heffez, D.S. and Blakemore, K.J. 1996. Acquired spinal cord injury in human fetuses with myelomeningocele. Pediatr Pathol Lab Med. 16:701-712.

Hutchins, G.M., Berman, J.J., Moore, G.W., Hanzlick, R. and the Autopsy Committee of the College of American Pathologists. 1999. Practice Guidelines for Autopsy Pathology. Arch Pathol Lab Med. 1999; 123:1085-1092.

Junor, E.J., Hole, D.J., McNulty, L., Mason, M. and Young, J. 1999. Specialist gynaecologists and survival outcome in ovarian cancer: a Scottish national study of 1866 patients. Br J Obstet Gynaecol. 106:1130-1136.

Kao, G.F. and Moore, G.W. 2000. Dermatopathology False Negative Terms in Unified Medical Language System (UMLS). Arch Pathol Lab Med. 124: (in press).

Klausner, R.D. 1999. The Nation's Investment in Cancer Resarch: A Budget Proposal for Fiscal Year 2001. National Cancer Institute. 51-55.

Kononen, J., Bubendorf, L., Kallioniemi, A., Barlund, M., Schraml, P., Leighton, S., Torhorst, J., Mihatsch, M.J., Sauter, G. and Kallioniemi, O.P. 1998. Tissue microarrays for high-throughput molecular profiling of tumor specimens. Nat Med. 4:844-847.

Kurman, R.J., Malkasian, G.D. jr., Sedlis, A. and Solomon, D. 1991. From Papanicoloau to Bethesda: the rationale for a new cervical cytology classification. Obstet Gynecol 77:779-782.

Light, R. 1997.Presenting XML. Sams.net Publishing.

Lilienfeld, D.E. and Stolley, P.D. 1994.Foundations of Epidemiology. Fifth Edition. Oxford University Press. 1994.

Mapp, T.J., Hardcastle, J.D., Moss, S.M. and Robinson, M.H. 1999. Randomized clinical trial: Survival of patients with colorectal cancer diagnosed in a randomized controlled trial of faecal occult blood screening. Br J Surg. 86:1286-1291.

Moch, H., Schraml, P., Bubendorf, L., Mirlacher, M., Kononen, J., Gasser, T., Mihatsch, M.J., Kallioniemi, O.P. and Sauter, G. 1999. High-throughput tissue microarray analysis to evaluate genes uncovered by cDNA microarray screening in renal cell carcinoma. Am J Pathol. 154:981-986.

Moore, G.W. and Hutchins, G.M. 1982. Consistency versus completeness in medical decision making: Application to 155 patients autopsied after coronary artery bypass graft surgery. Proc 6th Annu Symp Comput Appl Med Care. 805-811.

Moore, G.W., Boitnott, J.K., Miller, R.E., Eggleston, J.C. and Hutchins, G.M. 1988. Integrated anatomic pathology reporting system using natural language diagnoses. Modern Pathol 1:44-50, 1988.

Moore, G.W., Miller, R.E. and Hutchins, G.M. 1989. Indexing by MeSH titles of natural language pathology phrases identified on first encounter using the Barrier Word Method. In: Scherrer JR, Cote RA, Mandil SH, eds. Computerized Natural Medical Language Processing for Knowledge Representation. North-Holland. 29-39.

Moore, G.W. and Berman, J.J. 1994. Performance Analysis of Manual and Automated Systematized Nomenclature of Medicine (SNOMED) Coding. Am J Clin Pathol 101:253-256.

Moore, G.W., Berman, J.J., Hanzlick, R.L., Buchino, J.J. and Hutchins, G.M. 1996. A prototype internet autopsy database: 1625 consecutive fetal and neonatal autopsy facesheets spanning twenty years. Arch Pathol Lab Med. 120:782-785.

Moulton, G. 1999. Surveillance data take on a new statistical dimension. J Natl Cancer Inst. 91:671-673.

Mullick, F. 1997. The Center for Environmental Pathology and Toxicology at the Armed Forces Institute of Pathology. Hum Pathol. 52: 752-753.

Naber, S.P., Smith, L.L.,jr. and Wolfe, H.J. 1992.Role of the frozen tissue bank in molecular pathology. Diagnostic Molecular Pathology.1:73-79.

Nelson, S.J., Olson, N.E., Fuller, L., Tuttle, M.S., Cole, W.G. and Sherertz, D.D. 1995. Identifying concepts in medical knowledge. Medinfo. 8:33-36.

Nelson, R.L., Persky, V. and Turyk, M. 1999. Carcinoma in situ of the colorectum: SEER trends by race, gender, and total colorectal cancer. J Surg Oncol. 1999 Jun;71(2):123-129.

Payne, C. 1995. Developing a standard dataset for the NHS. Version 3 of Read Codes addresses many difficulties. BMJ. 311:951.

Peery, T.M. 1978. The autopsy data bank. A proposal for pathologists to contribute to the health care of the nation. Am J Clin Pathol 69 (Suppl): 258-259.

Read, J.D. and Benson, T.J.R. 1986.Comprehensive coding. Brit J Health Care Computing 1986; 3:22-25.

Rosai, J. and Ackerman, L.V. 1996. Ackerman's Surgical Pathology. Eighth Edition. C.V. Mosby.

Schmitt, A.O., Specht, T., Beckmann, G., Dahl, E., Pilarsky, C.P., Hinzmann, B. and Rosenthal, A. 1999. Exhaustive mining of EST libraries for genes differentially expressed in normal and tumour tissues. Nucleic Acids Res. 27:4251-4260.

Schneier, B. 1996. Applied Cryptography, Second Edition. Protocols, Algorithms, and Source Code in C. John Wiley & Sons

Simpson, A. 1996. HTML Publishing Bible, Windows 95 Edition. IDG Books Worldwide, Inc. 1996.

Smith, R.D., Benson, E.S. and Anderson, R.E. 1989. Some characteristics of the community practice of pathology in the United States. Arch Pathol Lab Med. 113:1335-1342.

Tersmette, K.W.F., Scott, A.F., Moore, G.W., Matheson, N.W. and Miller, R.E. 1988. Barrier word method for detecting molecular biology multiple word terms. Proc 12th Annu Symp Comput Appl Med Care.

U. S. Centers for Disease Control and Prevention. 1995. Manual of Procedures for the Reporting of Nationally Notifiable Disease to CDC. CDC.

U. S. Code of Federal Regulations. 1995. 45 CFR Subtitle A (10-1-95 Edition), part 46.101 (b) (4). U. S. Department of Health and Human Services. Office of the Secretary.

U. S. Code of Federal Regulations. 1999. 45 CFR Parts 160 - 164. Standards for Privacy of Individually Identifiable Health Information; Proposed Rule. Department of Health and Human Services. Office of the Secretary. Federal Register. 64:59917-60065.

http://aspe.hhs.gov/admnsimp/

U. S. Health Insurance Portability and Accountability Act. 1996. (HIPAA, Kennedy-Kassebaum Bill, H.R. 3103 of 104th U. S. Congress).

U. S. Government Documents at URL: http://thomas.loc.gov

U. S. National Bioethics Advisory Commission (NBAC). 1995.Executive Order 12975, October 3, 1995. Federal Register. 60:52063-52065.

http://bioethics.gov/general.html

Vigorita, V.J., Moore, G.W. and Hutchins, G.M. 1980. Absence of correlation between coronary arterial atherosclerosis and severity or duration of diabetes mellitus of adult onset. Am J Cardiol. 46:535-542.

Wagner, B.M. 1996. The future of environmental and toxicologic pathology. Human Pathol. 27:1003-1004.

Zhang, Q. 1981. Easy entry of Chinese character set symbols. 1981. Proc 5th Ann Symp Comp Appl Med 143-149.

Zipf, G.K. 1949. Human Behavior and The Principle of Least Effort. An Introduction to Human Ecology. Addison-Wesley Press.19-55.

5 A Data Clustering and Visualization Methodology for Epidemiological Pathology Discoveries

Doron Shalvi[1] **and Nicholas DeClaris**[1,2]
[1]College of Engineering
University of Maryland, College Park, U.S.A.
doron@eng.umd.edu
[2]School of Medicine
University of Maryland, Baltimore, U.S.A.
declaris@eng.umd.edu

In this chapter we introduce a methodology for hypothesis formation from clustering conventional Pathology data that leads to discoveries of epidemiological nature. It involves a medical Data Mining technique introduced previously which combines Unsupervised Neural Networks with Data Visualization (DeClaris et al. 1996). An application of this methodology on a set of traditional pathology data is presented. Inherent difficulties in the utilization of such data are overcome by a heuristic methodology based on a decision space that consists of the union of three pathology data feature subspaces identified as Topography, Morphology and Drugs / Substances. A series of Unsupervised Neural Networks were designed to study their potential to identify natural clusters of epidemiological pathology interest. Actual patient data were used and the underlying reasons for the resulting clusters (computer generated hypotheses) are examined. Promising results support the conclusion that the methodology presented and illustrated here yields discoveries and medical interpretations of epidemiological nature not otherwise possible.

5.1 Introduction

Data collection is often undertaken to monitor individual cases such as a patient in a hospital. This type of data is distinguishable from data sets collected for the purposes of studying a population; for example, determining which television programs are the most popular (DeClaris et al. 1996). Individual data sets may be gathered and studied collectively for purposes other than those for which the data sets were originally created; in such fashion new knowledge may be obtained while simultaneously eliminating one of the largest costs in developing knowledge, data collection. This approach is especially appropriate for medical data, which often exists in vast quantities in unstructured formats. Applying Data Mining techniques can facilitate systematic analysis.

Data Mining is the non-trivial process of identifying valid, novel, potentially useful, and ultimately understandable patterns in data (Fayyad et al. 1996). Thus Data Mining is a step in the knowledge discovery process essential for solving problems in a specific domain (Gonzalez and Dankel, 1993). Conventionally, data is gathered to test an existing hypothesis (a top-down search) (Krivda, 1995). Alternatively, the existing data is mined and allowed to form natural clusters (a bottom-up finding). Cluster detection may be employed through statistical techniques such as Bayes' Theorem (Maritz and Lwin, 1989; Thomasian, 1969) or non-statistical techniques such as unsupervised Neural Networks, which form clusters on the data set without knowing what the output clusters should model (Kohonen, 1990). In this chapter Kohonen Self-Organizing Maps (SOMs) and Adaptive Resonance Theory (ART) are used to cluster a specific medical data set containing information concerning the patients' drugs, topographies (body locations) and morphologies (physiological abnormalities); these categories can be identified as the three input subspaces. These subspaces are used to aid data dimensionality reduction leading to data preprocessing into a form suitable for network classification, and subsequently, clustering. The goal is to investigate whether these Data Mining techniques can be applied to pathology data to identify patient clusters that have unsuspected epidemiological pathology significance.

5.2 Understanding the Problem Domain

5.2.1 Objectives

A primary objective of medicine is to understand the nature of diseases. Clinical pathologists study diseases at the individual level in order to aid diagnosis and the evaluation of the effectiveness of any therapeutic intervention. Epidemiologists, on the other hand, attempt to understand diseases at the group level. Pathology data is collected at the individual level; sets of pathology data often have an implicit bias in the data set towards individuals exhibiting certain characteristics. Traditionally, epidemiologists usually study groups by applying statistical techniques to population data collected for a specific purpose; i.e., to evaluate a hypothesis. Because of biases in the data set statistical techniques may not work well if data sets are not appropriately collected; for instance, there may not be enough data to accept or reject hypotheses about under-represented populations. However, there may be enough data to study other groups which have not been identified a priori.

Data Mining techniques may be applied to pathology data sets with the possible realization of population groups that can be defined by meaningful criteria, even though they may not represent traditional epidemiological groups. Although there are many possible population groups of interest that can be chosen ahead of time to study, we will select the groups to study from what is available from the data. Applying Data Mining techniques will tell us if such groups are available. Our objective is to investigate whether these Data Mining techniques can be applied to pathology data to identify patient clusters that have unsuspected epidemiological pathology significance.

5.2.2 Project Plan

Our Data Mining project plan is as follows:

1. Use pathology domain knowledge to preprocess the data
2. Apply unsupervised Neural Networks to classify the data
3. Use data visualization to interpret cluster significance

A feature space will be defined that will allow us to use pathology domain knowledge in order to preprocess the data. This feature space is the union of three separate subspaces identified as Topography, Morphology and Drugs / Substances (hereinafter referred to as Drugs). These three subspaces encompass all pathology data enabling us to meaningfully prepare the data for Neural Network classification.

Unsupervised Neural Networks will be used to classify and organize the data. We will use and compare two techniques: Kohonen Self-Organizing Maps (SOM) and Adaptive Resonance Theory (ART). Both techniques are useful for organizing data where the target organization is not known.

Once the data has been organized by the SOM we will use data visualization techniques to further cluster the organized data. Data visualization allows us to apply heuristic judgments to identify clusters that may not be identified using unsupervised Neural Network techniques. The significance of any discovered clusters rests with the identification of common data attributes characterizing the cluster based on expert knowledge and/or intuition.

5.3 Understanding the Data

5.3.1 Data Collection

The data used in this study were extracted from the International Data Base for Toxic Lesions (INTOX) in animals and humans. INTOX is based on individual pathology findings, collected over a period of several decades, estimated in the tens of thousands of cases, and currently stored and retrieved on the basis of the Systematized Nomenclature of Medicine (SNOMED) architecture, described in the following section. INTOX is under continuing development by the American Registry of Pathology / Armed Forces Institute of Pathology (ARP/AFIP). The data used in our study are views (in the relational data model sense) of INTOX data selected to meet: 1) strict privacy requirements for the cases involved and 2) information content requirements imposed by our methodology discussed in the next section.

5.3.2 Data Description

Our data is a 'Working Data Set' (WDS) which in fact is a relational database constructed from INTOX selected 'views'. It consists of three tables, corresponding to the three mentioned subspaces:

1. DRUG contains 4258 patients, each with one to six drugs.
2. TOPO contains 4804 patients, each with one to six topographies.
3. MORP contains 2902 patients, each with one to six morphologies.

As is evident, there is not Drug, Topography and Morphology data available for all patients. If a patient data record appears in all three tables, it is at most 18-dimensional - containing one to six drugs, one to six topographies and one to six morphologies. However, 18 is the upper limit of dimensionality - not all tuples (patient data records) contain six drugs, six topographies and six morphologies. The minimum requirement for inclusion in the data set was one drug, one topography or one morphology. The mean dimensionality of a data record in this data set is about six.

The graph-based organization of the subspaces is based on the standard nomenclature and coding scheme of the Systematized Nomenclature of Medicine (SNOMED), available in (Cote, 1993) and at www.snomed.org. This coding scheme is organized as three hierarchical subspaces, identified as Drugs (Figure 1), Topography (Figure 2) and Morphology (

Figure 3). Each hierarchical subspace tree is several layers deep, providing ample opportunity for exploiting the trees' structure at various levels of depth. Each node in the tree is represented by both a code and a name (SNOMED termcode). Because of space limitations only the first two levels of each tree are displayed.

Each of the eighteen fields of a case in our Working Data Set either contains no data (null) or contains one of the thousands of leaf values within the subspace trees. This results in variable data dimensionality and occasionally repeated values. The data itself is of text ASCII format.

5.3.3 Data Quality

The Working Data Set is sparse but of high quality; of course, we did encounter the usual problems typically found in medical data: redundant and occasionally erroneous entries. A medication or condition may be commonly referred to by a variety of names; for example, "GI Bleeding", "Gi Bleed" and "Gastrointestinal Bleeding" all refer to the same condition. Some problems may well have been caused because of the way in which the Working Data Set was created. In any case errors and ambiguities were easily resolved.

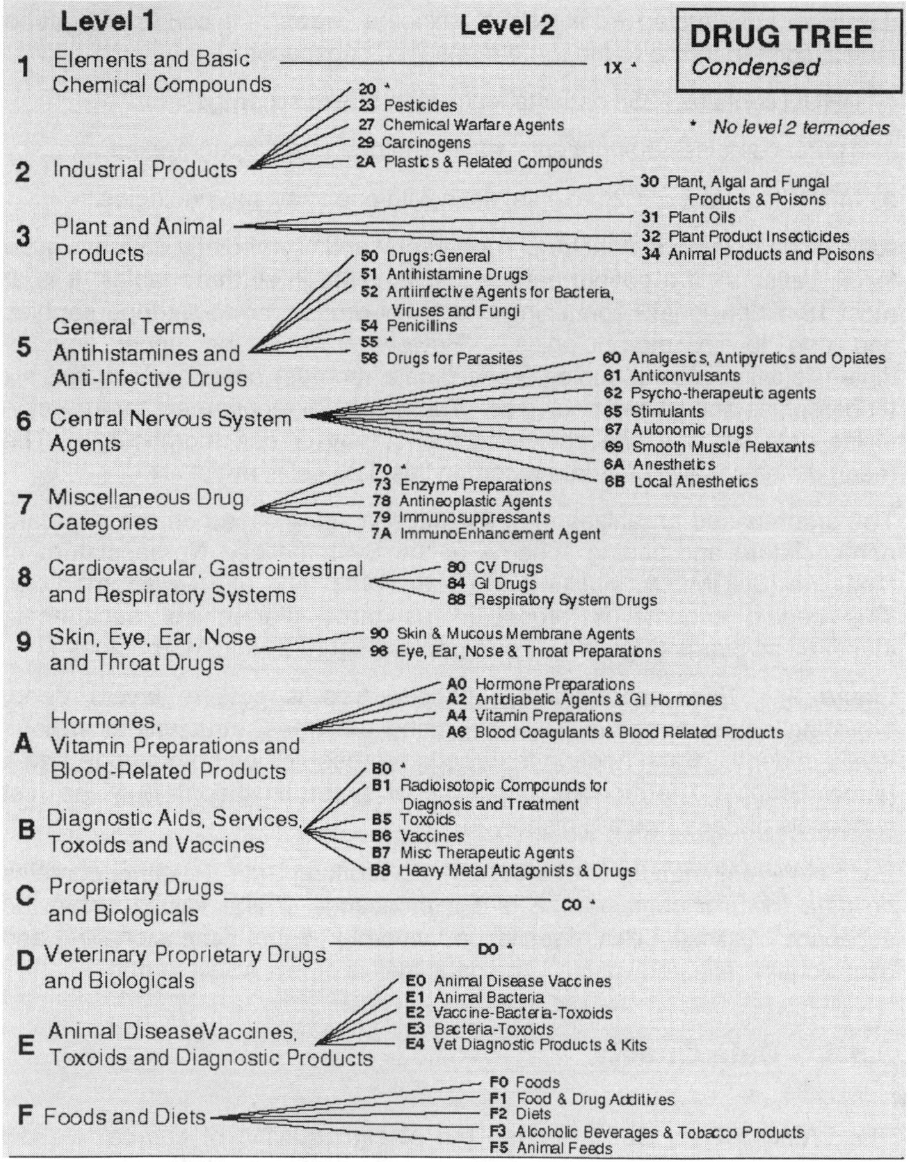

Figure 1. Drug Tree, condensed.

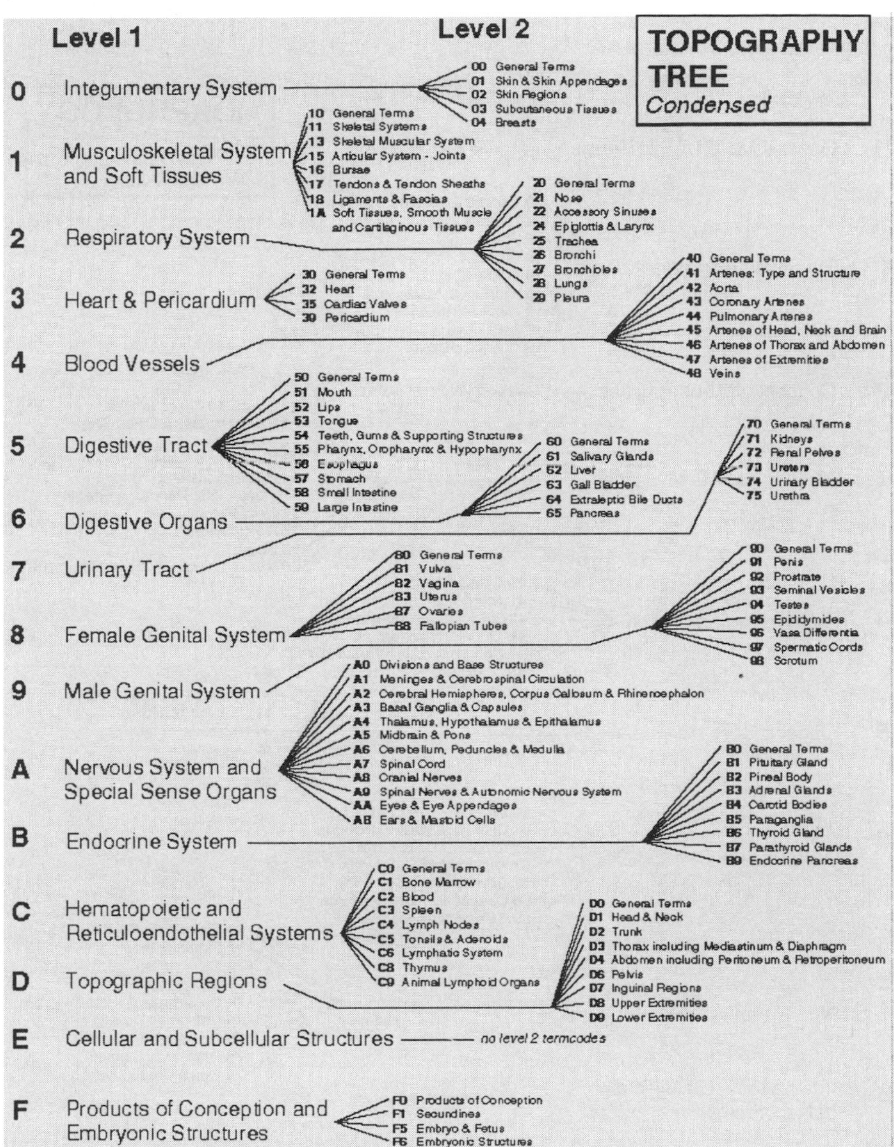

Figure 2. Topography tree, condensed.

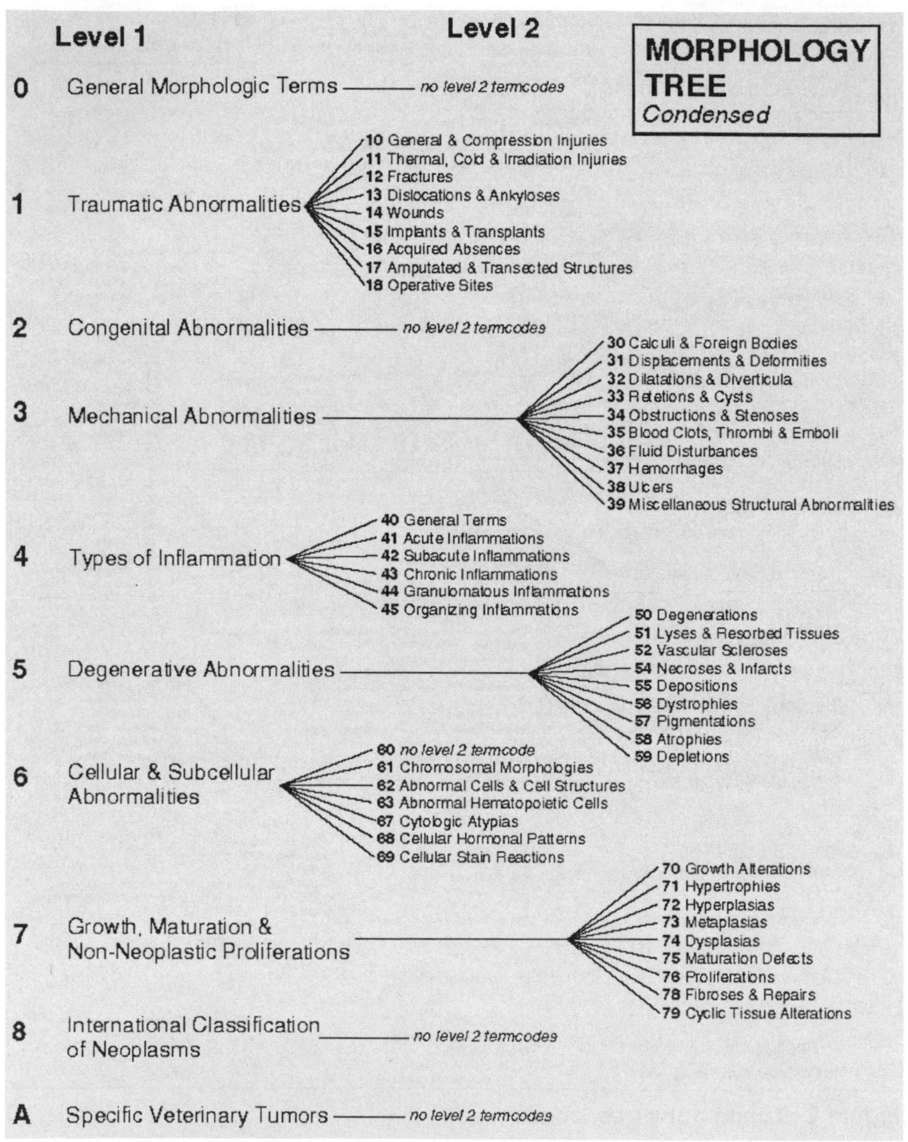

Figure 3. Morphology tree, condensed.

5.4 Preparation of the Data

5.4.1 Data Selection

As we are concerned with finding possible relationships between various drugs, topographies and morphologies we need only be concerned with patients for which there is data present in all three subspaces. A query was implemented to find the intersection of the three tables of our Working Data Set, yielding 2081 records. The output of the query is a table containing 19 columns: one column for the sequential case index, six columns for up to six drugs, six columns for up to six topographies and six columns for up to six morphologies. The sequential case index serves as a virtual patient ID encoded in a way that ensures patient confidentiality – a strict requirement for the use of INTOX. This table was then exported into a software data preprocessing tool.

5.4.2 Data Preprocessing

The objective in data preprocessing is to transform the raw input data into clean, consistent output data which is suitable for computationally intensive analysis (Stein, 1993; Lawrence, 1991). Standard techniques were employed to clean erroneous and redundant data.

Our Working Data Set contains data only at the leaves; each leaf node is present in only one or two tuples on average. This poses two problems: any conclusions formed would be statistically insignificant and the level of computation required for such an analysis would be exceedingly high due to the existence of roughly ten thousand different leaf nodes. To alleviate these problems the data was processed at the root level of each tree. At the root level each tree collapses into much fewer nodes; fourteen root level drugs, sixteen root level topographies and ten root level morphologies. By constraining all data to the root level the degree of differentiation has been greatly reduced from thousands to forty (14 + 16 + 10). The trade-off in cost is a great reduction in precision, while a benefit is the possibility of detecting trends within the data at a more general level.

In our Working Data Set, at the root level three of the forty nodes contained no data for any of the tuples (2081 total) that appeared in the intersection of all three tables. These three nodes are Drug D (Veterinary Proprietary Drugs and Biologicals), Drug E (Animal Disease Vaccines, Toxoids and Diagnostic Products) and Morphology A (Specific Veterinary Tumors).

Each node in the subspace trees, including the leaf level nodes, has a corresponding code which assisted in collapsing the subspaces to the root level. For instance, the drug Atropine, which is represented as a leaf in the drug tree, is given the code 67770, which is broken down in Table 11.

Tree level	Node Code	Node Name (SNOMED termcode)
1 (root)	6	Central Nervous System Drugs
2	7	Autonomic Drugs
3	7	Antimuscarinics and Antispasmodics
4/5 (leaf)	70	Atropine

Table 1. Node code and name representation of Atropine.

Atropine is a member of Antimuscarinics and Antispasmodics, which are types of Autonomic Drugs, which is one type of Central Nervous System Drug. We can break down drug node code 68010 (Albuterol) similarly, as shown in Table 22.

Tree level	Node Code	Node Name (SNOMED termcode)
1 (root)	6	Central Nervous System Drugs
2	8	Autonomic Drugs
3	0	no node name
4/5 (leaf)	10	Albuterol

Table 2. Node code and name representation of Albuterol.

These two examples illustrate some of the limitations in the available coding scheme. Not all intermediate nodes have a name descriptive of the node and all of its children; for instance, all drugs beginning with 680 lack a level 3 name. Note, however, that there are still drugs beginning with 680; the tree simply branches directly from level 2 to level 4/5 (leaf). Occasionally, a level two node does not have a name. Furthermore, node names may have more than one code; for example, Autonomic Drugs are assigned codes that begin with digits ranging from 67 - 68, as seen in the above examples. Lastly, while the coding scheme is primarily a hexadecimal system occasionally it reverts to a decimal system.

The effect of these limitations is that when collapsing a tree it is not sufficient to simply chop off the least significant digits of the ndoe. In the above examples, doing so would result in two different codes for Autonomic Drugs;

67 and 68. To overcome this problem a map was created within the preprocessing software so that any codes falling within the boundaries of a certain node would be assigned to a single code; thus, Autonomic Drugs was assigned strictly to code 67.

As the trees were collapsed to the root level the data was converted to bipolar format. For every record each of the 40 root level nodes was assigned a value of either 1 or -1 depending on whether any data existed for the leaves of that root node. The node is assigned a value of 1 if at least one data value is present at the leaves. The node is assigned a value of –1 if no data is at the leaves. In other words, only existence is preserved; quantity is lost. The end result for each record is a 40-dimensional bipolar array. The original data is at most 18-dimensional - containing one to six drugs, one to six topographies and one to six morphologies. Each dimension may contain one of thousands of values, and there is little structure to the data due to variable dimensionality and null (fields with no data) and repeated values. By contrast, every record of the transformed data contains 40 dimensions, each of which may take one of only two values, 1 or -1. The transformed data is much more consistent and lends itself to computationally intensive analysis such as Neural Networks.

5.5 Data Mining

In this section we discuss the use of two different types of unsupervised Neural Networks to classify the preprocessed data. An unsupervised Neural Network is one in which the desired output space is not known ahead of time; that is, there is no notion of 'right' or 'wrong' when classifying an input (Hagan et al. 1996). We will use and compare the Kohonen Self-Organizing Map (SOM) and Adaptive Resonance Theory (ART). These two architectures are both unsupervised in that we do not know what we want the output space to look like ahead of time. However, they have a fundamental difference – the SOM organizes the output into a spatially ordered map, such that spatial distance on the output map corresponds to degree of similarity of input (Kohonen, 1995). By contrast, the ART classifies inputs into distinct output categories, where there is no notion of degree of similarity between categories (Zurada, 1992).

We are using two different Neural Network architectures in order to detect whether the cause of any clustering is due to the nature of the data and its underlying subspace organization rather than the architecture employed.

If similar clusters are not detected using both the SOM and ART architectures than the basis of any clustering is due to network architecture. If similar clusters are detected then the basis for the clustering is the data and its structure.

In section 5.1 the SOM is used to organize the data. Data visualization techniques are presented in section 5.2 to further cluster the data organized by the SOM. The SOM output lends itself to visualization because the output is a 2-dimensional map where spatial distance represents degree of similarity. This will allow us to apply heuristic judgments to identify clusters that may not be identified using unsupervised Neural Network techniques. In section 5.3, the ART is used to cluster the same data. Subsequently, the two techniques are compared and contrasted.

5.5.1 Self-Organizing Map (SOM)

5.5.1.1 Description of the SOM

The Kohonen Self-Organizing Map (SOM) is an unsupervised Neural Network architecture; it does not know ahead of time what the target output that it is modeling looks like. The SOM organizes any k-dimensional input space into a 2-dimensional output space (typically $n \times n$) which preserves the spatial significance, or relative similarity, of the data (Kohonen, 1990). The output space can be thought of as a map consisting of $n \times n$ nodes, where a node is the finest resolution possible in the map. Subsequently, the SOM organizes each input data pattern into one and only one output node. An interesting and useful aspect of the SOM is that it tends to compact sparse data and expand rich data, dynamically using more of the output space to organize rich data (even if the rich data has very slight differences) and less of the output space to organize sparse data (even if the sparse data has large differences).

Classical Neural Network terminology refers to the output layer of the SOM as the Kohonen layer, consisting of nodes (Hagan et al. 1996). In this chapter we will occasionally use the terminology of a map consisting of squares since this description is more intuitive; a map preserves order, and direction (x, y axes) can be applied to it. Furthermore, the map is a grid composed of squares which can be completely described in terms of their location, an (x, y) coordinate pair.

Two layers comprise the classical SOM, an input layer and a Kohonen layer. Training patterns are presented at the input layer and the information is forwarded to the Kohonen layer through the connections between the two layers. Every node in the input layer is connected to every node in the Kohonen layer. Thus, with k Input layer nodes and n^2 Kohonen layer nodes there is a total of kn^2 connections between the two layers. Each connection is defined by a weight which describes the strength of the connection between the two nodes. In the typical implementation, which is used in this chapter, there are no connections between nodes in the same layer (Zurada, 1992).

The SOM is able to organize, compact and expand data by using a unique method of updating the weights. During training each input training pattern is randomly presented to the SOM and subsequently classified into exactly one of the n^2 Kohonen layer nodes; the winning node's weights are updated algorithmically to reflect the classification (Kohonen, 1990). Another way to think of this process is that the winning node learns the input pattern by adjusting its weight vector (containing k elements) so that it is closer to the input pattern vector (also containing k elements).

In general the weights of nodes very close to the winning node are also allowed to update their weights to reflect the input training pattern; this collection of close nodes is referred to as the neighborhood. The neighborhood is critical to creating and preserving order within the map. Since an entire region of the Kohonen layer is allowed to learn the input pattern that entire region is reflective of the input, thus neighboring nodes have extremely similar weight vectors. As training progresses the neighborhood size typically is reduced so that finer details of the input training set can be distinguished within the weight vectors. Thus broad trends within the data set are learned as training initiates with a large neighborhood and fine details are learned towards the end of training as a small neighborhood is employed. As training is completed the neighborhood is eventually reduced to one - only the winning node is allowed to update its weights.

One entire pass through the input training data set is termed an epoch. In the typical implementation data is randomly presented over many epochs to the SOM for training. Once the SOM is considered trained, one final pass through the data set is undertaken in order to determine the final classification (single winning node) for each input training pattern.

5.5.1.2 SOM Training

In order to implement the SOM algorithm an n x n SOM was constructed for n = 5, 7, 10 and 20. The Input layer consists of 40 input nodes, corresponding to the root layers of the three subspace trees: 14 Drug nodes, 16 Topography nodes and 10 Morphology nodes.

The following parameters were used to train the typical 10x10 SOM. The training period was set to 30 epochs which yields 62430 training iterations for 2081 input tuples. The learning coefficient α is initialized to 0.06. After approximately 7½ epochs α is halved to 0.03. After another 7½ epochs it is halved again to 0.015. For the final set of 7½ epochs it is halved again to become 0.0075. Thus, the network is trained relatively quickly at the beginning; as learning progresses training is reduced to fine-tuning. After 30 epochs no learning occurs.

Other network parameters are varied over time as well. The frequency estimation parameter β is initialized to 0.0005 and successively halved to 0.0001 for the final set of 7½ epochs. The conscience parameter γ is initialized to 1.0 and successively halved to 0.125 for the final set of 7½ epochs. The neighborhood shape is a square of variable width. The neighborhood width is reduced over time from 7 nodes to 1 node; this determines the portion of the network that learns after every iteration.

After the network is trained, it is used for one final pass through the input data set in which the weights are not adjusted. This network testing provides the final classification of each input data tuple into a single node in the 10 x 10 grid. The output is taken from the Coordinate layer as an *(x,y)* pair. Other *n=10* trials used similar parameters but different random initial weight values. For trials where *n=20*, the neighborhoods are larger throughout training. For trials where *n=5* or *n=7*, the neighborhoods are smaller throughout training. For all trials, the learning parameters mentioned above are very similar. The output of the SOM is a population distribution of tuples with spatial significance which may be decomposed into three subspace distributions representing the decision boundaries determined by the network. The population distribution may be visually aggregated into larger groups to provide clusters not distinguishable in a high resolution map. Such clusters can then be analyzed according to the subspace decomposition to determine significant patterns in the data.

Figure 4 displays the output data population distribution for one of the *n=10* trials. Other *n=10* trials produced similar data organizations once initial conditions are taken into account. This grid displays the number of tuples that were classified into each output layer node (square) during testing. Square (1,1) contains 180 tuples, by far the largest number of any square. Square (2,1) contains only one tuple and square (1,2) contains none. As SOMs tend to shrink or expand the output map as needed to fit the data these valleys suggest that the cluster at (1,1) is very sharp and well-defined.

y \ x	1	2	3	4	5	6	7	8	9	10
10	33	37	36	39	16	31	19	25	15	53
9	17	5	12	12	5	20	9	23	11	24
8	27	17	7	31	25	14	10	5	7	32
7	27	18	38	16	24	31	18	19	27	11
6	17	11	21	18	1	9	19	6	37	25
5	22	1	19	16	20	26	23	28	5	24
4	46	1	9	0	36	3	9	2	19	28
3	24	13	6	24	24	37	13	15	9	29
2	0	11	21	1	2	11	0	18	14	12
1	160	1	34	9	76	30	10	36	29	44

Figure 4. SOM Population output.

This hypothesis can be confirmed by looking at the raw data which upon examination reveals that every one of the tuples in square (1,1) contains root level data only for Drug 6, Topography 6 and Morphology 5. The tuple at square (2,1) contains these three root level nodes as well as Drug 7, a difference slight enough for the network to distinguish the tuple by classifying it one square away from (1,1). All of the 34 tuples in square (3,1) contain Drug 6, Topography D and Morphology 5 but only 29 of the 34 tuples contain Topography 6. Clearly the difference between square (3,1) and square (1,1) is greater than the difference between square (2,1) and square (1,1).

5.5.2 Data Visualization

5.5.2.1 Cluster Formation

The initial network organization of 100 squares is visually aggregated to form clusters that are spatially large; the outline of these areas was determined heuristically. Squares (represented by any coordinate pair) which have a population greater than 10 (an arbitrary threshold) were combined to form spatially large clusters, presented as a cluster map in Figure 5.

Cluster A is comprised of only one square, at (1,1); this is 1% of the output space. However, this cluster has a population of 180; or almost 9% of all the tuples! As SOMs tend to distribute the data over the entire 2-dimensional output space, this indicates that cluster A is very well-defined. Population and spatial considerations based on domain-specific knowledge were used to create this cluster map. Upon examination of the raw data within these clusters one finds similarities between the tuples indicative of medical relationships or dependencies. Numerous hypotheses may be formed regarding these relationships, many of which were not a priori known; these hypotheses require expertise from several medical specialties (i.e., Pathology, Pharmacology, relevant clinical practice, etc.).

The SOM groups together tuples in each square according to their similarity. The only level at which the SOM can detect similarities between tuples is at the root level of each of the three subspace trees since this was the level of differentiation presented to the SOM's input layer. Consequently we should expect that tuples in the same square often have the same root level drugs, topographies and morphologies. We can now drill down from the output map into the raw data to discover the source of the SOM's clustering.

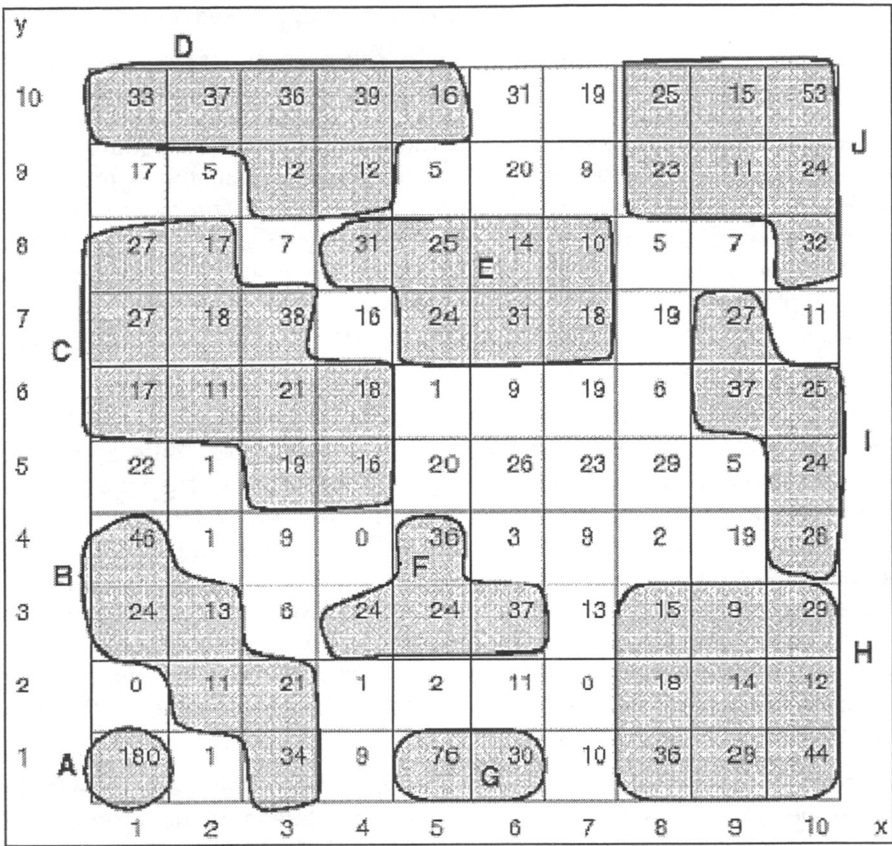

Figure 5. Population output clustered.

For instance, square (3,10) belongs to cluster D and contains 36 tuples. Drilling down into the data it is discovered that of the 36 tuples:

- 36 tuples (100%) contain Drug 2 (Industrial Products)
- 3 tuples (8%) contain Topography 5 (Digestive Tract)
- 13 tuples (36%) contain Topography 6 (Digestive Organs)
- 3 tuples (8%) contain Topography 7 (Urinary Tract)
- 12 tuples (33%) contain Topography A (Nervous System & Special Sense Organs)
- 1 tuple (2%) contains Topography B (Endocrine System)
- 5 tuples (13%) contain Topography C (Hematopoietic & Reticuloendothelial Systems)

- 2 tuples (5%) contain Topography D (Topographic Regions)
- 36 tuples (100%) contain Morphology 8 (International Classification of Neoplasms)

Clearly the presence of Drug 2 and Morphology 8 define square (3,10) since all of the tuples belonging to this square contain these root level nodes. For most squares, we discovered that there is one or at most two morphologies which can be found in all or roughly 95% of the tuples. If this arbitrary threshold level is dropped to 66% there is almost always one or two morphologies which will surpass the threshold. If the threshold level is raised to 100% the following morphology cluster map may be constructed; this appears as Figure 6.

The number inside each square in the morphology cluster map represents the root level code of the morphology tree. For example, there is a large cluster of squares in the bottom of Figure 6 that contain the label '5'. In each square labeled '5', 100% (the chosen threshold) of the tuples inside the square contain Morphology 5, Degenerative Abnormalities. These squares have been visually aggregated into a cluster. Occasionally 'holes' appear in the cluster; these holes represent squares in which not all of the tuples contain the root level code, even though most of them may. There are at least six distinct clusters in this graph. Clearly the morphology clusters are arranged in a spatially meaningful way by the SOM; one cluster flows into the next.

A comparison between Figure 4 and Figure 6 shows that there appears to be some relation between the Population clusters and the Morphology clusters. Population clusters A (Morph. 5), C (4), F (5), G (5) and J (3) are entirely enclosed by their respective Population clusters. Clusters D and H are almost entirely enclosed, while clusters B, E and I span two or more clusters; indicating that the Population clusters are not well formed with respect to the Morphology subspace.

The threshold level of 100% was chosen because in most squares, one or two morphologies are found in 100% of the square's tuples. If the threshold is dropped to 66%, the clusters somewhat expand in size, and the overlap between the Morphology and Population clusters increases. In particular, cluster H is now completely enclosed by Morphology 7, translating to a cluster in which 66% of the population contains Morphology 7.

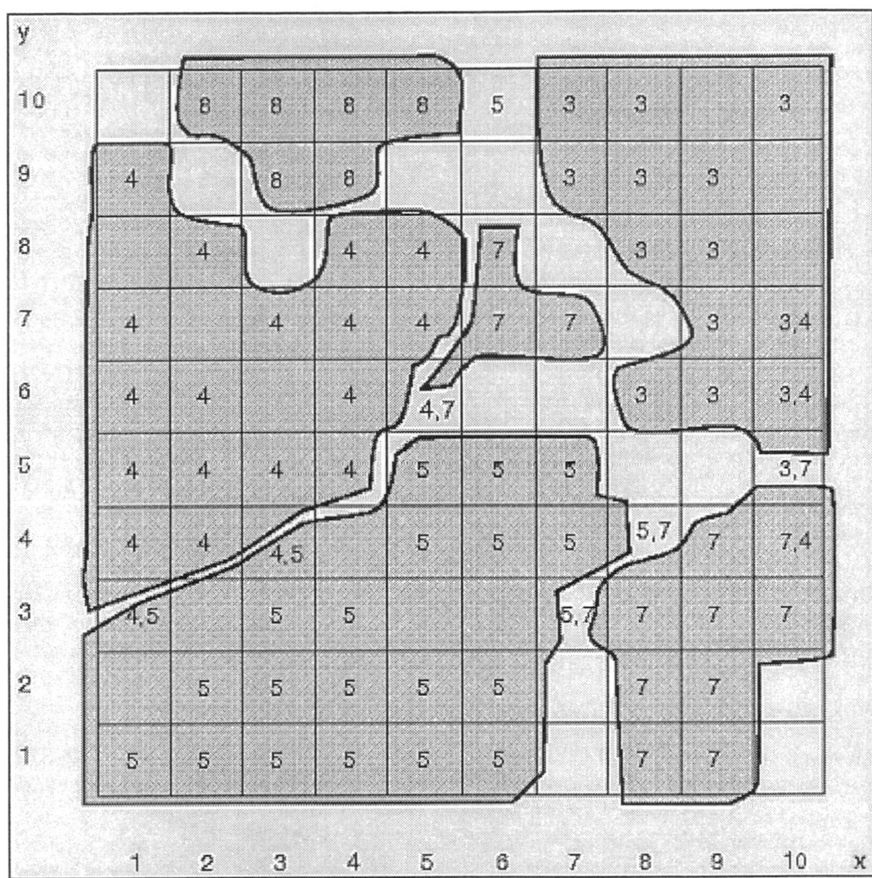

Figure 6. Morphology clusters.

A similar drill-down analysis is done for the Drug and Topography subspaces, yielding maps that can be used to explain many of the population clusters. These maps are presented in Figure 87 and Figure 8. SOM trials with other network dimensions and initial conditions yielded extremely similar results, with identical clusters identifiable to those presented above, indicating that the clustering of the data is independent of network size and training parameters. It is now possible to introduce several heuristics to rate the worthiness of the population clusters.

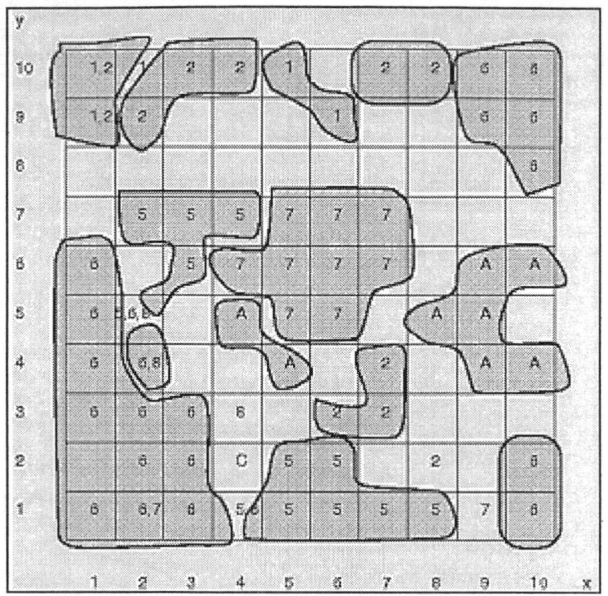

Figure 7. Drug clusters.

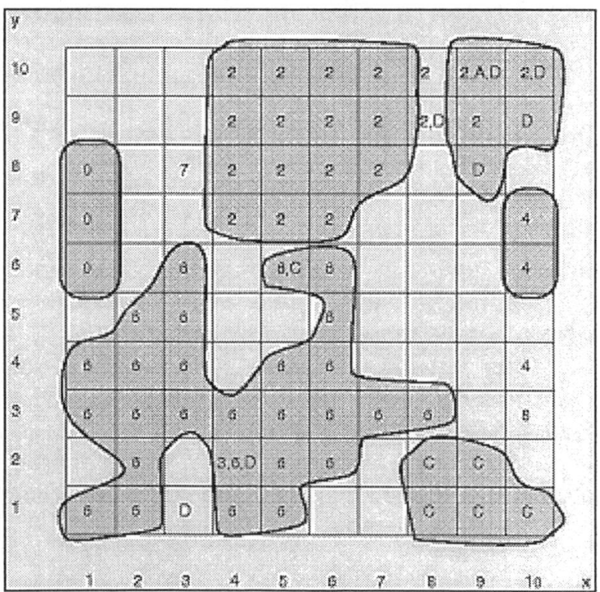

Figure 8. Topography clusters.

5.5.2.2 Cluster Assessment

The clusters delineated in the previous section were formed on the basis of population and spatial distribution alone. The worthiness of these clusters may be measured by the following parameters which make use of square tuple population, cluster square count and overlap with the three SNOMED subspaces trees. Subsequently, the population distribution is clustered again with a heavier emphasis placed on SNOMED subspace overlap.

We can estimate how well formed the Population clusters are by looking at the total number of tuples in each cluster compared to the average number of tuples expected for each square of that cluster in a random distribution. Table 3 displays this analysis.

Cluster	A	B	C	D	E	F	G	H	I	Av.
Population (Tuples)	180	149	229	185	153	121	106	206	141	165
Square Count	1	6	11	7	7	4	2	9	5	5.9
Tuples / Square	180	24.8	20.8	26.4	21.9	30.3	53	22.9	28.2	43.4
Cluster Intensity	8.6	1.2	1.0	1.3	1.1	1.5	2.5	1.1	1.4	**2.1**
Drug Inclusion	1	1	.27	.43	.43	.25	1	.22	.6	.59
Topo Inclusion	1	.67	.27	.43	.86	1	.5	.55	.4	.69
Morp Inclusion	1	.67	1	.86	.43	1	1	.77	.8	.85
Total Inclusion	3.0	2.33	1.54	1.71	1.71	2.25	2.5	1.55	1.8	2.1
Scaled Square Count	1.5	2.25	3.0	2.4	2.4	1.95	1.65	2.7	2.1	2.2
Relative Inclusion	4.5	5.3	4.6	4.1	4.1	4.4	4.1	4.2	3.8	**4.6**
Cluster Assessment	38.8	6.3	4.6	5.3	4.5	6.6	10.3	4.7	5.2	**9.5**

Table 3. Cluster assessment worksheet.

Tuples / Square reflects the average number of tuples per square for that particular cluster. A completely random distribution of the data would produce 20.81 tuples per square. A well-defined cluster should exhibit more; the Cluster Intensity value grossly reflects this; it is simply Tuples / Square divided by 20.81. Cluster E, which has an intensity of 1.1, is not a very well-defined cluster since a cluster chosen from a random collection of squares would on average produce the same intensity. By contrast cluster A, which has an intensity of 8.6, is extremely well defined. Note that the Cluster Intensity parameter does not incorporate the population of neighboring (border) squares. A very small population in the border squares, as is the case with cluster A, should translate to a more well-defined cluster; this factor is not accounted for in the definition and would be a useful parameter modification.

Most clusters exhibit an intensity slightly greater than 1, as would be expected. However, a cluster with an intensity of 1.5 (cluster F) is much more well-defined than a cluster with an intensity of 1.1 (cluster E); it contains 40% more tuples per square! Clusters A and G overshadow this significant difference.

Cluster evaluation becomes more accurate when the Drug, Topography and Morphology cluster maps are included in the analysis. The Inclusion parameters represent the percentage of each Population cluster that is encompassed in the most dominant Drug, Topography and Morphology cluster for that Population cluster, as defined by the 100% threshold. For example, cluster F is composed of 4 squares. One of the 4 squares (25%) is part of Drug cluster A, all 4 squares (100%) are part of Topography cluster 6 and all 4 squares (100%) are part of Morphology cluster 5. The Total Inclusion parameter is the sum of the 3 inclusion proportions; it is a relative measure of how well each Population cluster overlaps with the three SNOMED subspace map clusters. The Scaled Square count parameter resets the Square Count scale range, originally from 1 to 11, to a new range, 1.5 to 3.0. Relative Inclusion is simply Scaled Square Count multiplied by Total Inclusion. Square Count is scaled so that the new range has the same numerical impact (~1.5 to 3.0) as total inclusion on the derived parameter. In this fashion the dependence on cluster size is reduced.

In terms of Total Inclusion clusters A, B, G and J are notably sharp. This is impressive for large clusters such as B and J. This expectation is realized in the Relative Inclusion parameter for which clusters B (5.3) and J (6.2) have significantly higher values than all other clusters. Cluster C (4.6) also has a fairly large Relative Inclusion primarily due to its large size of 11 squares.

Finally, the Cluster Assessment parameter is an overall assessment of the quality of the cluster which combines Cluster Intensity (relative population) and Relative Inclusion (overlap with subspace clusters). As would be expected clusters A and G rate extremely well. Clusters B (6.3) and J (8.0) also rate fairly well, while cluster E rates very poorly. This can be attributed to cluster E's low intensity and inclusion.

These derived parameters are of course very subjective and only crudely attempt to rate a cluster. The sharpness of cluster boundaries is not included in the estimate and there is too great a reliance on cluster size. Nevertheless, the above numbers are still useful in rating the worthiness of heuristically determined clusters.

The following clusters were completely enclosed within two or more subspace root nodes:

- A: CNS Drugs; Digestive Organs; Degenerative Abnormalities
- B: CNS Drugs; Digestive Organs
- F: Digestive Organs; Degenerative Abnormalities
- G: General Terms, Antihistamines and Anti-Infective Drugs; Degenerative Abnormalities

These clusters are of particular interest since they relate root level nodes from different trees. Clusters A and F indicate a strong relationship between Digestive Organs and Degenerative Abnormalities; this relationship may simply be symptomatic of necrosis of the liver. A look at the raw data indicates that Cluster G contains many necroses and lipoid degenerations (forms of Degenerative Abnormalities) and the patient was often given Tetracycline or Isoniazid (penicillins, or Anti-Infective Drugs). This extracted relationship is a data nugget of a type that is discovered through Data Mining using graph-based similarity criteria. Many more types of relations can in fact be extracted by experts from medical specialties that use other types of similarity criteria. Evaluation of the significance of the resultant hypotheses in such cases are beyond the scope of this chapter. However, a very important aspect of the use of these types of relations will be mentioned in the conclusion of this chapter.

5.5.2.3 Generating Meaningful Clusters

Knowing that the original population cluster map is deficient we can re-cluster the network's output map using information gleaned from the subspace inclusion parameters. In Figure 9 a new cluster map is shown. Each square contains a code representing the root level nodes present for that square at 100%. For example, square (1,1) contains code 665, indicating that 100% of the tuples in (1,1) contain Drug 6, Topography 6 and Morphology 5.

This cluster map was heuristically constructed using clusters from the subspace maps as well as spatial configuration (use of the original SOM feature space to realize non-concave clusters) and population (to create larger clusters). The conflicting goals of cluster formation are cluster square size and dimensionality of cluster definition, given by the number of root level nodes which are contained by all of the tuples in the cluster. The increased specificity should enable detection of fine clusters perhaps indicative of unknown relations on the data which would likely be undiscovered with a broader clustered feature space.

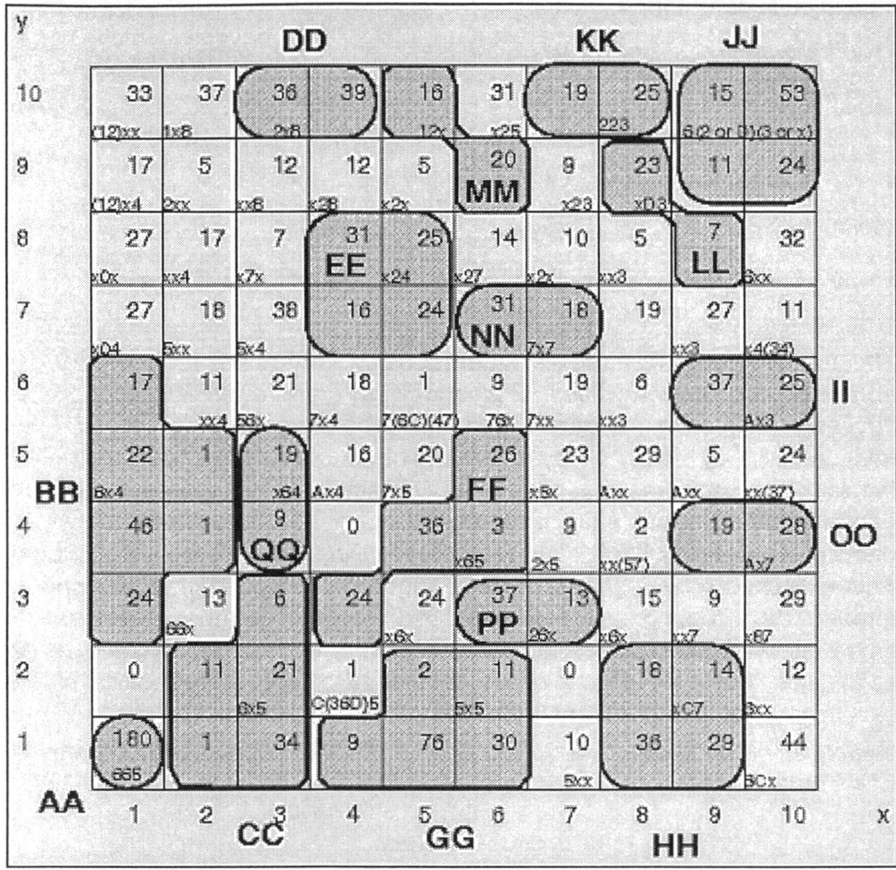

Figure 9. Population clusters regenerated.

All of the multiple square clusters contain at least two root level nodes from different trees. Many of the remaining single squares contain two root level nodes from different trees as well; for example, all 29 tuples in square (10,3) contain Topography 8 and Morphology 7 as indicated by the code "x87" within the square; the "x" denotes that no single drug was contained by 100% of the tuples. In summary, root level node frequency data allows construction of root level node clusters, individually by subspace and as an intersection of subspaces. This allows generation of more meaningful clusters using spatial, population and subspace correspondence considerations. Many of the clusters identified using the above method not only comprise multiple squares but often are defined by multiple root level nodes across the subspace trees. These clusters are a potential gold mine of data nuggets whose pathological significance can only be assessed by appropriate groups of specialists, as mentioned earlier.

5.5.3 Adaptive Resonance Theory (ART)

Adaptive Resonance Theory (ART) employs an unsupervised Neural Network architecture different from that of the SOM. Instead of organizing input tuples into a feature map ART classifies tuples into one of many possible output nodes each of which is defined by an exemplar vector. The output nodes contain no spatial significance but simply represent distinct categories. When a new tuple is presented to the network that is sufficiently different from previously presented tuples a new category is created; thus the number of output categories is not fixed as in a 10 x 10 SOM. The exemplar for each output node is stored as a tuple identical to the format of input tuples; for this study the exemplars have 40 dimensions. Each training tuple is compared to each output node's exemplar, and the one that is most similar is chosen as the winner if the measure of similarity exceeds a preset threshold vigilance. If the vigilance is not exceeded, the chosen node is eliminated from the current training iteration, and training is continued selecting a new output node using the same algorithm. If all current nodes are exhausted a new node is created to represent the category (Zurada, 1992). The measure of similarity is given as:

$$\frac{|P \cap E|^2}{|P|^2} \rangle vigilance$$

where P is the input training tuple and E is the exemplar tuple, each of which has 40 dimensions. Since ART defaults the bipolar inputs to binary inputs the vigilance threshold requirement reduces to a measurement of the number of common positive dimensions between the two vectors; this is the numerator in the above expression. Thus if an input tuple had four positive dimensions, three of which are present in the exemplar to which it is being measured against, the resultant ratio is 0.75. If this ratio is the highest among the exemplars of all nodes and it exceeds the vigilance then the tuple is classified into the exemplar's node.

The first implementation of ART used a vigilance of 0.6 and 20 nodes, setting an upper bound on the number of discrete categories. Only 50% of the 2081 tuples were classified indicating the need for a higher upper bound on the number of output nodes. The exemplars for this trial all had two positive dimensions out of 40 possible. This suggests that an input tuple with three positive dimensions, two common to an exemplar, would get classified with that exemplar (0.67 > 0.6), while an input tuple with four positive dimensions, two common to an exemplar, would not (0.5 < 0.6). As the mean positive dimensionality of the input tuples is 3.6 it is expected for ART to yield exemplars with two positive dimensions given a vigilance of 0.6.

The vigilance and upper bound on output nodes were varied to test network response and reliability; the varied parameters appear in Table 44. A vigilance of 0.6 is not very discriminatory as an input tuple need match only 60% of an exemplar. When the vigilance is increased to 0.7 the positive dimensionality of the exemplars increases to three since two is not enough discretion for most input tuples to exceed the vigilance (2/3 = 0.67 < 0.7). In this instance an input tuple with three (3/3 = 1.0 > 0.7) or four (3/4 = 0.75 > 0.7) positive dimensions would classify into an exemplar with three matching dimensions while an input tuple with five (3/5 = 0.6 < 0.7) would not. The upper bound on the output nodes was increased to 50 which still proved to be far too small as all 50 nodes were assigned exemplars; only 50% of the data in this case was classified. With 200 nodes classification increased to 75% indicating a drastic improvement; however, the upper bound of 200 was still realized. With 400 nodes 95% of the data was classified and all but five nodes were used, indicating that the network did not require further nodes to represent all the different categories it had found. Roughly half of the input tuples were classified into nodes that ended the final classification with less than ten tuples. It is unknown why roughly 100 tuples were left unclassified in this instance as five nodes were still available; unfortunately, the Neural Network software used does not allow an upper bound greater than 400 nodes.

Vigilance	Upper Bound on Nodes	Nodes Used	Input Classification %	Positive Exemplar Dimensions
0.6	20	20	50	2
0.7	50	50	50	3
0.7	200	200	75	3-4
0.7	400	395	95	3-4

Table 4. ART response to varied architecture parameters.

The clusters defined by the ART output nodes correspond exceptionally well to those realized from the SOM. The ART clusters which contain more than 20 input tuples are displayed in Table 5. The most populous ART cluster contains 193 tuples and is defined by root code "665" (Drug 6, Topography 6 and Morphology 5); these are the three positive dimensions of the cluster's exemplar. This cluster corresponds to cluster A in Figure 5, or square (1,1), which contains 180 tuples. The excess 13 tuples arise from tuples with four positive subspace root nodes, three of which match "665"; the exemplar matches these tuples at 0.75 which is higher than the 0.7 vigilance. The second most populous ART cluster contains 76 tuples and is defined by root code "6(2D)3" (both Topographies 2 and D); these are the four positive dimensions of the cluster's exemplar. This ART cluster corresponds fairly well to cluster J in Figure 5; a look at the preprocessed data reveals that this ART cluster is composed of tuples from squares (8,10), (9,10) and (10,10) from cluster J. Not all tuples in square (8,10) were classified with this particular exemplar since only 80% of these 25 tuples contained Drug 6, as seen in the preprocessed data and repeated in Table 5. Similarly, 93% of the 15 tuples in square (9,10) contain Morphology 3; the one tuple without this morphology could not have been classified with this exemplar.

The remaining ART clusters can easily be related to individual squares in Figure 9. This map relates particularly well to ART clusters since the map presents clusters that contain at least one root level node in each subspace; similarly, the ART exemplars contain three positive dimensions as set by the 0.7 vigilance. These dimensions most often relate one root from each subspace as expected due to the nature of the data.

In summary, the ART clusters correspond exceptionally well to the SOM clusters. The two methods are compared and contrasted at a general level in the following section.

DTM root code	ART 400 nodes Population	SOM Population	SOM Square
665	193	180	(1,1)
6(2D)3	76	25 (80% A6) (96% TD)	(8,10)
		15 (93% M3)	(9,10)
		53	(10,10)
565	74	76	(5,1)
6C7	37	44 (86% M7)	(10,1)
664	34	46	(1,4)
5C7	33	36	(8,1)
765	33	26	(6,5)
6(6D)5	27	34	(3,1)
865	27	24	(4,3)
A65	27	36	(5,4)
564	26	11 (81% M4) 21 (95% M4)	(6,2)
265	26	13	(7,3)
A47	24	28	(10,4)
727	23	31	(6,7)
228	23	39	(4,10)
66(45)	23	24	(1,3)
x(2D)3	20	23	(8,9)

Table 5. ART, SOM cluster comparison.

5.6 Evaluation of the Discovered Knowledge

Our objective in this study has been to investigate if our Data Mining techniques can be applied to routinely collected pathology data to yield epidemiologically meaningful groups, and to gain insight as to the kinds of hypotheses that generated the groups and how the formulation and evaluation of those hypotheses can be automated. Our findings with this particular Working Data Set amply demonstrate that meaningful groups can be extracted using our techniques.

In this regard there appears to be a choice - the SOM and ART models used in this study both proved to be effective; selection of one over the other depends on the data structure available and desired output space. If a notion of output similarity is desired the SOM is a better choice. The Data Visualization performed in conjunction with SOM organization proved to be the most powerful Data Mining technique in this study, permitting views of the data organization within the SNOMED subspaces. Further improvements in visualization techniques and cluster assessment would enhance the model used.

An advantage of the ART classification is that distinct clusters may be easily formed without requiring heuristic visual techniques or human processing. A disadvantage of this method is that it is heavily reliant on the vigilance, especially when the input tuples are active in only a very small fraction of their dimensions (here, 3.6 out of 40); tuples that overmatch the exemplars will not be included in the classification. For instance, a tuple with six positive dimensions, three of which match an exemplar with three positive dimensions, will not be classified with that cluster when in actuality the medical trend or pattern represented by that cluster may be present in the tuple.

By contrast, the SOM provides a spatially significant map which conforms to the data distribution, resulting in wasted nodes on populous clusters of very similar data that may be defined by only one ART node. Furthermore, an additional heuristic is generally needed to aggregate the spatial squares into independent clusters. However, the SOM excels in providing feature maps containing smooth transitions of data subspaces; this may lead to hypotheses not evident from an ART network that cannot delineate relative proximity of somewhat similar data. Neither the SOM nor ART architecture is clearly superior; both have their merits within specific domains.

The clusters detected in this study are valid because the same clusters were detected regardless of the clustering mechanism used. A wide variation in SOM size, learning parameters and initial conditions were employed, yet the same clusters were detected in all variations. Furthermore, a completely different architecture and algorithm (ART) also yielded the same clusters. This is significant because the ART network creates a new category (detects a cluster) only when it feels that the category is sufficiently unique to warrant its distinction. This indicates that our data organization and not the clustering mechanism is instrumental in cluster detection. The detection of identical clusters independent of the mechanism used validates the clusters detected.

The entire knowledge discovery process used in this study worked very well. The Working Data Set is common in size and format to those available in medium to large size hospitals and/or clinical laboratories. The level of cleansing and preprocessing required is also typical of studies of this nature. Using standard unsupervised Neural Networks and applying creative visualization techniques allowed discovery of groups that were immediately useful and recognizable to medical specialists. Moreover, many of these groups represent populations that have not been recognized in the usual epidemiological studies.

There are several areas in which the knowledge discovery process used in this study may be refined to improve performance. With sufficient data, data preprocessing may be performed at a higher level than the root level of each SNOMED subspace, permitting discovery of knowledge at more detailed levels than those outlined above. The involvement of medical specialists may assist further in the visualization and cluster formation process, targeting inter-subspace areas to visualize which may provide improved cluster and population recognition performance. Other classification schemes may be investigated for their applicability in this domain.

Since the completion of this work we have been studying the application of naturally extended methodologies which involve enlargement of the decision space by the union of additional data-feature subspaces from other relevant areas such as pharmacology, clinical practice and others.

5.7 Using the Discovered Knowledge

The groups discovered in this research are useful for the formation of epidemiological pathology hypotheses. Knowing that the probable causes of clustering can be extracted using the visualization techniques described above allows the epidemiologist to concentrate on particular courses of action for further investigation and research. Our technique has been clustering through use of dimensionality reduction and visualization. The extracted clusters generally are identified by signature common root nodes, representing the smallest possible dimensions by which a population may be identified. These broad-based data nuggets provide a starting point for the pathologist to continue investigation into the legitimacy and effects of the identified clusters by forming hypotheses based on the identified generalities and conducting tests tailored from the beginning to test the hypotheses. It is then useful to expand dimensionality by drilling down into the raw data used for the clustering, providing additional clues towards hypothesis formation. This methodology has not only allowed reuse of data collected for other purposes but it has generated hypotheses for investigations into areas that otherwise would have required much greater data collection.

The results presented in this chapter validate the methodology presented and encourage its application to other databases. We are currently investigating natural extensions of these methods whose significance will be indicated in the conclusion.

5.8 Conclusions

This study has shown that applying clustering and visualization techniques to preprocessed pathology data is useful in extracting clusters of medical significance by generating data-supported hypotheses not conceived a priori. The outcome of the network is heavily dependent on the preprocessing methodology which relies on structured subspaces. In the medical field such a structure is very subjective by nature and may not represent the best way to organize a subspace. As applied to this study the subspace proved adequate for Neural Network classification. An in-depth study of subspace implementation with regards to which tree slice is optimal is of extreme relevance to this approach and is material suitable for further research subject to the main obstacle of data availability. Effects of variance of SOM parameters have been studied by others (van Velzen, 1994) and would be an interesting study relevant to this research. However, the results presented here are fairly consistent across a variety of SOM parameters. Alternative implementations of ART networks, notably Fuzzy ART, are promising in regards to delivering similar and perhaps more disjoint tuple clusters (Brown and Harris, 1994).

Decomposition of the SOM output grid is straightforward and heavily dependent on subspace structure. Detailed features of the Drug, Topography and Morphology subspaces appear consistently. Heuristic aggregation of the output grid is very subjective and somewhat difficult to attain as the defined clusters overlap extensively. This is quite representative of smooth, analog transitions expected from the wide variety in real patient data. Increasing the network resolution aids in determining pocket clusters perhaps indicative of medical trends but at this fine level there is not sufficient data to form reasonable hypotheses except for the largest groupings. The underlying ideology of network classification of large groupings can be determined with respect to the subspaces and provides ample opportunity for suitable analysis by pathologists and/or medical specialists. Additionally, the described approach can be greatly automated to allow for creation of a knowledge-based system to aid medical hypothesis formulation and evaluation.

The utilization of a very high-dimensional decision space whose data feature subspaces can best be interpreted by highly experienced medical specialists is likely to have a major impact on how epidemiological studies (including clinical trials) will be undertaken in the future.

Acknowledgements

The application of the methodology discussed in this chapter was supported in part by the American Registry of Pathology / Armed Forces Institute of Pathology with a research grant awarded to the Department of Pathology, University of Maryland School of Medicine, N. DeClaris, Principal Investigator. The work was carried out in the Medical Informatics and Computational Intelligence Laboratories involving faculty, staff and student collaboration from the American Registry of Pathology in Washington, D.C., the Department of Pathology, School of Medicine in Baltimore and the Department of Electrical and Computer Engineering, University of Maryland in College Park. The P.I. acknowledges the significant contributions made to this effort by Dr. Donald King, ARP Executive Director and by Drs. Benjamin Trump, Chairman and G. William Moore, Professors in the Department of Pathology. Shah-An Yang, a graduate student in the Department of Electrical and Computer Engineering, aided in the programming implementation of the Adaptive Resonance Theory.

References

Brown, M. and Harris, C. 1994. *Neurofuzzy Adaptive Modeling and Control.* Prentice Hall

Cote, R. 1993. *SNOMED international: the Systematized nomenclature of human and veterinary medicine.* College of American Pathologists, American Veterinary Medical Association

DeClaris, N., Shalvi, D. and Tran-Luu, T.-D. 1996. Computational intelligence-based methodologies for population studies and laboratory medicine decision aids. *Proc. of the International Neural Network Society 1996 World Congress on Neural Networks*

Fayyad, U., Piatetsky-Shapiro, G. and Smyth P. 1996. From Data Mining to Knowledge Discovery in Databases. *AI Magazine*, 17(3):37-54

Gonzalez. A. and Dankel, D. 1993. *The Engineering of Knowledge-Based Systems.* Prentice Hall

Hagan, M., Demuth, H. and Beale, M. 1996. *Neural Network Design.* PWS

Kohonen, T. 1990. The self-organizing map. *Proceedings of the IEEE*, 78(9):1464-1480

Kohonen, T. 1995. *Self-Organizing Maps.* Springer-Verlag

Krivda, C. 1995. Data-Mining Dynamite. *Byte*, 10:97-103

Lawrence, J. 1991. Data Preparation for a Neural Network. *AI Expert*, 6(11):34-41.

Maritz, J.S. and Lwin, T. 1989. *Empirical Bayes methods.* Chapman and Hall

Stein, R. 1993. Preprocessing Data for Neural Networks. *AI Expert*, 8(3):32-37

Thomasian, A. 1969. *The structure of probability theory with applications.* McGraw-Hill

van Velzen, G.A., 1994. Instabilities in Kohonen's self-organizing feature map. *Journal of Physics A Mathematical and General*, 27(5):1665-1681

Zurada, J. 1992. *Introduction to artificial neural systems.* West

6 Mining Structure-Function Associations in a Brain Image Database

Vasileios Megalooikonomou[1] and Edward H. Herskovits[2]

[1]Department of Computer Science
Dartmouth College
Hanover, NH 03755
[2]Neuroimaging Laboratory, Division of Neuroradiology
Johns Hopkins University
Baltimore, MD 21287

In this chapter we present a data mining process for discovering associations between structures and functions of the human brain through the study of lesioned (abnormal) structures and associated functional deficits (disorders). We present the architecture of a Brain Image Database (BRAID) that integrates image processing and visualization capabilites with statistical analysis of spatial and clinical data. We demonstrate the use of the mining methods by applying them to epidemiological data and discovering clinically meaningful associations. Furthermore, we present a framework for the evaluation of the mining capabilities of BRAID. We show how to obtain measures of detection of known associations as a function of the number of subjects used, the strength and the number of associations in the model, the number of structures associated with a particular function, and the image registrtaion methods used.

6.1 Understanding the Problem Domain

Mining problems have been grouped in three categories (Agrawal et al., 1993): identifying classifications, finding sequential patterns, and discovering associations. Data mining is application-dependent and different applications usually require different mining techniques. In this chapter, we consider the problem of mining functional associations in the brain based on clinical data.

The discovery of associations between structures and functions of the human brain (i.e., human brain mapping), is the main goal of the Human Brain Project (Huerta et al., 1993). For this purpose, large brain image databases have been developed (Arya et al., 1996; Letovsky et al., 1998). These databases consist of 3-D images from different medical imaging modalities and capture structural (e.g., MRI[1] and/or functional/physiological (e.g., PET[2], fMRI[3]) information about the human brain.

Traditionally, two approaches have been employed for functional brain mapping. The first approach seeks associations between lesioned structures and concomitant neurological or neuropsychological deficits, where, for example, patients with trauma lesions and deficits like left visual field deficit are studied. The second approach utilizes specifically designed activation experiments where subjects are asked to perform a certain task and their brain activation is measured (by measuring, for example, the regional Cerebral Blood Flow (rCBF)).

The BRAin Image Database (BRAID) (Letovsky et al., 1998), was developed at the Johns Hopkins Hospital for the purpose of functional brain mapping through the study of lesioned structures and associated deficits. It is a large-scale archive of normalized digital spatial and functional clinical data with an analytical query mechanism.

6.2 Understanding the Data

The advent of widely available noninvasive methods for assessing macroscopic brain structure, particularly magnetic-resonance (MR) techniques, has dramatically improved neuroscientists' ability to perform lesion-deficit analysis with contemporaneous, accurate structural data to complement clinical functional assessment (Anderson, 1990). Large-cohort clinical studies have as a critical component neuroradiology variables.

---

[1] Magnetic Resonance Imaging: shows soft-tissue structural information.
[2] Positron Emission Tomography: shows physiological activity.
[3] Functional-Magnetic Resonance Imaging: shows physiological activity.

The Brain Image Database currently includes images and clinical information from over 700 subjects from two different studies: the Cardiovascular Health Study (CHS) (Bryan et al., 1994) and the Frontal Lobe Injury in Children (FLIC) study (Gerring et al., 1998). The first is an ongoing epidemiological study of cardiovascular risk factors. The second is a study that was designed to discover predictors of psychiatric sequelae after severe closed-head injury. BRAID also includes 5000 artificial subjects that were generated using a lesion-deficit simulator (Megalooikonomou et al., 2000) which is described in more details in Section 5. The artificial subjects are used to test not only the scalability of the mining methods but also to evaluate different lesion-deficit analysis methods as a function of the number of samples needed, the strength and complexity of lesion-deficit associations, the spatial distribution of brain lesions, and the registration method used.

The main objective in the implementation of a brain image database is to be able to manage image data from different modalities efficiently and transparently. This is a difficult task because of the different image-file formats, the spatial and contrast resolutions, and the large amount of space that image data need.

Although in principle lesion-deficit data could be analyzed using methods similar to those for activation studies (e.g., statistical parametric mapping (SPM) (Friston, 1995)), assumptions about the nature of the data (e.g., time series) has prevented investigators from applying this approach. BRAID uses several statistical methods to determine structure-function associations, such as chi-square analysis, log-linear analysis, logistic regression, and others, presented next.

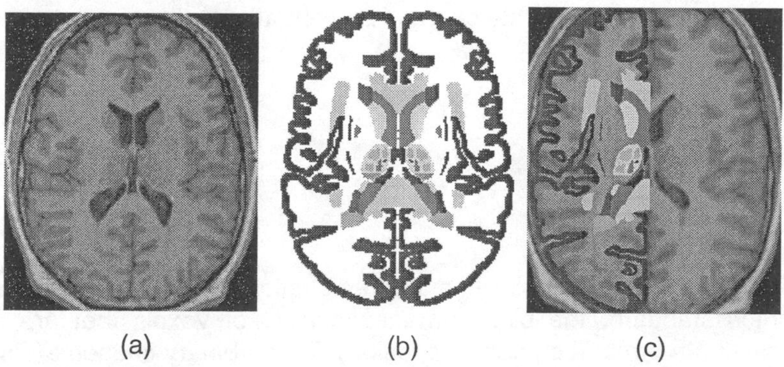

Figure 1. The (a) original MR image, (b) atlas, and (c) atlas image overlaid on the deformed MR image.

6.3 Preparation of the Data

After the 3-D MR image is collected for each subject, each lesion is delineated by a neuroradiologist as a region of interest (ROI) on each slice using thresholding and segmentation. Each ROI is reconstructed in three dimensions. The next step in the preprocesing phase is to make behavioral and image data comparable across subjects. In particular, for the image data, after lesions are identified (usually manually), image registration has to be performed to deal with the problem of morphological variability among subjects. This process maps homologous anatomical regions to the same location in a stereotaxic space, such as the Talairach anatomical atlas (Talairach and Tournoux, 1988). Several linear and nonlinear spatial transformations which bring the 3-D atlas and the subject's 3-D image into register, i.e., spatial coincidence, have been developed (Bookstein, 1989; Collins et al., 1994; Miller et al., 1993). We use a nonlinear method based on a three-dimensional elastically deformable model (Davatzikos, 1997). The effect of registration of an MR image to the Talairach atlas is presented in Figure 1.

In addition to patient 3-D image data, BRAID contains a set of anatomical atlases of the human brain that model the exact shapes and positions of anatomical structures. An MR image does not identify the structure to which each voxel (volume element) belongs, but an anatomical atlas can supply this information, with the accuracy of the registration methods, when overlaid on the image (see Figure 1). The atlases that are used at this time are the Talairach, Gyri, Brodmann, Damasio, and an artificial atlas containing regions of interest to us. However, here, for clarity of presentation, we concentrate on the Talairach atlas.

6.4 Data Mining

After the segmentation of lesions and registration of the binary images to a common standard, the binary images consist of voxels that are either normal or abnormal (i.e., part of a lesion). These binary images are stored in the database as line segments mainly to reduce the space requirements. This structural image data combined with the functional variables form the data for each patient. Mining methods for the discovery of the structure-function associations from this data can operate on a resolution range from the spatially distinct structures of an anatomical atlas (atlas-based analysis) to the voxel level (voxel-based analysis) (Megalooikonomou et al., 1999).

6.4.1 Atlas-Based Analysis

In the case where anatomical structures represent functional units, the atlas-based analysis is more sensitive than voxel-based analysis since the atlas provides significant prior knowledge. The first step in the atlas-based analysis is to calculate for each structure s_i and subject p_j, the fraction of lesioned volume, $f_{si,pj}$, which is defined as the volume of the lesioned part of s_i divided by the volume of s_i. These fractions form the continuous structural variables. Here, we present methods for both continuous and categorical structural variables. In the case of categorical variables, a structure is lesioned (abnormal) or not based on the fraction of it that is lesioned. For simplicity, in this case, a patient is treated as having a lesion in a structure if the intersection of all his lesions with the structure is at least one voxel. To remove the effect of thresholding, the atlas structures are analyzed as continuous variables, considering for each one, the fraction that is lesioned (abnormal).

In the case where the search of the model that explains the data observed can be directed through specific hypotheses or prior knowledge, the situation is easier. The hypotheses can be formed after using explorative visualization or other methods, and can be tested using statistical tests. An example where visualization helps to reduce the search space for a model is shown in Figure 4.1. If there is little preconception about the relationships between the variables, all the possibilities have to be explored. This exploratory, or data mining, analysis is presented below. There are two approaches one can follow: the bivariate (pairwise) and the multivariate analysis.

6.4.1.1 Bivariate Analysis

Let F be the number of functional and S be the number of structural variables respectively. In the case of categorical structural variables, $F \times S$ two-way contingency tables are constructed and for each one the Fisher exact test (Andersen, 1997) is computed. The associations between structures and deficits are sorted in increasing order of the p-values returned from the exact tests and the ones with the lowest p-values are reported. For continuous structural variables one can use the Mann-Whitney test and logistic regression analysis. The Mann-Whitney statistic is used because the distributions of the fractions of lesioned volumes are not Gaussian. In exploratory analysis of either categorical or continuous structural variables, computing a statistic for many pairwise tests creates the multiple comparison problem, i.e., certain portion of the tests to be positive by chance. A standard Bonferroni correction (Andersen, 1997) suggests to divide the significance threshold by the number of tests performed. However, this overestimates the number of independent tests performed in this case, since test results are correlated for neighboring structures because lesions usually extend to more than one neighboring structure. So, the Bonferroni correction leads to loss of sensitivity. A heuristic modification of the Bonferroni correction, the sequential Bonferroni correction (Andersen, 1997), is used to get more reasonable results. There, one sequentially increases the value of the significance threshold as hypotheses are evaluated.

6.4.1.2 Multivariate Analysis

Complex multivariate associations may not be found by multiple use of bivariate statistics. For example consider a deficit that is associated with two structures and appears only when both of them are lesioned. Also, multivariate analysis is free of the multiple comparison problem since it evaluates an entire model with one statistic. A multivariate extension of the chi-square test for categorical variables is the log-linear analysis. Logistic regression is another multivariate method that can be used to relate the log-odds of having a particular deficit to the fraction of lesioned structures. We use the stepwise logistic regression, where the algorithm that is used for discovering the model that explains the interactions, starts with no associations and a greedy approach is applied to add (or delete) associations based on their relative strength.

6.4.2 Voxel-Based Analysis

The atlas-based analysis results are as good as the atlas that is being used. Instead of imposing a model on the image data, one can analyze them on a voxel-by-voxel basis. A voxel can be either normal or abnormal so, in this case, the structural variables are categorical. Given that the number of voxels that are considered are on the order of 10^7, so many (i.e., 10^7) Fisher exact tests have to be performed for each of the functional variables that we examine. This procedure can be seen as clustering the voxels by functional association. For each deficit, d, two image files are created. Each voxel of the first (second) file is the sum of the corresponding voxels in the binary images for patients who have (do not have) the deficit. The calculation of the contingency table and of the Fisher exact test is computationally tractable if these two image files can be efficiently constructed. The multiple-comparison problem is even more intense here due to the large number of tests that are performed. However, in this case, it can be attacked with clustering analysis since random false positives will not tend to cluster.

Voxel-based regression analysis can also be used to determine whether voxels in a certain region are associated with a functional variable. One can construct a regression equation that relates lesions in a sphere of a given radius and center to a deficit. The "causal brain region" in which lesions are most strongly associated with that deficit can then be identified. Let l be a lesion, o be a sphere, v(r) denote the volume of a region r, and $i(r_1,r_2)$ denote the intersection of two regions r_1 and r_2. The identification of the causal region is done by calculating the optimal center and radius for the logistic regression equation:

$$\text{logit}(d) = \log(\text{odds}_d) = af_s + b$$

where

$\text{odds}_d = p_d(.)/(1-p_d(.))$, $p_d(.)$ is the probability of having a certain deficit d (e.g., ADHD), $f_s=v(i(l,o))/v(o)$ is the fraction of the sphere that is lesioned, a=(log odds of d)/(lesioned fraction of sphere volume), and b the prior log odds of deficit d.

Given the center (x,y,z) and the radius r of the sphere, solving this equation, one can find values for the parameters a and b such that the sum of squares of residuals is minimized. The goal is to optimize the sphere parameters (x,y,z,r) to obtain the best fit of the data to the regression line. We use simulated annealing for the optimization. The solution is the sphere that best discriminates between lesions that are and are not associated with deficit d. This nonlinear optimization procedure is computationally intensive. Another obvious problem of this approach is that it cannot describe multifocal functional associations.

6.4.3 Results from Mining BRAID

In this section we present results form the mining process (more details can be found in (Letovsky et al. 1998; Herskovits et al. 1999)). Visualization applied prior to the analysis procedure can help direct the analysis by choosing certain structures of the anatomical atlas to examine further using the statistical tests. Figure 2 shows the sum of images of all lesions over subjects that did and did not develop ADHD (ADHD+ and ADHD-, respectively). Based on these images and on previous research implicating a frontal lobe-basal ganglia-thalamic pathway, we choose the right putamen and the left thalamus (highlighted in Figure 2)[1] for further analysis using the Fisher exact test for categorical and the Mann-Whitney test for continuous structural variables (see Section 4). The p-values in Table 1 confirm that there is a strong association between lesions in the two structures and development of ADHD.

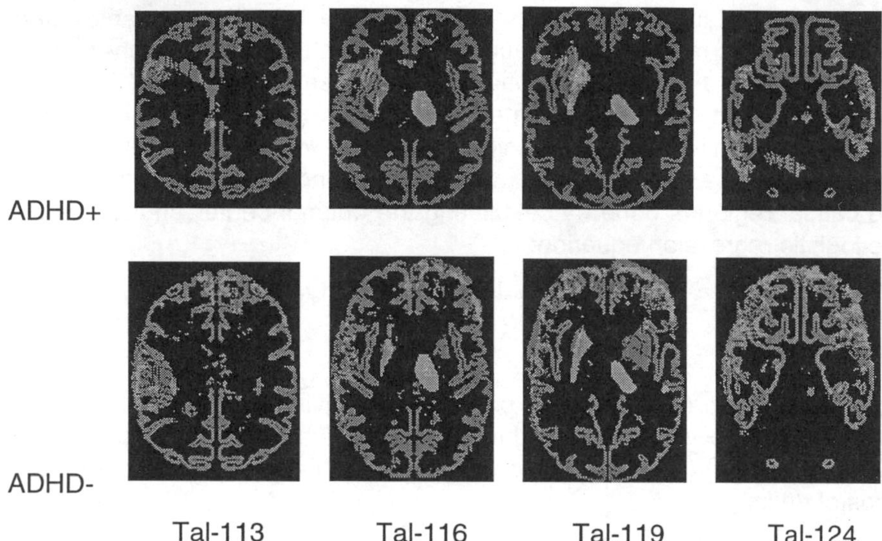

Figure 2. Sum of lesions for the ADHD+ and the ADHD- group of patients (3 slices of the Talairach atlas are shown for each group). The right putamen and left thalamus are also presented.

Structure	Fisher's exact p-value	Mann-Whitney p-value
R putamen	0.065	0.033
L thalamus	0.095	0.093

Table 1. Statistical analysis of selected Talairach atlas structures for association with ADHD (FLIC data set).

Testing the mining capabilities, one can run an exploratory analysis on the CHS data set (300 subjects) in which BRAID used the chi-square test to evaluate two-way contingency tables for all pairwise combinations of atlas

[1] Due to the compromised connections between the frontal lobe and these two structures, it is believed that the frontal lobe is not able to excert its normal oversight function to supress impulsive urges and behaviors. A common behavioral pattern in patients with ADHD is extreme impulsivity and lack of self-control.

structures (90) and functional variables (14) returning a sorted list (by p-value) of structure-function associations. The five most significant associations are presented in Table 2. Highly significant lesion-deficit associations detected by BRAID, such as visual field deficit and lesions in contralateral orbital or cuneate gyrus,are also consistent with current clinical knowledge (Bryan et al. 1997). The incorrect association between the left hippocampus and a right visual field deficit is due to registration error since the hippocampus is next to the optic radiations that are very well known to be correlated with a visual field deficit.

Structure	Function	Chi-square p-value	S-Bonf. Correct. p-value
R globus pallid.	R hemiparesis	0.00001	0.0039
L hippocampus	R visual defect	0.00001	0.0095
R gyri angular	L pronat. drift	0.00002	0.0195
R gyri orbital	L visual defect	0.00003	0.0225
R gyri cuneus	L visual defect	0.00003	0.0224

Table 2. The five most significant structure-function associations given by the chi-square analysis on the CHS data set.

Preliminary stepwise logistic regression analysis using continuous structural variables from the FLIC data set show similar results for the development of ADHD. This method identified the left SupCerebellarA (which is lateral to the left putamen area) as a strong predictor.

Results from a preliminary voxel-based analysis for the ADHD variable of the FLIC data set are presented in Figure 3. Each voxel represents the p-value for the association between the voxel being lesioned and the development of ADHD. Six slices of the Talairach atlas along with a grayscale bar that shows the correspondence between p-values and greyscale values are shown. A 3-D reconstruction is shown in Figure 4. The higher the intensity the lower the p-value, or the higher our confidence is that a certain location is associated with development of ADHD. In Figures 4(c) and (d) we present the Talairach atlas and a rendered image of the p-value volume where the brightness of each color associated with an atlas structure is scaled by a factor related to the inverse of the p-value so that parts of structures that are highly correlated with the development of ADHD appear more bright. These results are consistent with those of the atlas-based analysis.

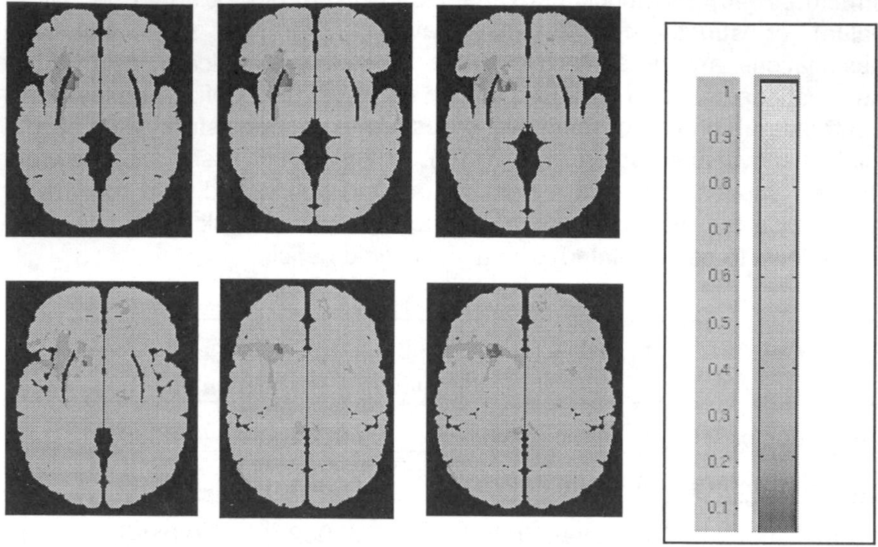

Figure 3. Voxel based analysis for development of ADHD.

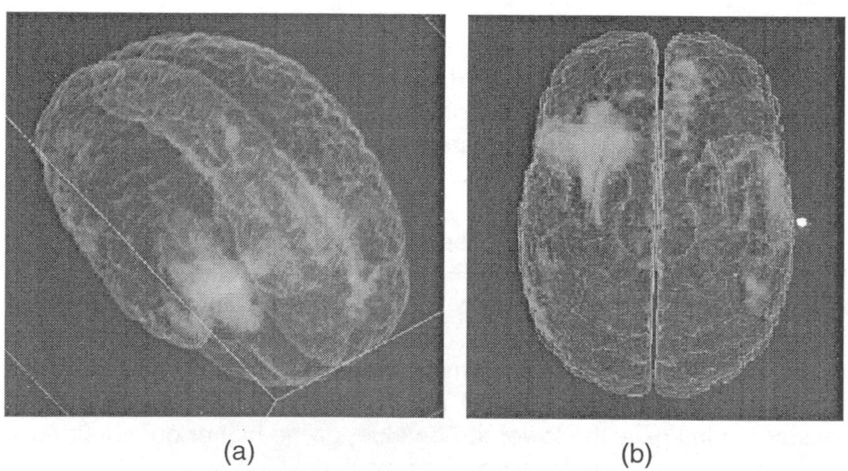

(a) (b)

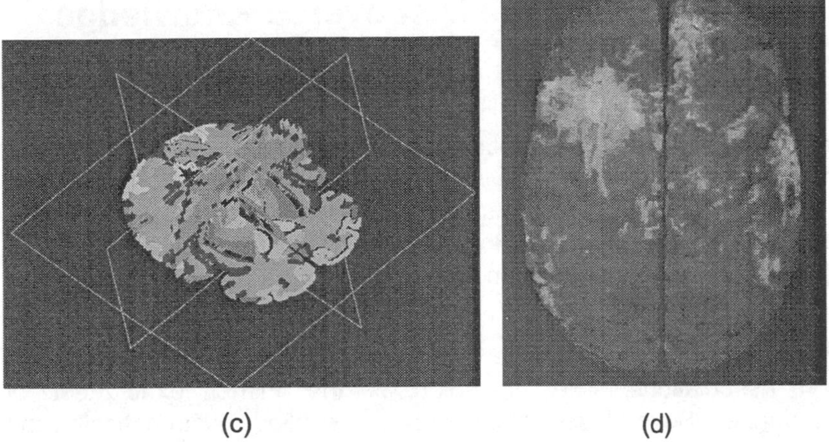

(c) (d)

Figure 4. Visualization of the voxel-based analysis p-value volume for development of ADHD.

Figure 5 shows the results of the voxel-based regression analysis for ADHD. Just one representative slice (119) of the Talairach atlas is displayed. Figures 5(a) and (b) show the sum of all lesions for patients that did and did not develop ADHD respectively. Figure 5(c) shows the optimal regression sphere that best discriminates between lesions that are and are not associated with the development of ADHD. These results are consistent with all the previous ones for ADHD.

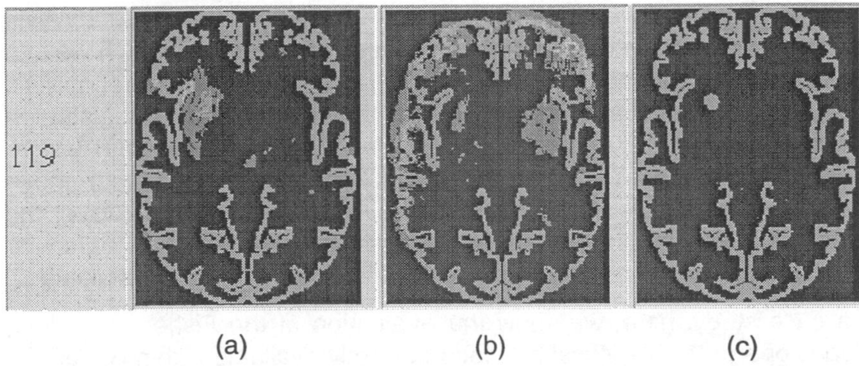

(a) (b) (c)

Figure 5. The optimal regression sphere (c) that best discriminates the (a) ADHD+ and (b) ADHD- groups.

6.5 Evaluation of the Discovered Knowledge

In the previous section we reported as findings associations between lesions in the visual cortex and visual deficits, and associations between basal ganglia lesions and subsequent development of Attention Deficit Hyperactivity Disorder (ADHD). However, the evaluation of the discovered knowledge and the structure-function analysis methods has not been addressed.

In BRAID several methods have been implemented to detect structure-function associations, one of which is the Fisher exact test of independence. Several researchers have studied systematically the problem of sample size corresponding to power for statistical tests such as the chi-square and Fisher exact tests of independence (Larntz, 1978; Fu and Arnold, 1992), and compare the relative power of different statistical tests of independence (Lee and Shen, 1994; Oluyede, 1994; Harwell and Serlin, 1997; Tanizaki, 1997). In addition, simulations have been performed to study the power of chi-square analysis in sample spaces of much higher dimensionality, as one would expect to find in many epidemiological studies (Osius and Rojek, 1992; Thomas and Conlon, 1992; Mannan and Nassar, 1995; Tanizaki, 1997). However, closed form power analysis do not exist that can account for the simultaneous effects of image noise and registration error, in addition to the characteristics of the statistical methods being employed.

Given the impossibility of a general closed-form solution for power analysis in this domain we have designed a lesion-deficit simulator in which we can generate a large number of artificial subjects, construct a probabilistic model of lesion-deficit associations, model the error of a given registration method and apply this nonlinear error to the image data, perform lesion-deficit analysis, and compare the generated associations with those detected by the analysis. The number of subjects required to recover the known associations reflects the statistical power of the particular combination of imgae-processing and statistical methods being evaluated.

As a case study, here, we show the evaluation of the Fisher exact test, which is one of the statistical methods currently available within BRAID for detection of associations. The effects of registration error due to our nonlinear image-registration algorithm on the power of lesion-deficit analysis within BRAID is also evaluated. The sensitivity and accuracy of the mining method as a function of the number of subjects in the sample, the strength and complexity of the associations, and the errors that arise due to imperfect registration, are quantified. This simulator can be seen as a test-bed for the subsequent development and evaluation of new methods for structure-function analysis; for determining the sample size required to detect an association of a given strength between a structure and a function for a given study; and for evaluating the effect of registration and other image-processing methods.

6.5.1 The Lesion-Deficit Simulator

We designed the LDS to generate a large number of artificial subjects, each consisting of lesions and deficits that conform to predefined distributions, which could then be analyzed within BRAID to determine lesion-deficit associations. Comparing the results of this analysis to the known lesion-deficit associations in our simulation model would allow us to quantify the performance of our system as a function of the parameters of the simulation. As a case study, we examined the Fisher exact test of independence, one of the statistical methods currently available within BRAID for lesion-deficit analysis.

The major components of the simulator are:

- generation of simulated lesions,
- modeling of registration error, and
- generation of simulated functional deficits.

To ensure that our simulator would generate a plausible data set, we obtained simulation parameters from data collected as part of the Frontal Lobe Injury in Childhood (FLIC) (Gerring et al., 1998) study. Previously, we reported the analysis of these data using BRAID, to determine whether there were associations among locations of lesions and subsequent development of ADHD (Herskovits et al., 1999).

6.5.1.1 Generation of Simulated Lesions

Because the data for the simulation parameters fit gaussian distributions with reasonable accuracy, we constructed gaussian distributions based on these data, although we could readily have used other functional forms had that been necessary. Thus, in order to construct the spatial distribution for brain lesions, we collected statistics from the sample data set that describe the number of lesions per subject, their sizes, and their locations. Then, for each subject, we sampled these distributions, generating the number of lesions, and, for each lesion, its centroid and size. For simplicity in the generation of the synthetic lesions, we assumed spherical shape.

Once we supplied the parameters for the LDS distributions with respect to the number, size, and location of lesions, the simulator generated the image data set. A representative example of the lesions for a simulated subject is presented in Figure 6.

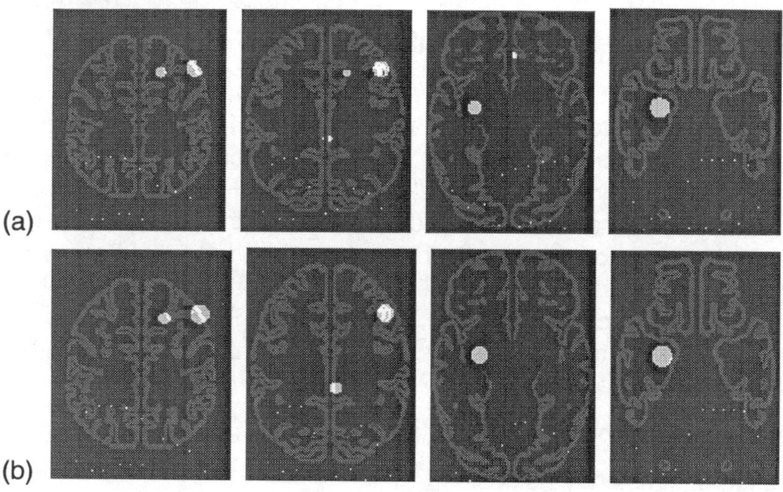

Figure 6. The artificial lesions of a simulated subject before (a) and after (b) taking into account registration error (slices 108, 110, 122, and 124 of the Talairach atlas are presented).

6.5.1.2 Modeling of Registration Error

As described in Section 3, image registration to a common standard is central to many systems for functional brain mapping. Within BRAID, the brain image data for all subjects are placed in the same coordinate system via an elastic-registration method. Although this procedure is very accurate, it is imperfect, i.e., it does not necessarily map corresponding regions to exactly the same location inTalairach space. Misregistration introduces noise, in the form of false-negative and false-positive associations. We quantified this important source of error by assuming that it follows a 3D non-stationary gaussian distribution. To determine this distribution, we collected data from 19 subjects and measured the registration error on 20 distinct anatomical landmarks, then interpolated the error at all other points in the brain. Figure 6(b) shows an example of the displaced lesions in Figure 6(a).

6.5.1.3 Generation of Synthetic Associations

The lesion-deficit-association model, with its conditional-probability tables and prior probabilities, describes the relationships among structures and functions. Because structure and function variables are categorical (i. e., normal/abnormal), we modelled these associations using Bayesian networks (BNs) (Pearl, 1988).

Briefly, a Bayesian network is a directed acyclic graph, in which nodes represent variables of interest such as structures or functions, and edges represent associations among these variables. Each node has a conditional-probability table that quantifies the strength of the associations among that node and its parents. Given the prior probabilities for the root nodes and conditional probabilities for other nodes, we can derive all joint probabilities (Pearl, 1988) over these variables. Note that this nonparametric model is general enough to represent any set of multivariate lesion-deficit associations. Furthermore, although in this paper we use discrete structure and function variables, BNs based on multivariate gaussian distributions, and mixed discrete-continuous distributions, have been constructed (Shachter and Kenley, 1989).

To use a discrete BN to model multivariate lesion-defict associations, we specified the numbers of structure and function variables, the number and strengths of associations among these variables, and a function mapping the fraction of an atlas structure that is lesioned to the probability that this structure will function abnormally.

To examine the effect of the strength of the lesion-deficit associations on BRAID's ability to detect them, we considered three cases presented in Table 3 that correspond to strong, moderate, and weak associations. Thus, a strong association between a structure s_i and a function f_j is denoted by conditional probabilities $p(f_j=A \mid s_i=N)=0$, $p(f_j=A \mid s_i=A)=1$, $p(f_j=N \mid s_i=N)=1$ and $p(f_j=N \mid s_i=A)=0$, where A means abnormal and N normal. We similarly defined moderate and weak associations as shown in Table 3.

Case	Association	Conditional probabilities for functions
1	Strong	0/1
2	Moderate	0.25/0.75
3	Weak	0.49/0.51

Table 3. The 3 cases of BNs considered.

To simplify the generation of conditional-probability tables, we used a noisy-OR model (Pearl, 1986). The noisy-OR model is a boolean OR gate with a failure function associated with each input line - there is a *leak* probability q_i that line i will fail. When no failure occurs, each line's input is passed to a boolean OR gate. This overall structure induces a probability distribution that is easily computed; the probability of no failure occurring is denoted by p^{nf}: $p^{nf} = 1 - \sum_{i \in M} q_i$, where M is the subset of lines with activated input. A boolean noisy-OR model with leak probability 0.25 for a function associated with two structures (parents) is shown in Table 4. Note that our framework allows us to specify arbitrary conditional-probability tables; we chose the noisy-OR model because it requires relatively few parameters to generate a well characterized conditional-probability table.

Structure 1	Structure 2	P(function=N)
N	N	0.75
N	A	0.25
A	N	0.25
A	A	0.06

Table 4. A noisy-OR gate with leak probability 0.25 for a function associated with 2 structures (N=Normal, A=Abnormal).

We calculated the prior probability of structure abnormality for each structure s_i, in each subject p_j, based on $f_{si,pj}$: the fraction of the volume of s_i that overlapped with lesions for p_j. The conditional probability $p(s_i | f_{si,pj})$ is expected to be a sigmoid function. One way to fit the sigmoid model is to compute $p(s_i | f_{si,pj})$ for various function and structure variables in our data set. This sigmoid function could differ for different structures. Computing this above conditional probability from our data set for the case in which the functional variable represents the absence or development of ADHD, and considering all of the Talairach structures and subjects from the FLIC study, demonstrated empirically that a step function with threshold fraction of 0.01 could be used in the simulations, instead of a sigmoid function. The threshold value 0.01 is also the mean of the optimal thresholds with respect to p-value, i. e., the mean of the thresholds that gave the smallest Fisher-exact p-value for all 132 Talairach structures and the functional variable that corresponds to the development of ADHD. Thus, for the FLIC data, we labeled each structure for which at least 1 percent of its volume overlapped with lesions as abnormal for that subject; the remainder of the structures were labeled as normal. Averaging over all subjects, we could compute a prior probability of abnormality for each structural variable.

For each simulated subject p_j and structure s_k, we sampled the prior-probability distribution and generated a binary vector S^K_j of dimension K (where $S_j[k]=1$ means that structure s_K is abnormal for subject p_j). By instantiating the states of all structure variables of the BN with S^K_j for subject p_j, we could determine the conditional probability for each function variable by table lookup, and use this probability to generate the binary vector F^M_j of dimension M for the function variables, where, $F_j[i]=0$ if function f_i was abnormal for subject p_j. The binary vectors S^K_j and , F^M_j for each subject p_j were then analyzed using the Fisher exact test of independence for each structure-function pair, as described earlier.

6.5.2 Results from the Evaluation of the Mining System

In this section, we describe how we used the LDS framework to characterize the performance of the Fisher exact test of independence for lesion-deficit analysis. We studied its behavior as a function of the number of subjects needed to discover the simulated lesion-deficit associations represented by a BN, the strengths of associations, the number of associations, the degree of the BN, i. e., the number of structures related to a particular function, and the prior probabilities for structure abnormality. We also examined the effects of registration error. Recall that the input to the simulator includes the number of structure nodes,the number of function nodes and the number of edges (associations) among them. The parameters we chose for the stochastically generated BN were the following unless otherwise stated: 132 structure nodes (corresponding to the Talairach atlas structures), 20 function nodes, and 69 edges from structures to functions. This BN has sufficient complexity to demonstrate the use of the simulator and help us reach meaningful results regarding the performance of the Fisher exact test and the effects of misregistration. The maximum degree, i. e., the maximum number of incoming edges to a given function node, was restricted to be 4; thus, a function could be associated to at most 4 different structures. Since the performance of any method for detecting associations depends on the characteristics of the conditional-probability tables, we examined the three cases of Table 3 to study this effect. The prior probability of abnormality for each structure was set to 0.5 to allow us to examine the behavior of the Fisher exact test for the optimal value of the prior probability (i. e., many examples of abnormal and normal structures would be available for analysis). To generate the conditional-probability table for those function variables that were related to more than one structure, we used a noisy-OR model (see Table 4 for a noisy-OR function that corresponds to the moderate case of Table 3, i. e., when the leak probability is 0.25). For the results that follow, we report the total number of edges (i. e., associations) detected, as well as the number of simulated (i. e., true-positive) edges found. The difference between these two numbers is the number of false-positive associations that were identified.

6.5.2.1 Experiment 1: Determining the p-value Threshold

Table 5 quantifies the statement that the lower the threshold for the p-value, the smaller the number of false positives and number of simulated edges detected (i. e., the more conservative the method). It presents the results for the case of moderate strength of associations (case 2 of Table 3); however, similar results were observed for the cases of strong and weak associations. In the following experiments we used the threshold 0.001 for the p-value, since this is a good trade-off between the number of simulated associations and the number of false positives detected.

	$p \leq 0.01$		$p \leq 0.001$		$p \leq 0.0001$	
# subjs	%true pos.	%false pos.	%true pos.	%false pos.	%true pos.	%false pos.
500	84	35	72	4	55	0
1000	100	45	99	1	90	0
1500	100	35	100	4	97	0
2000	100	32	100	1	100	0

Table 5. Percentage of simulated associations and false positives detected by the Fisher exact test for three values of the p-value threshold and for moderate strength of lesion-deficit associations.

6.5.2.2 Experiment 2: Effect of Conditional Probabilities

In Figure 5(a) we present the performance of the Fisher exact test ($p \leq 0.001$) for the cases in which all structure-function conditional probabilities were set to strong (case 1), moderate (case 2), and weak (case 3) associations as described in Table 3. The figures demonstrate the dramatic effects of the different conditional-probability distributions on the power of lesion-deficit analysis. Figure 7(a) demonstrates that, in order to discover 70% of the total number of simulated edges, we require approximately 180, 500, and 2000 subjects for the strong-, moderate-, and weak-association cases, respectively. As expected, the more samples are required to detect weak associations.

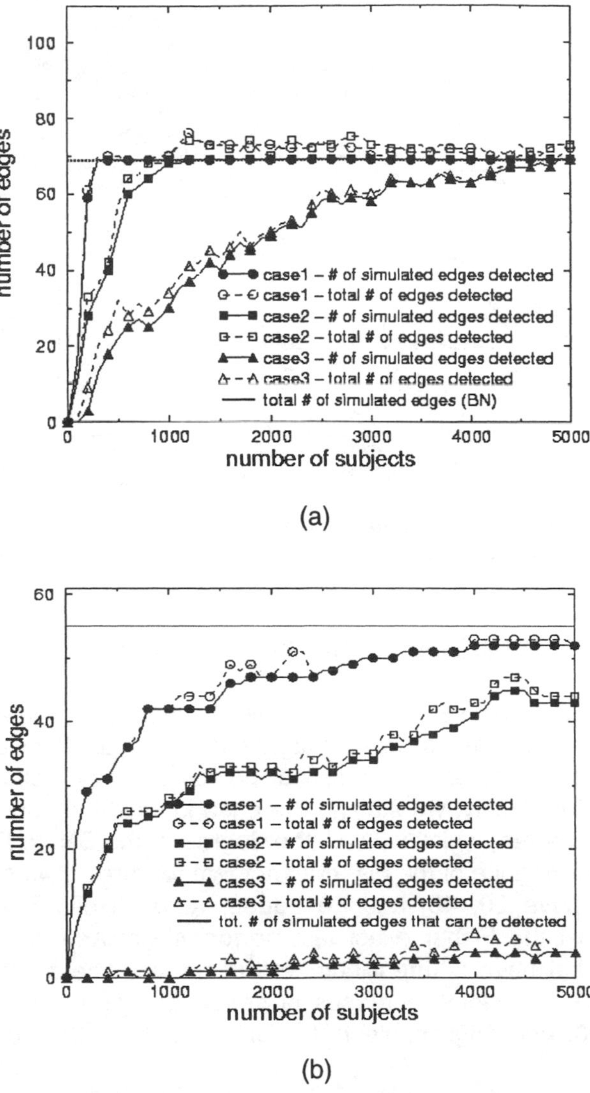

Figure 7. Performance of the Fisher exact test (p≤0.001) for (a) uniform (0.5) prior probabilities and (b) data-derived prior probabilities of structure abnormality, and for the 3 strengths of lesion-deficit associations from Table 3 that correspond to strong (case 1), moderate (case 2) and weak (case3) associations. The difference between the total number of associations detected, and the number of true associations detected is the number of false-positive associations detected ifor each case. The horizontal line in (a) represents the total number of simulated edges (69) and in (b) represents the total number of simulated edges that can be detected (55).

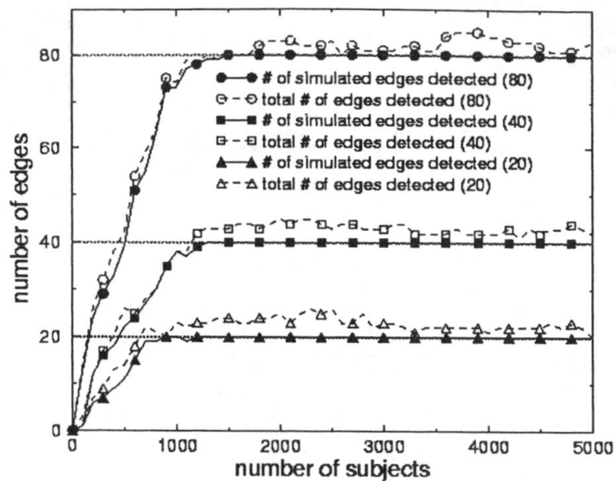

Figure 8. Performance of the Fisher exact test (p≤0.001) for BNs with degree 4, and with 20, 40 and 80 edges.

6.5.2.3 Experiment 3: Effect of Number of Associations

For this experiment, we selected the moderate case (i.e., case 2) for the conditional-probability tables, to investigate further the effect of the total number of associations on the statistical power of lesion-deficit analysis. Without loss of generality, we studied the case in which all function nodes have the same degree, which we call the degree of the BN. In Figure 8 we present the performance of the Fisher exact test for three BNs of degree 4. The networks have 20, 40, and 80 edges, respectively. These results demonstrate that the Fisher exact test performs similarly for BNs of the same degree that have different numbers of edges. The deterioration as the total number of edges increases is small. All edges are discovered after 900, 1300, and 1500 subjects for BNs with 20, 40, and 80 edges, respectively.

6.5.2.4 Experiment 4: Effect of Degree of the BN

For this experiment, we again selected the moderate case for the conditional-probability tables, to isolate the effect of the number of structures affecting a particular function, or the degree of the BN. Figure 9 shows the effect of increasing the degree of the BN while fixing the total number of edges. As expected, as the degree of the BN increases, more subjects are needed to detect the same number of associations. In particular, to discover 70% of the total number of simulated edges, we require approximately 500, 3700, and more than 8000 subjects for the cases of BNs that have degree 4, 6, and 8 respectively. As expected, the degree of the BN has a much greater effect on the performance of the Fisher exact test than does the total number of edges.

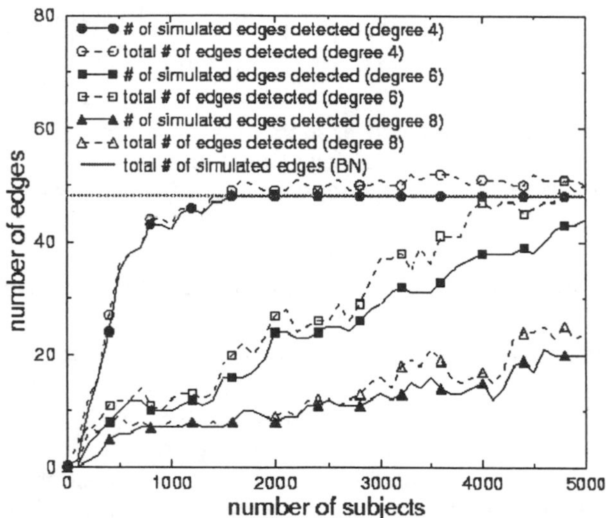

Figure 9. Performance of the Fisher exact test ($p \leq 0.001$) for BNs with 48 edges, and with degree 4, 6, and 8.

Since the parameters that most affect the performance are the conditional probabilities for the functions (i. e., strengths of associations) and the degree of the function nodes (i.e., number of structures related to a function), in Table 6 we present the percent of the associations detected by the Fisher exact test, as a function of these parameters for 1000 and 5000 subjects. These results confirm the profound effect of the degree of the BN on the power of lesion-deficit analysis.

	1000 subjects			5000 subjects		
cond. prob.	Deg. 4	deg. 6	deg. 8	deg. 4	deg. 6	deg. 8
0.0	100	100	17	100	100	58
0.1	100	48	15	100	100	44
0.2	94	25	15	100	94	42
0.3	79	19	15	100	83	42
0.4	63	17	15	100	71	38
0.5	52	17	15	100	63	35

Table 6. Percentage of simulated associations detected by the Fisher exact test ($p \leq 0.001$) as a function of the conditional probabilities for the structure-function associations, and of the in-degree of the function nodes.

6.5.2.5 Experiment 5: Using Priors from the Simulated Data Set

In the previous experiments, the prior probability of a given structure being abnormal was set to 0.5 for each structure variable, since our purpose was to evaluate the behavior of the Fisher exact test while manipulating the strengths and number of associations among the structure and function variables. For this experiment, we obtained the prior probabilities from the simulated data set. The number of edges that could actually be discovered is 55 (80%), since there were 14 edges from structures that did not intersect any lesions. The smallest nonzero prior probability for the structures is 0.0004, and only 5 out of the 132 Talairach structures have a prior probability of being abnormal that is above 0.2. Thus, in contrast to the experiments in which prior probabilities were uniform, most of the simulated cases in this experiment would not have abnormal structures.

Figure 7(b) demonstrates the performance of the Fisher exact test for the three cases of BN conditional probabilities (see Table 3). Comparing this figure with Figure 7(a), in which uniform prior probabilities were used, demonstrates that, as expected, more subjects are required to recover all associations when data-derived prior probabilities are used in the LDS, when compared to the case in which uniform prior probabilities were used to simulate abnormal structures. Even when all structure-function associations are deterministic (case 1), the number of subjects required to recover all 55 associations is close to 5000. To discover 70% of the total number of simulated edges (70% of 69 $\approx$ 48) would require approximately 2500, and more than 6000 subjects for the strong and moderate associations, respectively, instead of 180 and 500 in the case of uniform prior probabilities. As expected, the number of subjects needed is inversely proportional to the smallest prior probability. The detection of false-positive associations is due to the existence of associations among neighboring structures. These associations are due to lesions that intersect more than one structure. Additional false positives can be observed in the case where there are associations among the function variables, such as hemiparesis and upper-extremity weakness.

6.5.2.6 Experiment 6: Effect of Registration Error

Table 7 demonstrates the effect of registration error on the performance of the Fisher exact test, for two cases of conditional probabilities: strong (case 1) and moderate (case 2) strengths of lesion-deficit associations. As expected, registration error reduces the power of the Fisher exact test in detecting the associations, when compared with perfect registration. As shown in Table 7, on average our nonlinear registration method reduces the number of associations discovered by 13% for the same number of subjects.

	Strong associations		Moderate associations	
# subjects	% w reg. error	% w/o reg. error	% w reg. error	% w/o reg. error
500	43	49	30	35
1000	54	60	35	38
2000	57	68	39	46
3000	64	72	45	49
4000	65	75	48	58

Table 7. Percentage of detectable associations discovered by the Fisher exact test ($p \leq 0.001$) with and without registration error, for strong (case 1) and moderate (case 2) lesion-deficit associations (a maximum of 80% of associations can be discovered).

6.6 Using the Discovered Knowledge

We have considered the problem of mining lesion-deficit associations in a Brain Image Database (BRAID). Applying the mining capabilities of BRAID to epidemiological data from different studies we have discovered several clinically meaningful associations and drawn interesting conclusions about the functional mapping of the human brain and the effect of lesions (either traumatic or stroke lesions) in the development of neurological and neuropsychological deficits. Correlation of these results with the ones from task-activation studies (e.g., fMRI) can help reveal how functions remap to other brain locations in the presence of abnormalities.

Visualization helped us reduce the enormous search space by directing the analysis. Exploratory pairwise analysis produced reasonable results although one has to deal with the multiple-comparison problem. The preliminary voxel-based analysis that we presented shows encouraging results too. A future goal is to investigate more complex spatial analysis models and include clustering analysis in the voxel-based approach. The voxel-based regression analysis performs considerably well in cases other than multifocal functional associations. However, both of the voxel-based approaches are computationally intensive. The statistical simulations showed that more advanced mining methods and large sample sizes are required to determine lesion-deficit associations accurately, reducing the number of false positives. Towards this end, and in order to increase the number of subjects in BRAID, automation of the labor-intensive procedure of lesion detection and segmentation has to be performed. More robust mining methods that will reduce the number of false positive associations discovered have to be examined. Multivariate analysis methods like log-linear regression and logistic regression provide relatively simple methods for generating candidate models, usually relying on modifications of greedy search and making assumptions about cell frequencies or total number of samples that may not hold for rare lesions or deficits. A more promising approach generates models that consist of graphical structures along with statistical independence models, called bayesian networks (Pearl, 1986), scores each model and returns the most probable model that could have generated the data at hand (Cooper and Herskovits, 1992; Heckerman, 1997).

The analysis of simulated data was very important in demonstrating that the number of subjects needed to detect all the associations while reducing false positives has an inverse relationship to the strength of associations and the smallest prior probability of structure abnormality. The number of subjects required to detect all and only those associations in the underlying model (i. e., the ground truth) may be in the thousands, even for strong lesion-deficit associations, particularly if the spatial distribution of lesions does not extend to all structures. The more one descends from the 0.5 level for prior probabilities, the more difficult it becomes to discover associations. These results underline the necessity to develop large image databases, for the purpose of meta-analysis of data pooled from multiple studies, so that more meaningful results can be obtained. The degree of associations, i. e., the number of structures related to a particular function, has much greater effect on the performance of the Fisher exact test presented here, than does the number of associations to discover. This result implies that, for functions that are associated with many structures, identification of structure--function associations is difficult or requires a much larger sample size. The registration error also reduces (by 13% using our registration methods) the power of the statistical test in detecting the associations; a simulator like the one presented here, allows one to take into account this error when calculating the sample size needed for a particular experiment. The framework that consist of the lesion-deficit simulator and the testing procedure is very important since it can be used to characterize the power of methods used in BRAID to detect multivariate associations among lesions and deficits taking into account the effects of registration, noise, and lesion segmentation. This simulator can be used in the evaluation of log-linear, Bayesian, and other methods used for lesion-deficit analysis, as well as, to study the effect of different registration and lesion segmentation algorithms.

References

R. Agrawal, T. Imielinski, and A. Swami. Database Mining: A performance Perspective. *IEEE Transactions on Knowledge and data Engineering*,5(6):914-925, Dec. 1993.

E. Andersen. *Introduction to the Statistical Analysis of Categorical Data*. Springer Verlag, Berlin, 1997.

S. W. Anderson, H Damasio, et al. Neuropsychological impairments associated with lesions caused by tumor or stroke. *Arch Neurol,* 47(4):397-405, 1990.

A. Andres and I. Tejedor. On conditions for validity of the approximations to Fisher's exact test. *Biometrical Journal*, 39(8):935-954, 1997.

M. Arya, W. Cody, C. Faloutsos, J. Richardson, and A. Toga. A 3D Medical Image Database Management System. *Int. Journal of Computerized Medical Imaging and Graphics, Special issue on Medical Image Databases*, 20(4):269-284, Apr. 1996.

F. Bookstein. Principal Warps: Thin-Plate Splines and the Decomposition of Deformations. *IEEE Trans. on Patt. Analysis and Machine Intellig.*, 11(6):567-585, 1989.

R. Bryan, T.A. Manolio, et al. A method for using MR to evaluate the effects of cardiovascular disease of the brain: the cardiovascular health study.*American Journal of Neuroradiology,* 15:1625-1633, 1994.

R. Bryan, S. Wells, T. Miller, A. Elster, C. Jungreis, V. Poirier, B. Lind, and T. Manolio. Infarctlike lesions in the brain: Prevalence and anatomic characteristics at MR imaging of the elderly - data from the cardiovascular health study. *Radiology*, 202(1):47-54, 1997.

D. Collins, P. Neelin, T. Peters, and A. Evans. Automatic 3D intersubject registration of MR volumetric data in standardized Talairach space. *J. of Comp. Ass. Tomography*, 18:192-205, 1994.

G. F. Cooper and E. H. Herskovits. A bayesian method for the induction of probabilistic networks from data. *Machine Learning*, 9:309-347, 1992.

C. Davatzikos. Spatial transformation and registration of brain images using elastically deformable models. *Comp. Vision and Image Understand.*, 66(2):207-222, 1997.

K. Friston. Statistical parametric mapping: ontology and current issues. *Journal of Cerebral Blood Flow and Metabolism*, 15(3):361-370, 1995.

Y. X. Fu and J. Arnold. A Table of Exact Sample Sizes for Use with Fisher's Exact Test for 2x2 Tables. *Biometrics*, 48(4):1103-1112, Dec. 1992.

J. Gerring, K. Brady, A. Chen, C. Quinn, K. Bandeen-Roche, M. Denckla, and R. Bryan. Neuroimaging Variables Related to the Development of Secondary Attention Deficit Hyperactivity Disorder in Children who have Moderate and Severe Closed Head Injury. *Journal of the American Academy of Child and Adolescent Psychiatry*, 37:647-654, 1998.

M. Harwell and R. Serlin. An empirical study of five multivariate tests for the single-factor repeated measures model. *Communications in statistics - Simulation and Computation,* 26(2):605--618, 1997.

D. Heckerman. Bayesian networks for data mining. *Data Mining and Knowledge Discovery,* 1(1):79-119, 1997.

E. H. Herskovits, V. Megalooikonomou, C. Davatzikos, A. Chen, R. Bryan, and J. Gerring.Is the spatial distribution of brain lesions associated with closed-head injury predictive of subsequent development of attention-deficit hyperactivity disorder?: Analysis with brain image Database. *Radiology*, 213(2):389-394, November 1999,

E. H. Herskovits. *Computer-based probabilistic-network construction.* PhD thesis, Medical Informatics, Stanford University, 1991.

M. Huerta, S. Koslow, and A. Leshner. The human brain project: An international resource. *Trends Neurosci.,* 16:436-438, 1993.

K. Larntz. Small-Sample Comparisons of Exact Levels for Chi-Squared Goodness-of-Fit Statistics. *Journal of the American Statistical Association*, 73(362):253-263, June 1978.

C. Lee and S. Y. Shen. Convergence-rates and powers of 6 power-divergence statistics for testing independence in 2by2 contingency table. *Communications in statistics - Theory and Methods*, 23(7):2113--2126, 1994.

S. Letovsky, S. Whitehead, C. Paik, G. Miller, J. Gerber, E. Herskovits, T. Fulton, and R. Bryan. A brain-image database for structure-function analysis. *American Journal of Neuroradiology*, 19(10):1869-1877, 1998.

M. Mannan and R. Nassar. Size and power of test statistics for gene correlation in 2x2 contingency-tables. *Biometrical Journal*, 37(4):409-433, 1995.

V. Megalooikonomou, C. Davatzikos, and E. H. Herskovits. Mining Lesion-Deficit Associations in a Brain Image Database. In *Proceedings of the ACM SIGKDD International Conference on Knowledge Discovery and Data Mining, San Diego, CA*, Aug. 1999.

V. Megalooikonomou, C. Davatzikos, and E.H. Herskovits. A Simulator for Evaluating Methods for the Detection of Lesion-Deficit Associations. *Human Brain Mapping*, 2000. In press.

M. Miller, G. Christensen, Y. Amit, and U. Grenander. Mathematical Textbook of Deformable Neuroanatomies. *Proc. of the National Academy of Sciences*, 90:11944-11948, 1993.

B. O. Oluyede. A modified chi-square test of independence against a class of ordered-alternatives in an RxC contingency table. *Canadian Journal of Statistics*, 22(1):75-87, Mar. 1994.

G. Osius and D. Rojek. Normal goodness-of-fit tests for multinomial models with large degrees of freedom. *Journal of the American Statistical Association*, 87(420):1145-1152, Dec. 1992.

J. Pearl. Fusion, propagation and structuring in belief networks. *Artificial Intelligence*, 29:241-288, 1986.

J. Pearl. *Probabilistic Reasoning in Intelligent Systems: Networks of Plausible Inference.* Morgan Kaufmann, San Mateo, CA, 1988.

J. Talairach and P. Tournoux. *Co-planar Stereotaxic Atlas of the Human Brain.* Thieme, Stuttgart, 1988.

H. Tanizaki. Power comparison of non-parametric tests: Small-sample properties from Monte Carlo experiments. *Journal of applied statistics*, 24(5):603-632, Oct. 1997.

R. Thomas and M. Conlon. Sample-size determination based on Fisher exact test for use in 2x2 comparative trials with low event rates. *Controlled clinical trials*, 13(2):134-147, 1992.

7 ADRIS: An Automatic Diabetic Retinal Image Screening System

Kheng Guan Goh, Wynne Hsu, Mong Li Lee and Huan Wang

School of Computing
National University of Singapore
Singapore
{gohkg, whsu, leeml, wangh}@comp.nus.edu.sg

Diabetic-related eye disease is the most common cause of blindness worldwide. The most effective treatment is early detection through regular screenings. This produces a large number of retinal photographs for the medical doctors to review. In our work, we employ a combination of innovative image processing and data mining techniques to automate the preliminary analysis and diagnosis of diabetic-related eye disease from the digitised retinal photographs. Our experimental results show that we are able to accurately detect abnormal symptoms such as: abnormal optic disc to cup ratio, presence of exudates and tortuous blood vessels. With this, our system is able to classify the retinal images into normal and abnormal ones, thus cutting down on the number of retinal photographs a doctor needs to review.

7.1 Introduction

More than half (57.6%) of all newly registered blindness in Singapore is caused by retinal diseases, as reported by Lim (1999). Diabetic retinopathy (19.4%) is one of the main contributors. As Singapore has one of the fastest ageing population in the world and about 10% of Singaporeans are diabetic, as reported by Goh (1998), diabetic-related eye diseases are set to rise. Industrialised countries in the world are facing the same problem. For example, in the United States blindness has been estimated to be 25 times more common in people with diabetes than in those without the disease (Kahn and Hiller, 1974; Palmberg, 1977), and yearly 5000 new cases of blindness are reported as a result of diabetic retinopathy (Klein *et al.*, 1995; Javitt et al., 1989) In the United Kingdom, diabetic eye diseases are the most common cause of blindness in the country for the age group of 20 to 65 (Ghafour *et al.*, 1983).

The most effective treatment to combat these eye diseases is early detection through regular screening of the fundus to detect early signs of diabetic retinopathy, as reported by Singer *et al.* (Singer *et al.*, 1992). Early detection screenings consist primarily of obtaining fundus images through photography. However, with a large number of patients undergoing regular screenings, tremendous amount of time is needed for the medical professionals to analyse and diagnose the fundus photographs. As a result, this may delay the patients from being referred to ophthalmologist for further examination and treatment. Therefore, by automating the initial task of analysing the huge amount of retinal photographs for symptoms of diabetic retinopathy, the efficiency of the screening process can be greatly improved. At the same time, patients that require the attention of the ophthalmologist would be timely referred.

We have developed an Automatic Diabetic Retinal Image Screening system (ADRIS), which combines novel image processing techniques with data mining technique to analyse digitised diabetic retinal photographs. Based on the rules given by medical experts, the system classifies the retinal images into normal (healthy) and abnormal (unhealthy) ones. Once a diabetic retinal image is found to have any abnormal feature, the system would highlight it to the doctor for review. Initial studies indicate that the system can potentially reduce the number of retinal photos a doctor needs to review by more than 60%.

7.2 Understanding the Problem Domain

It has been estimated that to implement a regular screening programme for diabetic patients, 30,000 patients per million total populations would be involved (Retinopathy Working Party, 1991). Hence over the years, there have been quite a number of developments in automatic screening and detection of diabetic retinopathy and other age-related diseases. Gardner *et al.* (1996) concluded in their studies that a neural network program could be trained to detect retinal images with diabetic retinopathy features.

Numerous systems (Ward *et al.*, 1989; Spencer *et al.*, 1992; Spencer *et al.*, 1991; Katz *et al.*, 1988; Katz *et al.*, 1990) reported some successes in the automatic detection of glaucoma, exudates, microaneurysm and maculopathy in diabetic retinopathy. However, an application in automatic diabetic retinal screening has yet to be developed and implemented.

Cox *et al.* (1991) used grey level information around the vicinity to automatically extract the boundary of the optic disc with initial approximate location given by the user input. Morris *et al.* (1994) employed dynamic contour to map out the boundary of the optic disc. Their approach is dependent on image pre-possessing where there is a heavy emphasis on enhancing the image contrast.

Phillips *et al.* (1993) used simple thresholding method to detect and quantify exudates. Global and local thresholding levels are used for extracting large and small exudate respectively. However, their straightforward approach generated some false-negatives due to the presence of exudates with low grey level intensity. Leistritz *et al.* (1994) acquired retinal images through scanning laser ophthalmoscope with monochromatic illumination to detect exudates with the highest contrast. However, images have to be captured with a suitable wavelength for this approach to be reliable.

Zhou *et al.* (1994) used match-filtering approach with *priori* knowledge to automatically extract and track retinal vessel in digital fluorescein angiograms. Zana *et al.* (1997) used mathematical morphology and linear processing techniques that include Laplacian filter and curvature differentiation to extract retinal blood vessel in retinal angiography. Both approaches are targeted at retinal angiograms. Capowski *et al.* (1993) employed *relative length variation* (arc/chord information) to ascertain the tortuousity of retinal blood vessel manually.

7.2.1 Data Mining Applications on Medical Data

The prevalence of large databases created a need to devise new tools that can sift out useful and interesting knowledge from these data. As a result, a new research area, data mining and knowledge discovery is rapidly gaining popularity.

Data mining is the application of specific algorithms for extracting interesting patterns from data, (Fayyad *et al.*, 1996). Large databases contain vast amount of data which is most often left hidden from the user. These hidden data might harbour some very useful relationships (e.g. in the diabetic retinal screening database patients of certain race with a minimum number of years of illness might have a certain percentage of likelihood that eye disease may develop within a certain number of years), trends (e.g. the deterioration of a particular eye disease might localise around a certain race or gender based on patient's lifestyle and age of employment) and prediction (e.g. based on past data, a prediction of certain accuracy can be made on whether a new patient is going to develop diabetic-related eye disease), etc.

Classification-Based on Association (CBA, Liu *et al.*, 1998) is a data mining tool that combines classification rule mining and association rule mining to take advantage of the benefits of both methods. Classification rule mining separates the data into different classes based on a small set of rules in the database. And the target of classification rule mining is pre-determined. In association rule mining, constraints such as minimum confidence and minimum support are used to discover all the rules in the database. And the targets in association rule mining are not pre-determined.

Some of the research and applications carried out using knowledge discovery techniques in medical domains (notably medical diagnosis) includes oncology, Elomaa and Holsti (1989); liver pathology, Lesmo *et al.* (1984); urology, Bratko and Kononenko (1987) ; thyroid disease diagnosis, Hojker *et al.* (1988); rheumatology, Kern *et al.* (1990); neuropsychology, Muggleton (1990); abdominal pain diagnosis, Provan *et al.* (1996) and gynaecology, Nunez (1990).

In our system, we use an association based data mining classification tool developed by Liu *et al.* (1998) to discover the association rules between the different curvature definitions of retinal blood vessels.

7.3 Understanding the Data

Figure 1 shows a healthy normal fundus image which has the following features:

I. Optic Disc

Colour:	Red-yellow; the yellowish colour (optic cup) is more pronounced on the temporal and the nasal side part may appear pale.
Form and size:	Round to oval with diameter ranging from 1.5mm to 1.7mm.
Margins:	Sharply outline.

Vessels: They originate within the perimeter of the disc and both the arteries and veins appear distinct.

II. Vessels

Colour: Arteries appear light red while veins appear dark red.

Form and size: Largely straight with gentle curves. The arteries appear somewhat narrower than the veins, with an average ratio of 2:3 between arteries and veins. Average diameter of veins is 125μm.

Margins: Generally more sharply outline in the centre than at the peripheral.

III. Macular

Colour: Appears darker than the surrounding retina.

Form and size: Lies in the optic axis of the eye and is situated about 2 disc (3 ~ 4 mm) diameter temporal from the optic disc.

Margins: Not clearly defined in normal illumination. Marginally visible in red free illumination.

IV. Choroid

Colour: Reddish colour.

Margins: Normal even appearance throughout the inter-vascular space.

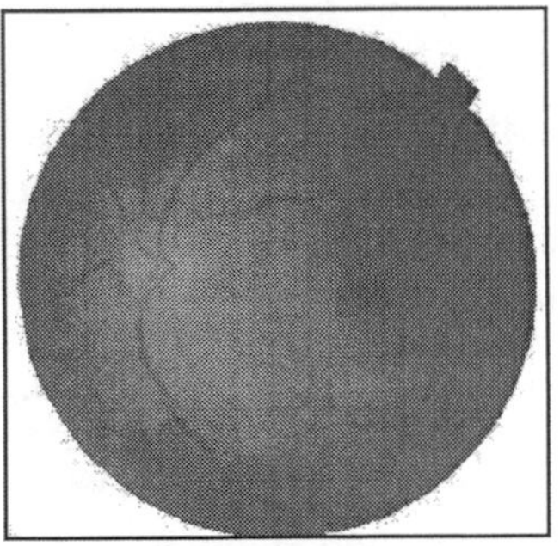

Figure 1. Sample of a healthy normal fundus image.

On the other hand, a diabetic retinopathy fundus will exhibit some of the following symptoms as shown in Figure 2:

i. Abnormal Optic Disc and Cup Ratio

The centre of the optic disc has a small white depression, optic cup (physiologic excavation). Under normal healthy circumstances, the size of the optic cup is about 40% or less compared to the optic disc. Abnormal condition appears when the optic disc is not visible, the outline is not circular, or it appears completely white (only the optic cup is visible).

ii. Presence of Exudates

Exudates show up as random white patches around the inter-vascular region. They vary in shapes and sizes.

iii. Tortuous Vessels

Normal retinal blood vessels appear largely straight or gently curved. In some diseases, the blood vessels become tortuous, i.e. they become dilated and take on a wavy path.

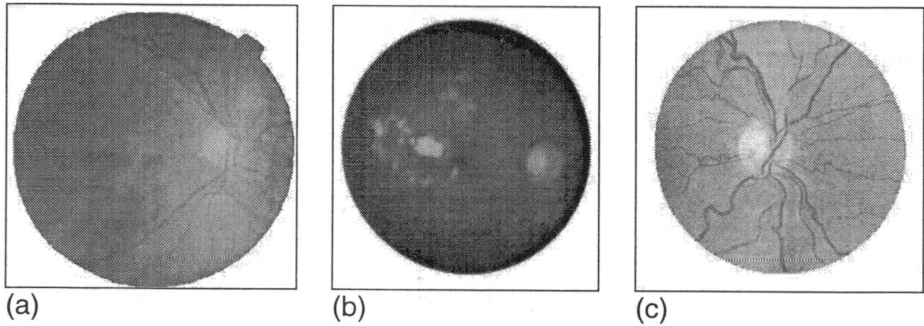

Figure 2. Sample of unhealthy retinal images. (a) Abnormal disc/cup ratio, (b) Presence of exudates, (c) Tortuous vessel.

The specifications of the types and conditions of diabetic retinopathy are identified and defined into rules. These rules are built into the algorithm to detect the normal healthy features of the ocular fundus and common symptoms of diabetic retinopathy.

In order to determine whether a retinal image is normal or not, we employ image processing techniques to extract the features of the fundus. The extraction of optic disc seems relatively simple, as the disc is usually the brightest region on retinal images. However, we find that simple edge detection and thresholding image processing techniques do not yield the expected results. Figure 3 shows that the optic disc is inaccurately detected due to the presence of comparatively bright regions near the optic disc.

(a) 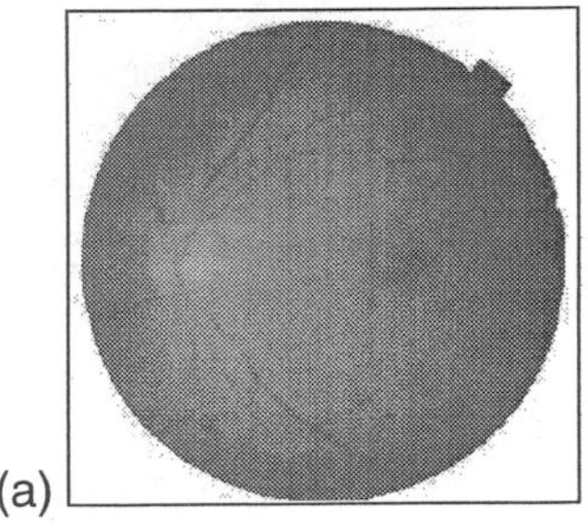 (b) 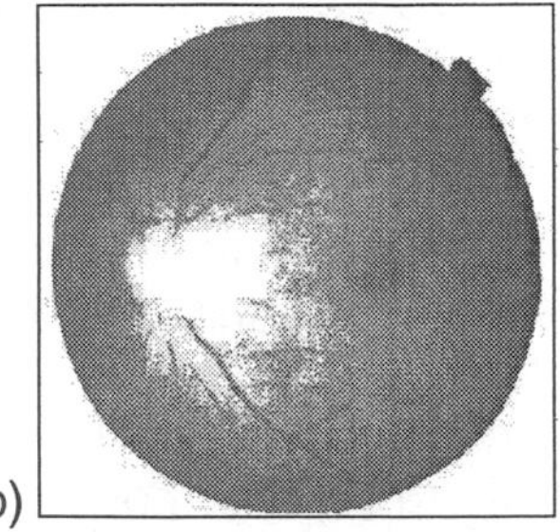

Figure 3. Detecting optic disc using simple thresholding techniques. (a) Original image, (b) Inaccurately detected optic disc.

7.4 Preparing the Data

A whole range of different image processing techniques is used to detect the main features of retinal images as well as the clinical symptoms that indicate the presence of diabetic retinopathy. The following subsections describe each of them in detail.

7.4.1 Optic Disc and Cup Detection

The optic disc is the region on the fundus where optic nerves and blood vessel emerge. It appears relatively brighter than the rest of the choroid due to the absence of retina layer. It ranges from round to oval in shape and has an average diameter size of 1.5 to 1.7mm. The optic cup is situated near the centre of the disc and is more pronounced on the temporal half as opposed to the nasal half. The optic cup appears brighter than the optic disc and usually covers less than 40% of the optic disc, although its position, shape and size may vary.

In our approach we employ a combination of the various image processing techniques to accurately detect the optic disc and cup. These include: Sobel edge extraction, varying ellipse fitting, neighbourhood accumulation, and histogram thresholding.

I. Sobel Edge Extraction

An edge is the boundary between two regions of different constant intensity (or grey level). An edge detector looks for regions in an image where the grey levels are changing too quickly to be a random effect, and some look for changes in a specific direction. Basically, locating an edge involves detecting points that fall on the edges. However, the edge points detected at this stage are discrete points and they do not directly show up as an edge. Therefore, a special algorithm is necessary to group all the similar edge points into boundaries. In recent years, many edge point detection algorithms (Davis 1975) have been developed. The most common edge detection method is to analyse the change of intensity gradient where an edge point is said to be present when the magnitude of the gradient exceeds a pre-defined threshold.

Sobel is one of the most well known edge detectors in sensing gradient variation in an image because of their low computation costs and easy implementation, as pointed out by Pitas (1993). Figure 4 shows the convolution masks of the edge detector. *Convolution* is accomplished by a simple multiplication, followed by an addition, and then finally a shifting operation. Sobel edge detector is efficient for different types of edges, including the "sudden step" edge 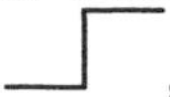 , the "slanted step" edge 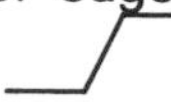 , the "roof" edge 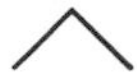 and the "planar" edge .

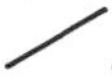

-1	0	1
-2	0	2
-1	0	1

x

1	2	1
0	0	0
-1	-2	-1

y

Figure 4. Sobel edge detector mask of 3 × 3.

The principal approach of the Sobel operator, $G(x, y)$ is to compute the magnitude of the gradient at each pixel location using the relation,

$$G(x,y)=\sqrt{G_x^2+G_y^2} \qquad (1)$$

where G_x and G_y are the first-derivative operators at any point (x,y) which are defined as

$$\begin{aligned} G_x = &[f(x+1,y-1)+2f(x+1,y)+f(x+1,y+1)] \\ &-[f(x-1,y-1)+2f(x-1,y)+f(x-1,y+1)] \end{aligned} \qquad (2)$$

and,

$$G_y = [f(x+1, y-1) + 2f(x, y+1) + f(x+1, y+1)] \\ -[f(x-1, y-1) + 2f(x, y-1) + f(x-1, y+1)] \quad (3)$$

where *f* is the mask value.

In Figure 4, the left mask represents the column gradient while the right mask represents that of the row gradient of the Sobel filter. Sobel filter combines both the row and column gradients to create two orthogonal directions in an image. The mask values of Sobel operator enable it to be more sensitive to both the horizontal and vertical edges.

In our system, the colour retinal image is converted to grey level image before using the simple and fast Sobel edge filter to extract the edges. This filtering operation produces a binary image where the positive (black) data represents edges and the negative (white) data represents uniform texture. The edges detected could be the outline of the optic disc, blood vessel, macular, or any abnormal lesion in the retinal.

II. Ellipse Fitting

Since the shape of a normal optic disc varies from round to oval, it makes sense to generate a range of ellipses and try to fit them to the edges extracted as described above. The ellipse that has the highest fit is considered to be the optic disc outline. However, we observe that the top and bottom regions of a normal retinal disc rim usually contain main blood crossings from which blood supply is transported to the retina. Therefore it would not be easy for the ellipse fitting function to obtain a perfect fit to the extracted optic disc outline. Hence, some percentage of minimum fit would have to be imposed so that the badly fitted ellipse would not be passed off as the detected optic disc. The numerical figure of the minimum fit is described next.

III. Neighbourhood Accumulation

The fitting of the ellipse is done by running the generated ellipse over extracted optic disc outline and accumulating the pixel values along the way when the ellipses' outline coincide with optic disc outline. To increase the accuracy of the fitting, the accumulation of edge pixel (those pixels that coincide with the ellipses' outline pixels) points includes the neighbouring pixels around the edge pixel. Varying the horizontal and vertical radii of the ellipse generates a range of different sizes of the fitting ellipse. The ellipse that returns the maximum response of accumulated pixel points is regarded as the boundary of the detected optic disc. If the maximum response of accumulated pixel points is lower than the minimum fit then the algorithm have failed to find a normal optic disc; such retinal images would be classified as abnormal.

The minimum fit figure is arrived at by averaging over all the maximum accumulated pixel points of each positively and negatively detected optic disc from a specially chosen set of 20 test retinal images. This set of test images are chosen to give a good measure of the average good fit and bad fit of the ellipse to the extracted optic disc outline.

The range of horizontal and vertical radii of the ellipse is selected so that it is greater than the average normal size of the optic cup to prevent falsely detecting the optic cup as that of the optic disc. Figure 5 shows samples of the optic discs detected.

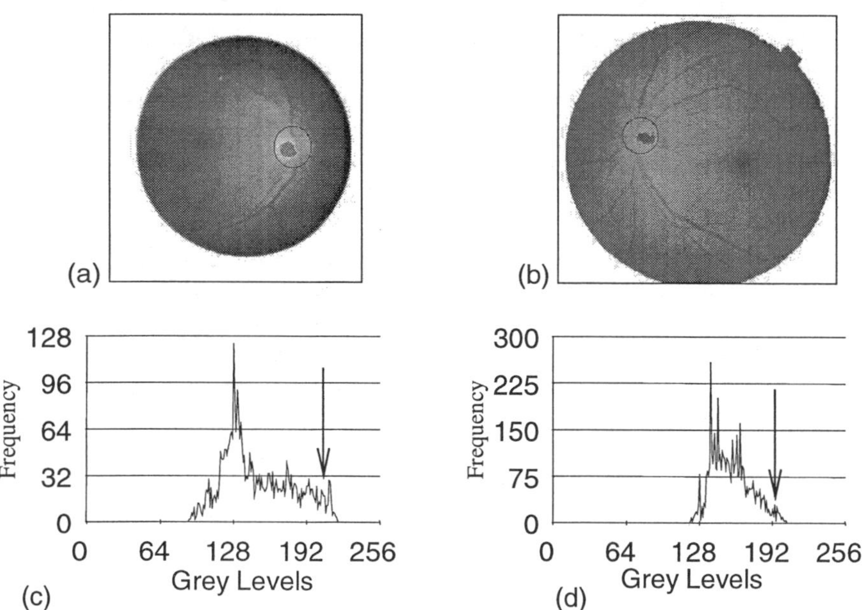

Figure 5. Detection of optic disc and cup. (a), (b) Sample of extracted optic disc and cup. (c), (d) Histograms of the corresponding optic disc showing the threshold grey level (arrow) where the optic cup is segmented from the optic disc.

IV. Histogram Thresholding

The optic cup is defined to be the brightest region within the optic disc. In the detection of the optic cup, a survey of the histogram distribution of the optic disc region reveals an interesting pattern. When a threshold is set at the second highest 'peak' of grey levels in the histogram with respect to the maximum grey level (walking from the right side of the histogram of 256), a reliable and accurate optic cup region is extracted.

Thresholding is used in image processing to separate an object's pixels from the background pixels. This technique converts a multi-grey level image into a binary image containing only two distinct grey levels. The threshold operation may be defined as

$$g(x, y) = \begin{cases} Go & \text{if} \quad f(x, y) > T \\ Gb & \text{if} \quad f(x, y) \leq T \end{cases} \tag{4}$$

where $f(x, y)$ is the original image, $g(x, y)$ is the threshold-processed image, T is the threshold value, G_O is the object grey level value after thresholding operation, and G_b is the background grey level value after the thresholding operation. The objects in an image can be separated effectively from a background by grouping the pixels that share common grey levels.

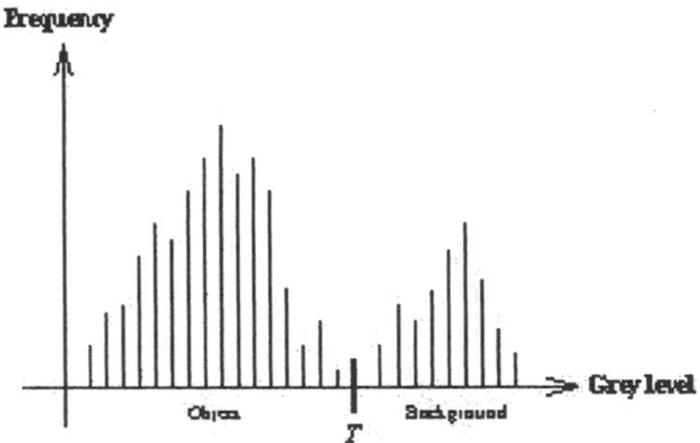

Figure 6. Principle of thresholding a grey level histogram.

In Figure 6, a dark object in an image $f(x, y)$ can be extracted from a light background by choosing a suitable threshold T (a particular intensity level) between the two grey regions. Then, any point (x, y) in the image that has a grey level lower than the value of T is considered an object point; otherwise, the point is called a background point. In other words, the objective is to generate a binary image $g(x, y)$ containing only the object points as defined in (4). The ratio of the optic cup to disc is calculated as the pixel area of the detected optic cu p to the corresponding area of the detected optic disc.

7.4.2 Exudates Detection

The presence of exudates indicates retinal disorders and is associated with patches of vascular damage. Exudates usually show up as white patches (in grey images; yellowish in colour images) of varying sizes and shapes scattered randomly in vascular spaces. Simple thresholding techniques do not give a satisfactory result as some smaller exudates have about the same intensity as the background of the retinal. Hence, we used a more effective method that employs the minimum distance discriminant (Kressel U and Schurmann, 1997; Castleman, 1996) to detect the exudates.

7.4.2.1 Minimum Distance Discriminant

Each pixel in colour digital image consists of three basic spectrum features (or colour features) in red, green and blue planes and each plane has its own illuminance. In general, different types of objects in digital images have their own range of spectrum features so that they appear in various colours and form different clusters (or classes) based on their spectrum features in the RGB colour space. In general, the greater the spectrum distance between the centres of different classes, the easier it is to identify the boundaries of different objects that belong to different clusters.

Utilising Bayes' theorem (Bayes, 1763) we can reliably carry out the classification of different objects belonging to each class. Bayes' theorem states the rule for updating belief H given state of evidence E, and background knowledge (context) I:

$$p(H|E,I) = p(H|I)^{*}\, p(E|H,I) \,/\, p(E|I) \qquad (5)$$

The term $p(H|E,I)$ is called the posterior probability, and it gives the probability of H after considering the effect of evidence E in context I. The $p(H|I)$ term is just the prior probability of H given I alone; that is, the belief in H without the evidence E being considered. The term $p(E|H,I)$ is called the likelihood, and it gives the probability of the evidence assuming H and background knowledge I is true. The last term, $1/p(E|I)$, is independent of H, and can be regarded as a normalising or scaling constant. The information I is a conjunction of all of the other statements relevant to determining $p(H|I)$ and $p(E|I)$.

Let $\mathbf{C}_i(c_r, c_g, c_b)$ be the mean value vector of spectrum feature of class i in RGB space, where i=1,2,...N and N is a class number in an image. Let $\mathbf{X}(x_r, x_g, x_b)$ be the measurement vector of pixel X, that is, X's illuminance in RGB space. Let $F_i(\mathbf{X})$ be the discriminant function for classifying pixel X into class i.

Let $p(\mathbf{C}_i/\mathbf{X})$ be the conditional probability (posterior probability). It represents the probability of **X** belonging to class i using the particular pixel's spectrum feature vector $\mathbf{X}(x_r, x_g, x_b)$. If it is found that $p(\mathbf{C}_i/\mathbf{X}) > p(\mathbf{C}_j/\mathbf{X})$, where j=1,2,...N and j≠i, then it can be concluded that **X** belongs to class i.

According to Bayes' theory, $p(\mathbf{C}_i/\mathbf{X})$ can be expressed as:

$$p(\mathbf{C}_i/\mathbf{X}) = p(\mathbf{C}_i) * p(\mathbf{X}/\mathbf{C}_i) \,/\, p(\mathbf{X}) \tag{6}$$

Where $p(\mathbf{C}_i)$ is the priori probability of class i in the image to be classified. $p(\mathbf{X}/\mathbf{C}_i)$ indicates the class specific probability distribution of **X**.

In (6), $p(\mathbf{X})$ is independent of class i so it can be safely discarded here. So the discriminant factor can be defined as,

$$F_i(\mathbf{X}) = p(\mathbf{C}_i) * p(\mathbf{X}/\mathbf{C}_i) \tag{7}$$

Here it is reasonable to assume $p(\mathbf{X}/\mathbf{C}_i)$ is a normal distribution,

$$p(X/C_i) = \frac{1}{\sigma^{1/2}\sqrt{2\pi}} \exp\left(-\frac{(X - C_i)^T}{2\sigma}\right) \tag{8}$$

Where σ is the covariance and is defined as

$$\sigma = \sum_i^N (X - C_i) \tag{9}$$

and $p(\mathbf{C}_i)$ is constant for i=1,2,...N.

It can be further assumed that the covariance σ is almost constant for all classes. So the

simplified discriminant $F_i(\mathbf{X})$ is redefined as

$$F_i(X) = X^T X - 2C_i^T X + C_i^T C_i \tag{10}$$

where X^T and C_i^T refer to the matrix component of illuminance X and feature spectrum C_i of class i, respectively. Finally the concept of "minimum distance" is used to replace the maximum discriminant $F_i(\mathbf{X})$,

$$D_i(X, C_i)^2 = -F_i(X) = 2C_i^T X - X^T X - C_i^T C_i \tag{11}$$

The minimum distance discriminant from (11) is the classification function that is used to detect exudates in retinal images.

7.4.2.2 Extraction of Exudates

We observe that a colour retinal image consists of two main classes, yellowish patches (exudate) and reddish vessel and background. The spectrum feature centre, C_{exdt} and C_{bkgrnd} of the two classes can be easily obtained by selecting a small window in the exudates region and the background region respectively in the training samples. The training samples are specially chosen from a set of retinal images that contain exudates. Then the mean illuminance of the two windows can be tabulated and stored as prior information as $C_{exdt}(C_r,C_g,C_b)$ (ie. C_{exdt}) and $C_{bkgrnd}(C_r,C_g,C_b)$ (ie. C_{bkgrnd}), respectively.

During the processing of retinal images, for each pixel $X(x_r,x_g,x_b)$, the distance $D(X,C_i)$ from itself to class center C_i (C_{exdt} and C_{bkgrnd}) is calculated. If $D_{exdt}(X,C_{exdt})$ is smaller than $D_{bkgrnd}(X,C_{bkgrnd})$, then the pixel X is classified as exudates otherwise it is being classified as background pixel. Figure 7 shows a sample of detected exudate.

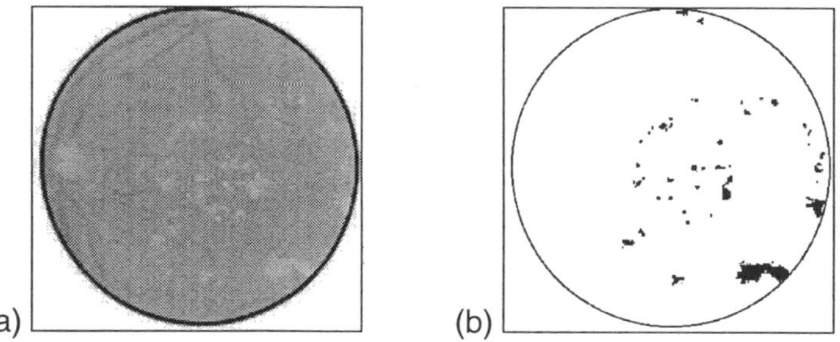

Figure 7. Detection of exudate. (a) Original image, (b) Detected exudate.

7.4.3 Vessel Detection

The cross section profile of the retinal blood vessel resembles a 'ridge' with the points running through the centre of the vessel having the highest intensity and these intensity levels tend to taper off toward the boundaries of the vessel. Figure 8 shows the cross section profile of a typical retinal blood vessel. Chaudhuri *et al.* (1989) used a two-dimensional matched filter, approximated by Gaussian fitting function to detect the retinal blood vessels. *Gaussian kernel* is a popular filter used for smoothing or fitting function as it models after 'bell' shape characteristics. Our approach to detect retinal vessel is adapted from this method.

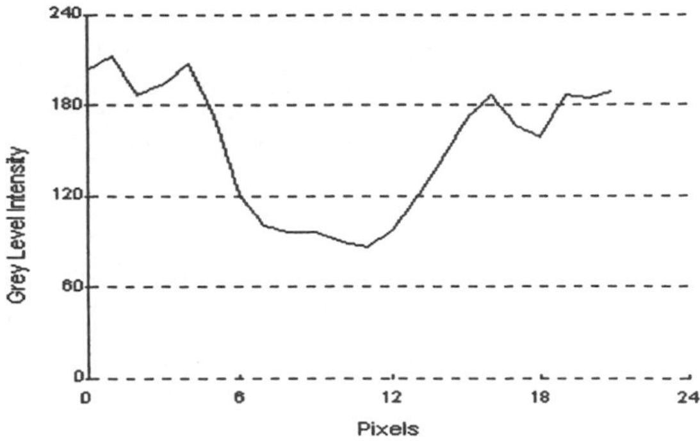

Figure 8. Cross section profile of a typical retinal blood vessel.

We investigated the properties of retinal blood vessels to develop image processing algorithms to detect the outlines of the vessels precisely. The main properties observed are:

If the vessel is divided into segments along its length, then the segment direction will vary continuously. The change of direction between segments is a smooth continuous function.

The width of the segment varies continuously. There is no abrupt step change in the width of the vessel segments and there is always a smooth transition between adjacent segments.

The density distribution of a blood vessel cross sectional profile can be estimated using Gaussian shaped function. The density distribution is smooth and never exhibits any step-like appearance.

Our vessel detection algorithm is as follows:

I. Smoothing

The input grey image is smoothed by a 5×5 mean filter to reduce the spurious noise effects. Low pass spatial filters are used to smooth high spatial frequencies and accentuate low spatial variations in an image. These filters are characterised by positive values in their masks, which clearly yields an additive, hence smoothing effect between neighbourhood pixels during the convolution process. The overall effect is to smooth noisy edges and they are also known as *smoothing filters*. Neighbourhood can be achieved using the relation,

$$q(x,y)=\frac{1}{N}\sum_{S}p(x,y) \tag{12}$$

where $p(x,y)$ and $q(x,y)$ are the original and smoothed images respectively, S is a set of co-ordinates of points in the neighbourhood of (x,y), and N is the total number of pixels in the neighbourhood. Each pixel is replaced with the average of itself and its neighbours.

II. Matched-filter Convolution

The smoothed-image is convolved with a set of two-dimensional matched filters. The two-dimensional matched filters are approximated with the Gaussian fitting function, as its profile matches the cross-sectional profile of a typical vessel. The filters consist of twelve different kernels, with each kernel specifically rotated to optimise for a different vessel angular direction. The angular difference between each kernel is chosen to be 15°. Hence, a total of twelve kernels are needed to accommodate the 180° of possible vessel directions. Each kernel is a set of 15×15 matrix-floating points. Each pixel of the smoothed-image is convolved with the twelve filters and only the maximum response of each convolution is retained.

III. Histogram Thresholding

The matched-image is then converted into a histogram and an automatic thresholding algorithm, where the threshold is selected to be the highest few percentage of response, is applied to retrieve the enhanced vessels from the background.

Figure 9 shows an example of the original retinal image and extracted vessel.

(a) 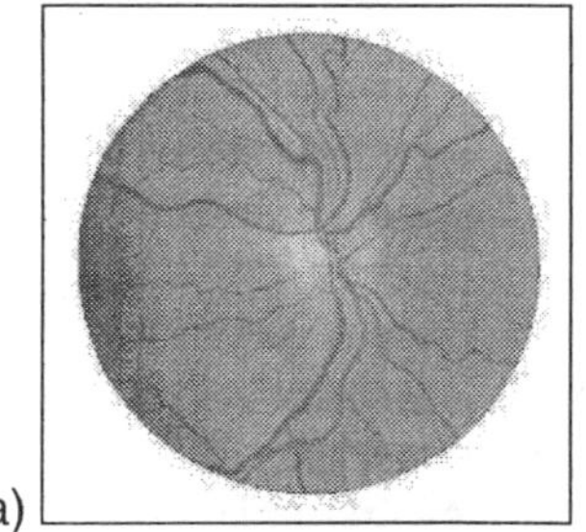

(b) 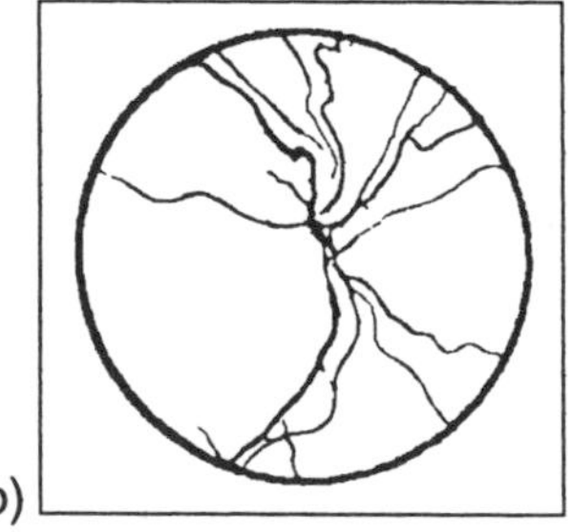

Figure 9. Detection of retinal vessel. (a) Original image, (b) Extracted vessel.

7.4.3.1 Vessel Tortuosity Detection

One of the symptoms of diabetic retinopathy is the presence of new vessel formation, often appears as tortuous vessel. Hence, the detection of tortuous vessel is important in the screening of diabetic retinopathy. In our system, a skeletonisation algorithm is used to extract the centre line of the vessel points. The resulting output contains only the centre line pixels outlining the extracted blood vessel, as shown in Figure 10. The *Skeletonisation* operation involves thinning an image to remove extra redundant pixels until it produces a simpler image. The characteristics of a skeletoned image are: (i) it should consists of thin regions of one pixel wide; (ii) the pixels that make up the skeleton should lie near the centre of a cross section of the region; and (iii) the skeletonisd pixels must be connected to each other to form the same number of regions as in the original image.

(a) 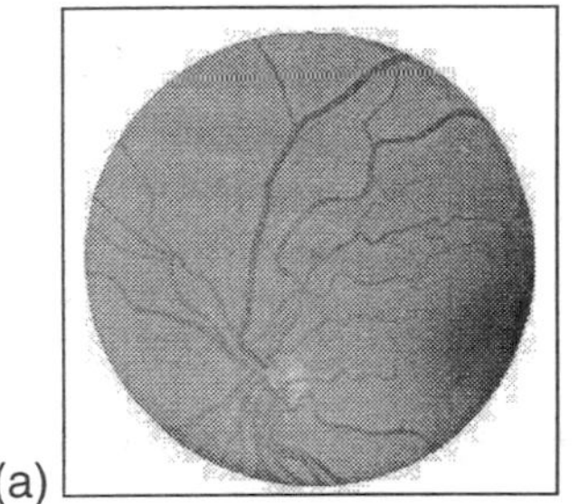 (b) 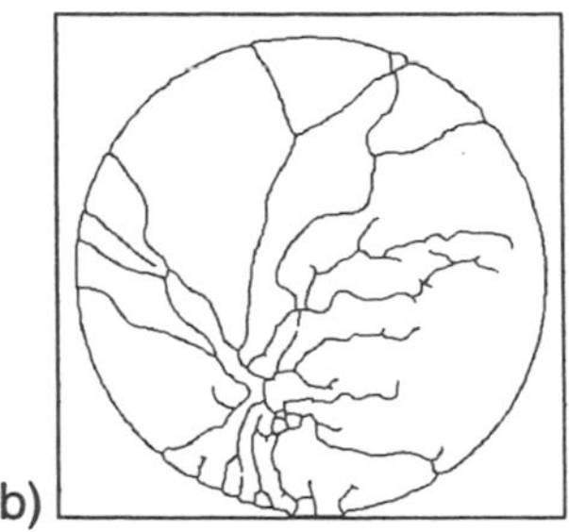

Figure 10. (a) Original image with tortuous vessel. (b) Centre line pixel outline of the extracted vessel of (a).

The detection of tortuous vessel is carried out by walking along the centre line of the extracted vessel and tabulating the curvature of the outline. Curvature can be defined in a number of ways which we will describe in the following subsections.

7.4.3.2 Absolute Direction Change

When tracking a centre line of a chosen segment of the blood vessel, each direction change along the path can be accumulated. At the end of the tracking, the number of direction changes indicates how tortuous is the segment. The direction change, hereby refer to as *DirChg*, of each pixel of the centre line is calculated by drawing an imaginary line from the fifth pixel point prior to the current pixel to the fifth pixel point ahead. The direction of this imaginary line is differentiated with the imaginary line collected from the previous pixel point. This differentiation value determines that there is a *DirChg* if the angle difference between the two imaginary lines is greater than a fixed angle, in this case it is chosen as 30°. The integration of all the *DirChg* of all the pixel points along the centre line of the segment of blood vessel gives a measure of tortuosity of this segment of the vessel. However, this *DirChg* only gives an indication of a measure of curvature at localised regions along the segment and it does not give an indication of how straight the segment is just before or after the *DirChg*. It can be seen in Figure 11 that both segments of the vessel contain almost the same curvature of *DirChg*. However, if the range of pixel points near the *DirChg* pixels is taken into account, then the segment of vessel in Figure 11b can be observed to be more tortuous than that in Figure 11a. This is due to the fact that the vessel in Figure 11a has a gradual curve while that of Figure 11b has a more abrupt curve.

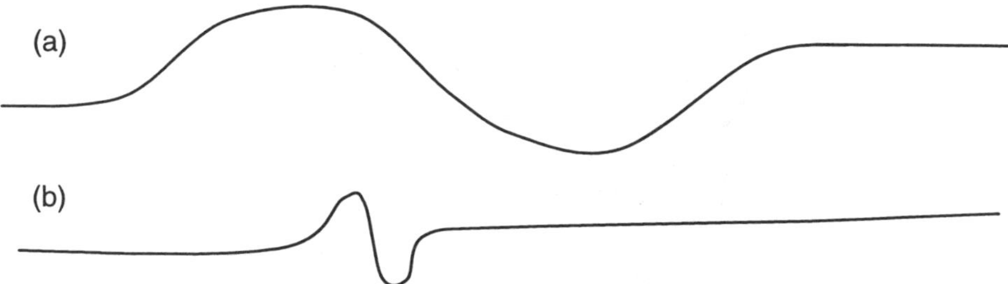

Figure 11. Curvature as a measure of *DirChg*. (a) Gradual change of direction. (b) Localised abrupt change of direction.

7.4.3.3 Arc to Chord Ratio

Another definition of curvature is the simple arc to chord ratio, hereby known as *ACurve*. If a segment of the vessel is chosen which contains some degree of curvature, then this curvature can be calculated by taking the arc length and dividing it by its chord length, as shown in Figure 12. The arc length is the length of the blood vessel while the chord length is the Euclidean distance between the start and end point of the blood vessel. The greater the ratio is, the higher is the curvature or tortuosity of the blood vessel. The arc to chord ratio can be normalised with respect to the arc length and the chord length to give an average value over the length of the vessel, known as *ACURVEarc* and *ACURVEchord* respectively. However, this measure of tortuosity is accurate only if the start and end point of the segment of vessel contains a single arc. This measure of tortuosity of a segment of a blood vessel only indicates whether a segment contains any curves and would not indicate what degree of curvature the segment holds (Figure 12b).

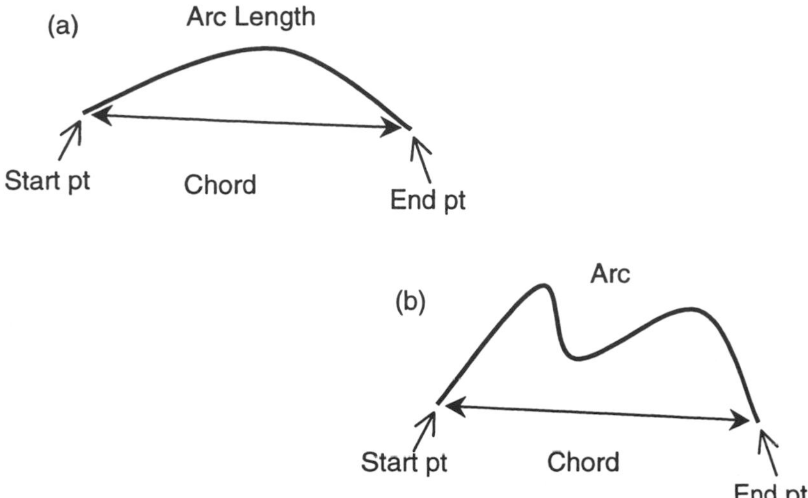

Figure 12. Curvature as a measure of arc to chord ratio. (a) Start and end point containing single arc. (b) Start and end point containing multiple arcs.

7.4.3.4 Curvature Based on Paths

Mokhtarian and Mackworth (Mokhtarian and Mackworth, 1986) introduce the curvature of a particular point on a line with respect to its x and y components as,

$$k(t) = \frac{x_0(t)\, y_1(t) - x_1(t)\, y_0(t)}{\left(x_0(t)^2 + y_1(t)^2\right)^{\frac{3}{2}}} \qquad (13)$$

where $k(t)$ is the curvature measure at point t, $(x_0(t), y_0(t))$ is the pixel co-ordinates at point t, $(x_1(t), y_1(t))$ is the co-ordinates chosen to be five pixels ahead of point t. $k(t)$ is hereby referred to as *kCurve*. The normalised version of *kCurve* is *kCurvearc* and *kCurvechord*, where the former is normalised with respect to the total segment's arc length and the latter is normalised with respect to the total segment's chord length.

7.4.3.5 Curvature Based on Line Fitting

Anderson *et al.* (1984) and O'Gormann (1988) propose an alternate definition of curvature estimation of a particular point on a line which is based on the angular difference between two straight lines fitted to the curve at some fixed pixels apart. Then the curvature point t can be defined as,

$$K(t)=\frac{d\alpha}{ds}(t) \tag{14}$$

where $K(t)$ is the curvature measure at point t, α is the difference of the angle of the two tangent lines at point t, s is the arc length between the tangent line at point t and the other tangent line, which is chosen to be five pixel ahead of point t. $K(t)$ is hereby referred to as *αCurve*. The normalised version of *αCurve* is *αCurvearc* and *αCurvechord*, where the former is normalised with respect to the total segment's arc length and the latter is normalised with respect to the total segment's chord length.

7.5 Data Mining

The above definitions of curvature do not individually give a reliable and consistent indication of the overall measure of tortuosity of the vessel segment under consideration. However, we observe that if some of the attributes of the different curvature definitions are used collectively, then the degree of reliability and accuracy in measuring the curvature of a particular segment of the retinal vessel is increased. In ADRIS, we combine all the data of the 12 attributes associated with the four curvature definitions and feed the data into an association based data mining classification tool, CBA. The output of CBA consists of a set of association rules governing the relationship between the 12 attributes that reliably and accurately classify the input vessel segment.

The rules generated by CBA are incorporated into the vessel tortuosity detection algorithm. Each of the rules generated indicates the association between the tortuosity measure given by each curvature definition. Collectively, when these rules are applied to each unseen segment of the vessel under consideration, the algorithm would classify whether the vessel is tortuous or otherwise.

7.6 Evaluation of the Discovered Knowledge

In Singapore, all diabetic patients are required to undergo an annual eye screening in Government-run medical clinic. We obtained a total of 310 retinal photographs from this screening exercise and digitised them to generate the retinal images. These images are used in our experiments to detect the optic disc and cup, and exudate. In addition, more than 1000 vessels are automatically extracted for the vessel detection experiment.

There are two types of retinal images, normal and abnormal. Normal retinal images shows healthy retina. Abnormal retinal images contains symptoms of diabetic retinopathy or age-related disease such as cataracts and glaucoma where the former causes the retinal image to appear hazy or opaque, and the latter exhibits high optic cup to disc ratio.

There are three main phases in the development of the ADRIS: (1) image preparation, (2) image processing and (3) review. The first phase includes digitising the retinal photos and pre-processing them. The second phase consists of processing those images which involve medical expert input to specify the features that discriminate normal and abnormal retinal images. Any abnormal retinal images are presented to the doctor for review in the last phase. We discuss each of these phases in detail:

I. Image Preparation

The inputs to the system consist of a pair of digital fundus images obtained from a colour fundus camera for each patient. The images are converted from high-resolution Polaroid colour photographs to digital format through an image scanner device. These digital images are expected to exhibit a relatively distinct outline of the main features of a healthy retina, namely the optic disc, optic cup, main blood vessels and macular. For unhealthy retina, symptoms of the corresponding eye diseases must be clearly visible and distinctly detectable with human vision. The resolution of the digital images are scanned with a minimum of $1k \times 1k \times 24$ bits.

This phase is also known as the pre-processing phase where the images are digitally prepared prior to feeding them to the next processing phase. Pre-processing operations include removal of noise and artefacts (introduced during digitising process) with smoothing filter, and re-sizing the digital image to a standard size of $400 \times 400 \times 24$bits.

II. Image Processing

Retinal digital images are first filtered through the specifications of *Normal* (healthy) retina. The initial phase detects the optic disc and cup, followed by the presence of main blood vessel of a minimum total length and average width. The next phase detects symptoms of diabetic eye diseases which includes abnormal optic cup to disc ratio and the presence of exudates and tortuous vessels. The choroid intervascular region should contain only uniform background and should not contain any patches of variation.

III. Review

This last phase classifies the retinal images into *Normal* and *Abnormal* cases. Input images with healthy fundus features and with no detected abnormal conditions are classified as *Normal.* Otherwise, the images are classified as *Abnormal.* Abnormal images are highlighted for the doctor's attention.

7.6.1 Optic Disc and Cup Detection

Out of 310 retinal images used for this experiment, 252 images has visible and normal optic disc to cup ratio, 58 images has poor visibility and/or blur optic disc outline, 75 images has poor visibility of optic cup and/or incorrect optic cup to disc ratio. The experimental results of optic disc and cup detection are discussed separately in the following two subsections.

7.6.2 Optic Disc Detection

The optic disc processing algorithm is able to correctly classify 227 images with disease free optic disc as *Normal* (true-positives), 25 images with disease free optic disc as *Abnormal* (false-positive) and all the 58 images with symptoms of irregular optic disc as *Abnormal* (true-negatives). In other words, the detection performance is 90.1% for true-positive, 9.9% of false-positive, and 100% of true-negative. An image is considered to be true-positive when the automatically detected optic disc outline is visually compared with the visually detected ellipse outline and the difference between the two centres of the ellipses is found to be less than 5 pixels apart. That means with an image resolution of 400×400 pixels, the maximum error rate is 6.25% (100%*5*5/400). Figure 13 shows examples of false-positive and true-negative detections. 25 images with normal optic disc are detected as abnormal because of poorly defined outline of optic disc.

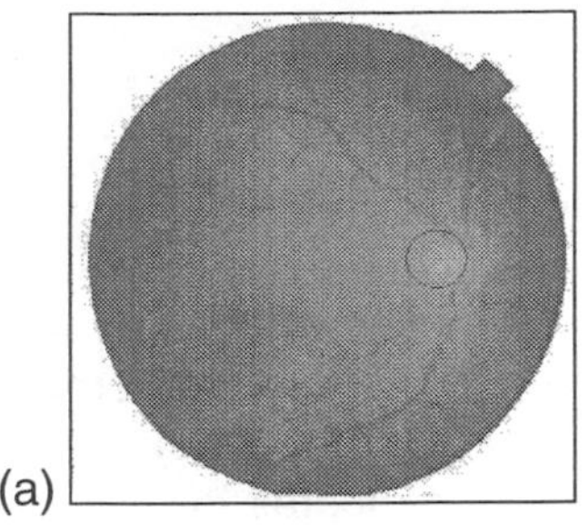

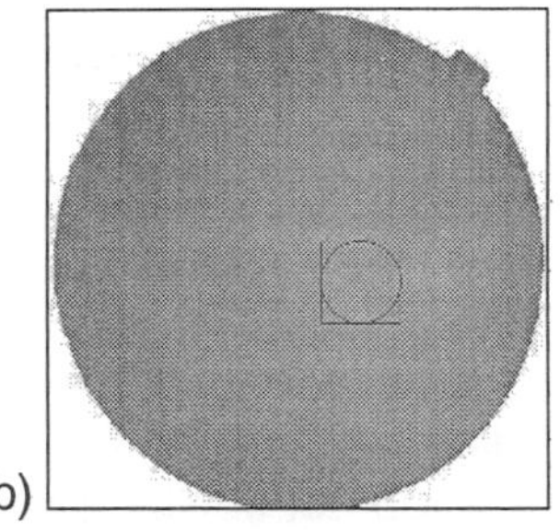

(a) (b)

Figure 13. Detection of optic disc. (a) False-positive due to ill-defined optic disc outline (circle registers falsely detected optic disc), (b) True-negative (square-enclosed-circle represents the approximate disc area which the algorithm identified as abnormal optic disc due to normal disc area not found → disc area larger than normal).

7.6.3 Optic Cup Detection

The optic cup processing algorithm correctly classifies 204 images with disease free optic disc as *Normal,* 31 images with disease free optic cup as *Abnormal* (false-positive) and 75 images with symptoms of irregular optic cup to disc ratio as *Abnormal* (true-negative). In other words, the success rate is 86.8% of true-positive, 13.2% of false-positive, and 100% of true-negative. Part of the reason that there are 31 images being wrongly classified as false-positives is due to incorrect detected optic disc, as shown in Figure 14. The other reason for false-positives is the poor contrast brightness of the optic cup and disc, inherent in the retinal photographs. The optic cup is considered to be correctly detected by comparing the automatically extracted cup with the manually extracted one.

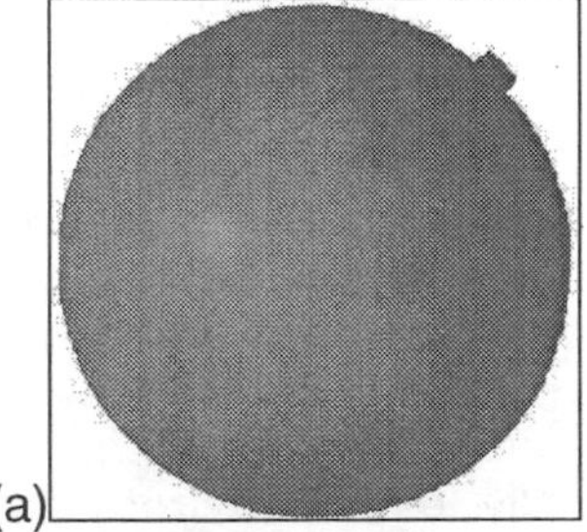

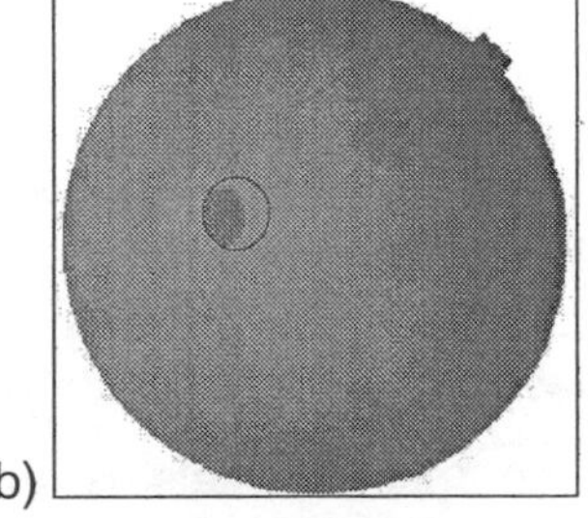

(a) (b)

Figure 14. Alse-positive detection of optic cup. (a) Original image. (b) The wrongly detected optic cup (black region within the circle) where it's location is not in the middle of the inaccurately detected disc (circle).

7.6.4 Exudates Detection

A total of 23 images with visible exudates are identified by medical expert. ADRIS is able to correctly classify 23 of the images that contain exudates as *Abnormal* (100% true-negatives), 75 images with no presence of exudates as *Abnormal* (26.1% of false-negatives) and the remaining 212 with exudate free images as *Normal* (73.9% true-positives). There are 75 images that do not contain any symptoms of exudates but are incorrectly classified as having exudates. These errors are due to the presence of relatively bright patches of variation scattered around the choroid regions and as a result, the algorithm incorrectly identified them as having the same spectrum features as that of exudate. These relatively bright patches of variation are mainly due to artefacts introduced during the fundus photography or digitisation process. Figure 15 shows an example of incorrectly detected images (false-negatives).

(a) 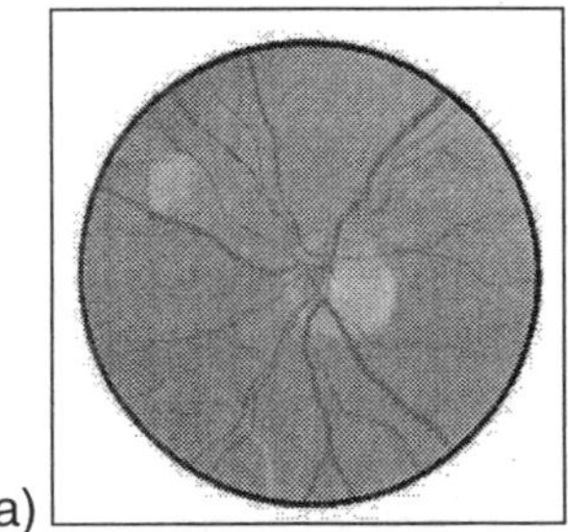

(b) 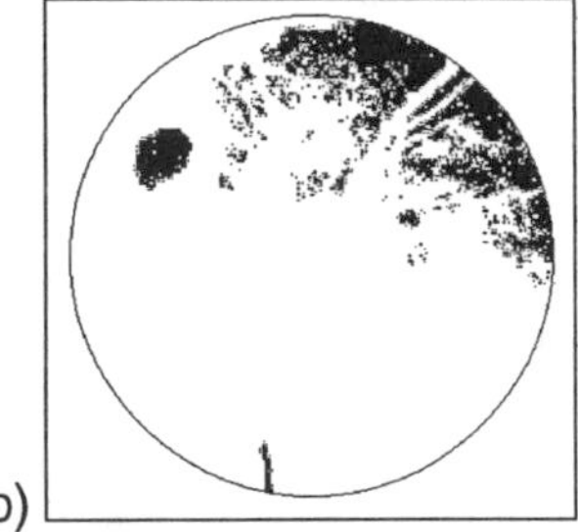

Figure 15. Errors in exudate detection. (a) Original image. (b) False-positive reflected on the upper right region (black pixels) due to the its relative brightness (same spectrum features as the exudates).

7.6.5 Vessel Processing

The processing of retinal vessels consists of two stages. First, the main vessels, those with average width greater than 90μm (5 pixels) and average length greater than 30 pixels (540μm) are extracted. Second, these extracted vessels are processed into single pixel width of connected lines from which the tortuosity of the vessel is measured.

Each of the main vessels is automatically extracted from the retinal images. On average about 4 vessel segments are successfully extracted from each image and they are visually verified. In Figure 16, an example of tortuous vessel is highlighted.

(a) 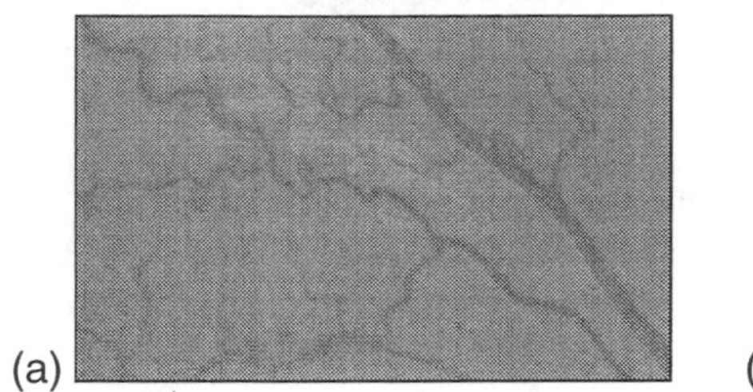

(b) 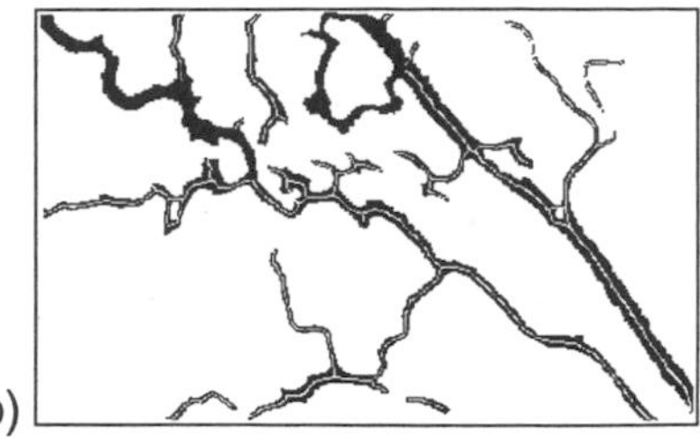

Figure 16. Detection of tortuous vessel. (a) Original image, (b) Some of the detected tortuous vessel (darken portions).

Out of the total 310 images, 35 of them contain almost featureless image, possibly caused by cataracts. A total of 1205 main vessel segments are automatically extracted. The vessel tortuosity detection algorithm extracted 12 attributes (Sections 3.4.1 to 3.4.4) from each vessel segment and fed them into the CBA classification tool. We configure CBA to mine at 35% minimum support[11], 50% minimum confidence[22], 30% of data used as training cases and 10 times cross validation[33]. CBA generated 11 association rules with a cross-validation error rate of 12.1%.

[1] Minimum support refers to a constraint in classification technique whereby it gives a minimum percentage of the number of transactions in the data set that supports a rule.

[2] Minimum confidence is a constraint that gives the minimum percentage of confidence that the number of transactions in the data set satisfy both the left-hand-side and right-hand-side items in an association rule. For example in an association rule, $X \Rightarrow Y \mid C$ implies that X (a set of items in data set T) is associated to Y (a single item in T and which is not present in X) has a confidence that C% of transactions in T that satisfy X also satisfy Y.

[3] Cross-validation is a way to test how accurate is the classification. It is done through executing the system over a number of folds (or times) over the data which is being split into training case and testing case. The output of cross validation gives the average error rate accumulated after applying the classification rules on the unseen test data.

7.7 Using the Discovered Knowledge

We used these association rules to determine whether a vessel is normal or tortuous. If a retinal image contains at least one tortuous vessel, then it will be classified as abnormal. In total, the rules detected 95 vessels as tortuous.

7.8 Conclusion

In this paper, we have shown that images captured from Diabetic Retinopathy Screenings can be fed into a computer system for automatic classification. ADRIS can detect symptoms such as the size of optic disc and cup, and its ratio; exudates or unspecific lesion in the intervascular region; and the presence of tortuous main vessel. Experimental results show that the basic features of the retina and diabetic retinal disease can be detected.

The performance of the optic disc and cup detection algorithm as well as its ratio calculation is found to be up to expectation, as verified by the various doctors working with us on this system. Likewise the detection of the exudate and the detection of tortuous vessel is within expectation. We also found out that a large proportion (74%) of the retinal images obtained from the screening exercise is normal, where only 80 retinal images are abnormal out of the total 310 images.

Most importantly, the occurrence of false-negatives, where the presence of abnormal features fails to be detected by the system does not happen in ADRIS.

Our future works include identifying more advanced diabetic retinopathy symptoms with an ophthalmologist's input.

Acknowledgement

We would like to thank Dr. S. C. Emmanuel, Director of Family Health Services, Ministry of Health, Singapore, for her commitment to the development of ADRIS. We are also indebted to Dr. Jonathan Phang from the Institute of Health Polyclinic for initiating this collaboration and giving us much of his time and invaluable medical domain knowledge.

References

Lim KH, 'Registration of New Blindness in Singapore for 1985-1995', *Singapore Medical Journal*, vol. 40, no. 2, Feb 1999.

Goh LG, 'A Diabetes Centre In The Community', *Singapore Medical Journal*, vol. 30, no. 3, Mar 1998.

Kahn HA, Hiller R, 'Blindness caused by diabetic retinopathy', *Am. J. Ophthal.*, vol. 78, pp. 58-67, 1974.

Palmberg PF, 'Diabetic Retinopathy', *Diabetes*, vol. 26, pp.703-709, 1977.

Klein R, Klein Bek, Moss SE, Cruickshanks KJ, 'The Wiscousin Epidemiologic study of diabetic retinopathy. XV. The long term incidence of macular edema', *Ophthal.*, vol. 102, pp.7-16, 1995.

Javitt JC, Canner JK, Sommer A, 'Cost effectiveness of current approaches to the control of retinopathy in type I diabetics', *Opthal.*, vol. 96, pp.255-264, 1989.

Ghafour IS, Allan D, Foulds WS, 'Common causes and blindness and visual handicap in the west of Scotland', *Brit. J. Ophthal.*, vol. 67, pp.209, 1983.

Singer DE, Nathan DM, Fogel HA, Schachar AP, 'Screening for diabetic retinopathy', *Ann. Intern. Med.*, No. 116,, pp.660-671, 1992.

Retinopathy Working Party, 'A protocol for screening for diabetic retinopathy in Europe', *Diabetic Med.*, no. 8, pp.263-270, 1991.

Gardner GG, Keating D, Willaimson TH, Elliot AT, 'Automatic detection of diabetic retinopathy using an artificial neural network:a screening tool', *Brit. J. Ophthal.*, vol. 80, pp. 940-944, 1996.

Ward NP, Tomlinson S, Taylor CJ, 'Image analysis of fundus photographs. The detection and measurements of exudate associated with diabetic retinopathy', *Ophthal.*, vol. 96, pp. 80-86, 1989.

Spencer T, Phillips RP, Sharpe PF, Forrester JV, 'Automatic detection and quantification of microaneurysm in fluoresceins angiograms', *Graefe's Arch. Clin. Exp. Ophthal.*, vol. 230, pp 36-41, 1992.

Spencer T, Phillips RP, Sharpe PF, Ross T, Forrester JV, 'Quantification of diabetic maculopathy by digital imaging of the fundus', *Eye.*, vol. 5, pp 130-137, 1991.

Katz N, Goldbaum M, Nelson M, Chaudhuri S, 'An image processing system for automatic retina diagnosis', *SPIE.*, vol. 902, pp. 131-7, 1988.

Katz N, Goldbaum M, Nelson M, Hart LR, 'The discrimination of similarly colored objects in computer images of ocular fundus', *Invest. Ophthal. Vis Sci.*, vol. 31, pp. 617-627, 1990.

Cox MJ, Wood CJ, 'Computer-Assisted optic nerve head assessment', *Ophthal. Phy. Opt.*, vol. 11, pp. 27-35 , 1991.

Morris T, Wood I, 'On the Automatic Identification of the Optic Nerve Head', American Academy of Optometrists Biennial Meeting in Europe, Presentation, 1994.

Phillips RP, Sharpe PF, Forrester JV, 'Automatic detection and quantification of retinal exudate', *Graefe's Arch. Clin. Exp. Ophthal.*, vol. 231, pp 90-94, 1993.

Leistritz L, Schweitzer D, 'Automated detection and quantification of exudate in retinal images', *SPIE: Appl. Digital Image Proc. XVII*, vol. 2298, San Deigo, July 94.

Zhou M, Rzeszotarski S, Singerman LJ, Chokreff JM, 'Detection and quantification of retinopathy using digital Angiogram', *IEEE Trans. Medical Imaging*, vol. 13, no. 4, pp. 619-626, 1994.

Zana F, Klein JC, 'Robust segmentation of vessels from retinal angiogram', *Proc. DSP*, pp. 1087-1090, 1997.

Capowski JJ, Kylstra JA, Freedman SF, 'A numeric index based on spatial-frequency for the tortuousity of the superficial femoral artery in early atherosclerosis, *J. Vasc. Res.*, vol. 30, pp. 181-190, 1993.

Elomaa T, Holsti N, 'An experimental comparsison of inducing decision tress and decision lists in noisy domain', *Proc. 4th Europ. Work. Session on Learning*, Montpeiller, pp. 56-69, Dec 1989.

Lesmo L, Saitta L, Torasso P, 'Learning of fuzzy production rules for medical diagnosis', In Gupta MM, Sanchez E(eds.*), Approx. Reasoning in Decision Analysis*, North Holland, 1982.

Brako I, Kononenko I, 'Learning Rules from incomplete and noisy data', in B Phelps(eds.), *Interaction in AI and Stat. Methods*, Hampshire: technical press, 1987.

Hojker S, Kononenko I, Jauk A, Fidler V, Porenta M, 'Expert's system development in the management of thyroid diseases', *Proc. Europ. Congress for Nuclear Med.*, Milano, Sept 1988.

Kern J, Dezelic G, Tezak-Bencic M, Durrigl T, 'Medical decision making using inductive learning program', *Proc. 1st Congress Yugos. Med. Info.*, Beograd, pp. 221-228, Dec 1990.

Muggleton S, 'Inductive acquisition of expert knowledge', Turing Institute Press and Addison-Wesley, 1990.

Provan GM, Singh M, 'Datamining and model simplicity: a case study in diagnosis', *Proc. 2nd Int. Conf. KDD.*, pp. 57-62, Oregon, Aug 1996.

Nunez M, 'Decision tree induction using domain knowledge', in Wielinga B et al. (eds.), *Current Trends in Knowledge Acquisition*, IOS Press, 1990.

Liu B, Hsu W, Ma Y, 'Integrating Classification and Association Rule Mining.' *Proc. 4th Int. Conf. KD. and DM.* (KDD-98, Plenary Presentation), New York, USA, 1998.

Davis LS, 'SURVEY: A Survey of Edge Detection Techniques,' *Computer Graphics and Image Processing*, vol. 4, pp. 248-270, 1975.

Pitas I, 'Digital Image Processing Algorithms', Prentice Hall, ISBN 0-13-145814-0, 1993.

Kressel U, Schurmann J, 'Pattern classification techniques based on function approximation', In 'Handbook of character recognition and document image analysis', Bunke H, Wang PSP (eds.), ISBN : 981022270X, *Singapore : World Scientific*, 1997.

Castleman KR, 'Digital image processing', ISBN : 0132114674, Englewood Cliffs, N.J. : Prentice Hall , c1996.

Bayes, Rev. T., "An Essay Toward Solving a Problem in the Doctrine of Chances", Philos. Trans. R. Soc. London 53, pp. 370-418 (1763); reprinted in Biometrika 45, pp. 293-315 (1958), and Two Papers by Bayes, with commentary by W. Edwards Deming, New York, Hafner, 1963.

Chaudhuri S, Chatterjee S, Katz N, Nelson N and Goldbaum M, 'Detection of Blood Vessels in Retinal Images Using Two-Dimensional Matched Filters', *IEEE Transaction on Medical Imaging*, vol. 8, no. 3, Sept 1989.

Mokhtarian F, Mackworth A, 'Scale-based description and recognition of planar curves and two dimensional shapes', *IEEE Trans. Pattern Anal. Mach. Intell.*, vol. 8, pp.34-43, 1986.

Anderson IM, Bezdek JC, 'Curvature and deflection of discrete arcs:A theory based on the commentary of scatter matrix pairs and its application to vertex detection in planar shape data', *IEEE Trans. Pattern Anal. Mach. Intell., vol.* 6, pp. 27-40, 1984.

O'Gormann, 'An analysis of feature detectability from curvature estimation', *Proc. IEEE Conf. Comp. Vis. Pattern Reco.*, Ann Arbor, M1, pp. 235-240, 1988.

Fayyad U, Piatetsky-Shapiro G, Smyth P, 'Knowledge discovery and data mining:toward a unifying framework', *KDD96*, pp. 82-88, 1996.

8 Knowledge Discovery in Mortality Records: An Info-Fuzzy Approach

Mark Last[1], Oded Maimon[2] and Abraham Kandel[1]

[1]University of South Florida,
Tampa, FL 33620, U.S.A.
[2]Department of Industrial Engineering
Tel-Aviv University
Tel-Aviv 69978, Israel

In this chapter, we analyze a data set, which has been provided by the Israel Ministry of Health. It includes the records of all Israeli citizens who passed away in the year 1993. The death cause (medical diagnosis) of each person is defined by the international, 6-digit code (ICD-9-CM). We start the chapter with the description of the data pre-processing operations, such as transformation and cleaning of the original attributes. An information-theoretic data mining algorithm, developed in our previous work, is applied to the pre-processed dataset. The algorithm includes discretization, dimensionality reduction, and rule extraction. The original dataset is extended to a fuzzy relational table by adding a new, fuzzy attribute: the reliability degree of the recorded diagnosis. Our approach to the calculation of the reliability degree is based on the Computational Theory of Perception (CTP). Most records having the lowest reliability degree are shown to represent exceptional and possibly inaccurate information.

8.1 Introduction

Causes of death are a constant subject of medical and demographic research. The issues of interest include the change of the leading causes over time, geographical patterns of deadly diseases, life expectancy, tracking diseases to genetic factors, and many others (Blij and Murphy, 1998). The importance of these studies goes beyond the area of medical research and health care industry. For example, the life insurance companies have to analyze mortality data in determining the terms of their policies.

Unfortunately, the tools used in the research on death causality have been so far limited to the standard statistical techniques, like summarization, regression, analysis of variance, etc. In the last decade, more advanced methods of finding patterns in data have become known under the general name of "data mining", and a formal framework for the entire process of knowledge discovery has been suggested (see Fayyad et al. 1996). In this chapter, we are making one of the first attempts (to the best of our knowledge) of applying several data mining techniques to knowledge discovery in a set of mortality data.

The methods implemented by us in the different stages of this project are based on two approaches to knowledge discovery, developed in our previous work: *information-theoretic connectionist model* (Last and Maimon, 1999; Maimon et al. 1999) and *automated perceptions* (Last and Kandel, 1999a). The information-theoretic model is used to find a minimum set of attributes associated with the cause of death and to represent the discovered patterns in the form of disjunctive rules. The methods of automated perception are applied to several pre- and post-processing tasks, like detection of outliers and assessment of data reliability.

This chapter is organized as follows. In section 2, we describe the problem domain and set the main objectives for our project. The obtained set of mortality records, along with other available information, is represented in section 3. Manual and automated data preparation activities are covered by section 4. Section 5 describes the construction of an information-theoretic network, based on the pre-processed data. The network output is evaluated in section 6, followed by an overview of the entire project (section 7). The chapter is concluded by section 8, which represents possible directions for the future studies of mortality data.

8.2 Understanding the Problem Domain

The Ministry of Health of the State of Israel bears the primary responsibility for the health of the Israeli citizens. According to the Law of the State

Medical Insurance (effective since January 1995), the Ministry of Health is the only medical insurance company in the country (the law outline is posted on the Ministry official web site [http://www.health.gov.il/]). The health budget, based on the taxes paid by the citizens, is distributed to hospitals, clinics, and other public health care providers, according to the number of patients, types of provided treatments, and other criteria. The Ministry of Health is also responsible for the constant improvement of the health services, including the support of the medical research activities.

Causes of death can have a significant impact on the budget priorities of the Health Ministry. Higher frequency of certain cause in a distinct population group (defined by gender, age, origin, etc.) can increase the budget, aimed at reducing the death rate of that group. The portion of a cause in the entire population may be used as another important criterion: preventing the leading causes of death should obtain a higher priority.

The complete demographic and medical data on all deceased citizens is contained in the Israel Registry of Deaths (see next section). The current studies of this data, based on the traditional statistical methods, have concentrated on identifying the leading causes of death and testing the association of single factors (like gender, age or continent of birth) with certain diseases. Some examples of this analysis are posted on the Ministry web site (see above). However, no complex models (involving more than one factor) have been built. Moreover, some of available attributes (like place of residence and time of death) have been considered unimportant and, thus, completely ignored by most studies. The current studies have also assumed total correctness of the Registry data, without attempting to clean it from possible errors.

We have determined the following objectives of the data mining process:

- Automated cleaning of the original dataset by detecting outliers in the values of each database attribute.
- Dimensionality reduction of the original data by finding the minimum set of features associated with the recorded diagnosis (cause of death).
- Extracting single-attribute and multi-attribute patterns (rules) from the selected set of features.
- Identifying possible errors in the recorded diagnosis codes by using the extracted patterns.

The project plan has been coordinated with the Computing Division of the Ministry of Health. The project has been designed to include the following stages:

- Selecting a pilot data set

- Obtaining the data file and the metadata
- Defining the target and the input attributes
- Data pre-processing (missing values treatment, transformation, data cleaning, etc.)
- Finding the significant input attributes
- Extracting informative rules
- Data post-processing (identifying lowly reliable values, etc.)

The Computing Division has promised to provide all the data and the metadata. Detailed discussions have been planned with the Division representatives, following the completion of each stage and the representation of the results.

8.3 Understanding the Data

8.3.1 Extended Database Model

To discover informative patterns (rules) in a relational database, we use the following partition of the relation scheme (Maimon et al. 1999):

- A subset $C \subset R$ of *candidate input* attributes ($|C| \geq 1$). This is a subset of attributes that *can be* used to predict the values of *target* attributes (see next).
- A subset $O \subset R$ of *target* ("classification") attributes ($|O| \geq 1$). We assume that an attribute cannot be both a candidate input and a target ($C \cap O = \emptyset$). However, some attributes (e.g., the key ones) may be out of both subsets ($C \cup O \subseteq R$).
- I_m -a subset of *m input* attributes selected by the dimensionality reduction procedure from a subset of *candidate input* attributes ($I_m \subseteq C$).

8.3.2 Main Data Table

Dimensionality. The data set, provided by the Computing Division, includes the 33,134 records of all Israeli citizens who passed away in the year 1993. Each original record has 19 attributes, some of them being defined as irrelevant for the analysis purposes (like the date of immigration to Israel). During the pre-processing stage, we have used a number of additional tables, listed in the next sub-section.

Key Attributes. The original file, stored by the Israel Register of Deaths, has a complete identifying information about each person, including the first and the last name + personal ID number (parallel to the SSN in the US). All the identifying attributes have been removed from the file by the Computing Division representatives before the start of the knowledge discovery process. Each record has been identified by a mere serial number (starting with 0).

Candidate Input Attributes. The candidate input attributes include the following:

- *Age.* The age of the deceased person. In the original database, the age of a late person has been represented by three digits, the first digit standing for the time unit (days, months or years) and the succeeding two digits denoting the age itself. Thus, an infant's age could be 120 (20 days) and the age of a grown-up person could be 360 (60 years). The age of 100 years and more has been defined as a special "time unit".
- *Date of Death.* Represented by three fields (day, month, and year).
- *Gender.* A binary-valued code.
- *Area of Residence.* The code of the administrative area (similar to county in the US), where the late person lived (e.g., Tel-Aviv, Haifa, etc.). Israel is partitioned into 20 areas.
- *Religion.* The ethnicity of Israeli citizens is recorded as their religion (Jew, Muslim, etc.) 14 different codes of religion are used in the file.
- *Country of Birth.* The origin of a citizen is recorded as the country of birth. Each country has a unique code. A significant percent of Israeli population consists of Jewish immigrants from other countries. A country of origin may be associated with certain genetic heritage.

Target Attribute. The target attribute is the medical diagnosis, encoded by the international, 6-digit code (ICD-9-CM). The code is entered by a medical encoder – the person who reads the complete report prepared by a doctor. Only one code can be assigned to each death case. The 6-digit codes provide highly detailed information on the diseases: the 1993 file includes 1,248 distinct codes.

8.3.3 Additional Data Tables

The following additional tables have been obtained from the Ministry of Health:

- *Regions Table.* The list of regions in Israel. Israel is partitioned into seven regions (e.g., Center, North, etc.).
- *Areas Table.* The list of administrative areas. There is a one-to-many relationship between the Regions Table and the Areas Table. The Areas table includes a foreign key: the code of the corresponding region for each area.
- *Religions Table.* The list of existing religion codes. Each record in the table has been added a flag field: Jew / Non-Jew. This is because the majority of population is Jewish, with Muslims being the largest minority.
- *Continents Table.* The continents of birth have been defined as Israel, Asia, Africa, Europe-America, and Other (unknown). The purpose of this grouping is to make a distinction between Israeli-born people and immigrants from certain parts of the World.
- *Countries Table.* The list of the countries of birth. There is a one-to-many relationship between the Continents Table and the Countries Table. The Countries table includes a foreign key: the code of the corresponding continent for each country.

8.3.4 Data Quality

Generally, the data in the Register of Deaths is based on highly reliable sources of information (like the Register of Population, maintained by the Ministry of Interior). However, the following problems have been indicated / detected with respect to the recorded diagnoses:

- *Data Errors.* The medical diagnosis code may be erroneous in some records, due to data entry errors.

- *Missing Values.* There are 898 records with missing diagnosis code. No particular reason for non-recorded diagnoses is known.

8.4 Preparation of the Data

8.4.1 Data Transformation and Reformatting

The following transformation and reformatting operations have been applied to the original attributes in the main data table:

- *Encoding Target Attribute.* The first three digits of the original ICD-9-CM code (the "prefix") have been used for grouping the medical diagnoses into 36 sets of similar diseases / causes of death. The Ministry of Health representatives have defined corresponding groups for individual prefixes and prefix intervals (see Table below). Some groups include more than one interval (e.g., group no. 2, "Other Malignant Neoplasms"). A small conversion procedure has been written in C language for encoding the original 6-digit diagnosis codes.
- *Decoding Age Attribute.* In the original database, the age of a late person has been encoded by three digits (see above). We have used years as a time unit for all persons, including infants who died at the age of "zero" (less than 12 months).
- *Calculating Region of Residence.* The attribute "Area" and the region code in the Areas Table have been used to calculate the region of residence for each person.
- *Decoding Religion Code.* The attribute "Religion" and the flag attribute (Jew / Non-Jew) in the Religions Table have been used for representing the religion (ethnic origin) for each person.
- *Calculating Continent of Birth.* The attribute "Country" and the continent code in the Countries Table have been used for calculating the origin of birth for each person.

8.4.2 Treatment of Missing Values

As previously indicated, the main data table includes 898 records with missing diagnosis code. These records have been treated as the group "Other", having a code of “0" (see Table below).

Code	**Group Intervals**	**Group Description**	**No of Cases**	**Probability**
0	Missing Code	Other	898	0.0271
1	001 - 139	Infectious and Parasitic Diseases	506	0.0153
2	140-152, 155-161, 163-173, 175-184, 186-203	Other Malignant Neoplasms	3667	0.1107
3	153-154	Malignant Neoplasm of colon-rectum	973	0.0294
4	162	Malignant Neoplasm of trachea etc.	1050	0.0317
5	174	Malignant Neoplasm of female breast	752	0.0227
6	185	Prostate	367	0.0111
7	204-208	Leukemia	309	0.0093
8	210-239	Non-Malignant Neoplasms	328	0.0099
9	240-249, 251-279	Other Endocrine Diseases	185	0.0056
10	250	Diabetes	862	0.0260
11	280-289	Diseases of Blood	129	0.0039
12	290-319	Mental Disorders	592	0.0179
13	320-389	Diseases of the Nervous System	523	0.0158
14	390-409	Other Diseases of the Circulatory System	569	0.0172
15	410-414	Ischaemic heart disease	6689	0.2019
16	415-429	Diseases of pulmonary circulation	3045	0.0919
17	430-438	Cerebrovascular disease	3325	0.1004
18	439-459	Other Diseases of the Circulatory System	297	0.0090
19	460-479, 488-489, 497-519	Diseases of the Respiratory System	263	0.0079
20	480-487	Pneumonia and Influenza	399	0.0120

Code	**Group Intervals**	**Group Description**	**No of Cases**	**Probability**
21	490-496	Chronic obstructive pulmonary disease	982	0.0296
22	520-579	Diseases of the Digestive System	973	0.0294
23	580-599	Diseases of the Urinary System	879	0.0265
24	600-629	Diseases of the Genital Organs	32	0.0010
25	630-639	Abortion	1	0.00003
26	640-679	Pregnancy etc.	3	0.0001
27	680-709	Diseases of the Skin	83	0.0025
28	710-739	Diseases of the Muscoloskeletal System	89	0.0027
29	740-759	Congenital Anomalies	322	0.0097
30	760-779	Prenatal period	345	0.0104
31	780-799	Symptoms and Ill-defined Conditions	1899	0.0573
32	800-809, 820-949, 970-999	Other Accidents	949	0.0286
33	810-819	Motor Vehicle Traffic Accidents	452	0.0136
34	950-959	Suicide and Self-inflicted injuries	277	0.0084
35	960-969	Homicide	120	0.0036
Total			33,134	1.00

Table 1. Target Attribute – Grouping of Diagnoses.

8.4.3 An Automated Approach to Data Cleaning

As emphasized by Pyle (1999), isolating outliers is an important step in cleaning a data set before any kind of data analysis. The first reason for isolating outliers is associated with data quality assurance. The exceptional values may represent mistakes. In that case, the outliers should be replaced with correct values or treated as missing values. Otherwise, they may cause a bias in the results of the data mining process.

The outliers can also have a dramatic impact on the efficiency of the knowledge discovery process. Unlike continuous attributes, which can be discretized to an arbitrary small number of intervals (e.g., two), each value of a discrete attribute is treated separately by most data mining algorithms (like decision trees, Bayesian methods, etc.). Thus, each additional value, no matter how rare it is, increases the space and the time requirements of a data mining program, up to the point of complete uselessness.

In (Last and Kandel, 1999a; 1999b), we have developed a novel approach to the automated detection of outliers in discrete and continuous attributes. The approach is based on modeling the human perception of exceptional values by using the Computational Theory of Perception (CTP). The automated perception of an outlying (rare) *discrete* value is determined in (Last and Kandel, 1999a; 1999b) by the number of records where the value occurs, the total number of records, and the number of distinct attribute values. For *continuous* attributes, the number of distinct values is irrelevant, but an additional criterion, the distance between subsequent values, is used. In the next sub-section, we are describing the application of the perception-based approach to cleaning the data set, provided by the Ministry of Health.

8.4.4 Detecting Outliers in the Main Data Table

The summary of the automated procedure for outliers detection is represented in Table 2 below. For each attribute, we represent its type (discrete / continuous), the total number of distinct values existing in the dataset, the number of outlying values (detected by the perception-based method) vs. the number of conforming values, and the number of records having outlying values vs. the number of conforming records. The analysis of the procedure results is performed below:

- *Age, Gender,* and *Religion.* No outliers have been detected in these attributes. For example, the ages of the people vary between 0 and 100 years, which is quite reasonable.
- *Month.* Surprisingly enough, the perception-based method has revealed four records, where *Month* = 0. These are clear outliers, representing, probably, non-recorded dates.
- *Region.* There is one region having exceptionally small number of records – only 178, out of 33,134. This is not a mistake: the region does exist, but it is populated by a relatively small number of citizens. Including this exceptional value in the data mining process may deteriorate the results.
- *Continent of Birth.* There is one continent code (Other), where only 70 people have been born. Again, the data is correct, but its inclusion in the data mining process may be inappropriate.

- *Diagnosis.* Six diagnosis groups (no. 24 -28 and no. 35 in Table above) have been found to have an exceptionally small number of cases, though they have been defined as separate groups by the Ministry representatives. Thus, there is only one death case, related to abortion (code no. 25). Due to its exceptionality, the case itself may be *very* interesting, but no statistical patterns can be discovered, based on just one record.

The detected outlying values can be treated in different ways, from ignoring the entire records to "rectifying" each individual outlier (Pyle, 1999). If an outlying value is either erroneous, or representing an exceptional phenomenon in the dataset, then a data mining method can treat it as a *missing* value. At his stage, we are storing two versions of the dataset: the "original" version (including all the outlying values) and the "cleaned" version, where each outlier is denoted by a special code. For the target attribute (diagnosis), the outlier code is identical to the code of a missing value ("0"). The comparison between mining the original and the cleaned data is a subject of our next section.

Attribute Name	Type	Total Values	Outlying Values	Conforming Values	Outlying Records	Conforming Records
Age	Continuous	101	0	101	0	33134
Month	Continuous	13	1	12	4	33130
Gender	Discrete	2	0	2	0	33134
Region	Discrete	7	1	6	178	32956
Religion	Discrete	2	0	2	0	33134
Continent of Birth	Discrete	5	1	4	70	33064
Diagnosis	Discrete	36	6	30	328	32806

Table 2. Outliers Detection – Summary.

8.5 Data Mining

8.5.1 Information-Theoretic Approach to Data Mining

An information-theoretic connectionist approach to data mining and knowledge discovery (Last and Maimon, 1999; Maimon et al. 1999) is aimed at maximizing the available information on a target attribute (e.g., diagnosis) by reducing dataset dimensionality (number of input attributes) and extracting highly informative patterns (rules). It provides us with a ranked list of the significant input attributes, associated with the target (see the extended database model in sub-section 3.1 above). The association between the input attributes and the target attribute are represented in the form of an information-theoretic connectionist network, which is constructed by a greedy search algorithm. Continuous input attributes are *discretized* (partitioned into disjoint intervals) in the process of the network construction. Irrelevant and redundant attributes are excluded from the network, leading to the dimensionality reduction of the original dataset. An information-theoretic connection weight is assigned to each rule extracted from the network. As shown by Maimon et al. (1999), the sum of rule scores (connection weights) is equal to the estimated mutual information between the input attributes and the target attribute.

We have chosen the information-theoretic approach as our data mining method in this project for the following reasons:

- The method is applicable to data sets of mixed nature (comprising continuous, ordinal, nominal, and binary-valued attributes). In this dataset, we have two continuous attributes (*Age* and *Month*), two binary-valued attributes (*Gender* and *Religion*), and three nominal attributes (*Region*, *Continent of Birth*, and *Diagnosis*).
- The dimensionality reduction procedure finds a minimum set of significant input attributes. In this case, the data user (Ministry of Health) is interested only in the factors associated with the target (*Diagnosis*). Irrelevant and redundant attributes can be removed from the user database.
- The multi-layer information-theoretic connectionist network explicitly represents associations of any order between predictive attributes and the target attribute. Finding complex relationships (involving more than one attribute) is one of the project objectives (see section 2 above).

- The Information-Theoretic Network can be constructed without assuming anything on the probability distributions of the database attributes. Most statistical models (like the regression methods) are applicable only to certain types of probability distributions.
- The network construction is based upon statistical significance tests, eliminating the need in a separate "testing" set for building a valid model. The resulting model is more accurate, since *all* the available data is used for training.
- No set of perfect data is required to construct the network. The information-theoretic approach is robust to noise, both in the input attribute values and in the target attribute values. Medical information is known to include a considerable amount of noisy data.
- The running time of the algorithm has been shown quadratic-logarithmic in the number of records and quadratic polynomial in the number of initial candidate input attributes (Last and Maimon, 1999). The poor scalability, with respect to the number of records, is a serious limitation of many data mining algorithms (e.g., Artificial Neural Networks). The construction of the Information-Theoretic Network from the Mortality Dataset (having more than 33,000 records) has taken only about 30 seconds of CPU time on a desktop PC, with a Pentium-II microprocessor.
- Disjunctive association rules, extracted from the network connections, can be scored in terms of their contribution to the overall mutual information, which is a general measure of association between random variables. According to the well-known Pareto principle, a small number of rules are expected to explain a major part of the association between the input attributes and the target. This can significantly reduce the number of rules, represented to the user (Ministry of Health).

The application of the information-theoretic procedure to the Mortality Dataset is described in the next sub-sections.

8.5.2 Dimensionality Reduction Procedure

We start with applying the information-theoretic algorithm to the original ("unclean") dataset. Only three out of six candidate input attributes (*Age, Month, Gender, Region, Religion,* and *Continent of Birth*) have been identified as significant and included in the Information-Theoretic Network. The selected input attributes and the degree of their association with the target attribute (*Diagnosis*) are represented in Table 33 below.

Iteration	Attribute Name	Mutual Information	Conditional MI	Conditional Entropy
0	**Age**	**0.300**	**0.300**	**3.918**
1	Gender	0.361	0.062	3.856
2	Month	0.381	0.019	3.837

Table 3. Dimensionality Reduction Procedure (Original Data).

Table 3 shows three information-theoretic measures of association between the input attributes and the target attribute: Mutual Information, Conditional Mutual Information, and Conditional Entropy. All these parameters are based on the notion of *Entropy* (see Cover, 1991), which represents the uncertainty degree of a random variable. The entropy is measured in *bits*. Thus, the entropy of the target attribute *Diagnosis* is equal to 4.218 bits. Information on input attributes, associated with the target, can decrease the uncertainty and the resulting entropy. In the ideal case, there is no uncertainty left and the entropy becomes equal to zero.

The column "Mutual Information" shows the cumulative association between a subset of input attributes, selected up to a given iteration inclusively, and the target attribute. The three selected attributes together are contributing only 0.381 bits of information (0.381/4.218 = 9% of the overall entropy). This means that the dataset of mortality records is extremely noisy. The next column, "Conditional MI (Mutual Information)" shows the net decrease in the entropy of the target attribute "Diagnosis" due to adding each input attribute. The first input attribute (*Age*) alone reduces the entropy by 0.3 bits, which are about 80% of the overall mutual information (0.381 bits). This attribute is shown in bold. The next two input attributes (Gender and Month) contribute 15% and 5% respectively. The first two selected attributes represent the well-known fact that a person age and gender are usually related to his / her death cause. However, the third input attribute (*Month of Death*) is less expected and it has never been considered by the Ministry of Health analysts. Three other attributes (*Region, Religion,* and *Continent of Birth*) have been found irrelevant or redundant. The last column ("Conditional Entropy") is equal to the difference between the unconditional entropy (4.218 bits) and the estimated mutual information. It represents the uncertainty of the target, given the values of the input attributes.

In (Last and Kandel, 1999b), we have enhanced the information-theoretic algorithm to ignore values, marked as "outliers", without discarding the values of other attributes in the same record. The results of applying the enhanced algorithm to the "cleaned" version of the dataset are shown in

Table 44 below. The first two input attributes selected by the algorithm have not changed: they are still *Age* (the major factor) and *Gender*. However, the third input attribute (*Continent of Birth*) is new: the algorithm has discarded it before the cleaning process. One value of this attribute has been detected as an "outlier" by the automated cleaning procedure (see sub-section 4.4 above). Consequently, the cleaned attribute *Month* (also having one outlying value) has been moved to the less "respectful" fourth place.

The overall results of mining the cleaned dataset seem better in terms of explaining the uncertainty: the total mutual information has increased from 0.381 to 0.387 bits. However, the efficiency of these results is lower: the ratio of the mutual information to the number of input attributes is now 0.097 only vs. 0.127 with the original data. Thus, we have decided to keep the first model (represented in Table 33) for the subsequent stages of the discovery process.

Iteration	Attribute Name	Mutual Information	Conditional MI	Conditional Entropy
0	**Age**	**0.286**	**0.286**	**3.882**
1	Gender	0.344	0.058	3.823
2	Continent of Birth	0.374	0.03	3.794
3	Month	0.387	0.013	3.78

Table 4. Dimensionality Reduction Procedure (Cleaned Data).

8.5.3 Discretization of Continuous Attributes

As mentioned above, the construction procedure of the information-theoretic network includes automated discretization of continuous input attributes. The Mortality Dataset contains two continuous attributes: *Age* and *Month*. The discretization schemes of these attributes are shown in Table5 and Table6 below.

Each interval in these tables represents a consistent set of patterns (association rules). A new interval is generated by the information-theoretic procedure, when there is a change in the rules explaining the target attribute. Thus, the death causes of infants (*Age* = 0) are different from children between the ages of one to three (see Table5). From looking at interval no. 2 in the same table, one can see that there is a stability of diagnoses for children of four to sixteen years old. The intervals can be used for monitoring the causes of death over years and for other purposes.

The intervals of the attribute *Month* (see Table6) are also interesting. They represent seasonality patterns, which may be related to weather conditions and other seasonal factors. For example, January, February, March, and April are the typical winter months in Israel and May to August is the time of summer (the transitional period is very short). The seasonality of diagnoses can be studied more accurately by analyzing data of several years. Unfortunately, the mortality records of other years (besides 1993) were not available in the time of our project.

Interval No.	Years Included	Number of Records	Mean Age
0	0	918	0
1	1 - 3	185	1.77
2	4 - 16	294	9.99
3	17 - 22	319	19.78
4	23 - 27	225	25.01
5	28 - 32	231	30.18
6	33	59	33.00
7	34 - 38	324	36.15
8	39 - 46	830	42.92
9	47 - 56	1559	52.19
10	57 - 60	1178	58.57
11	61 - 68	4091	64.88
12	69 - 71	2435	69.99
13	72 - 74	2600	72.98
14	75 - 79	4800	77.28
15	80 - 84	6209	81.97
16	85 - 87	2886	85.89
17	88 - 93	3138	90.00
18	94+	853	96.41

Table 5. Discretization Scheme - *Age*.

Interval No.	Months Included	Number of Records	Mean Month Number
0	January - April	12490	2.46
1	May - August	9847	6.50
2	September - November	7829	10.03
3	December	2968	12.00

Table 6. Discretization Scheme - *Month.*

8.5.4 Rule Extraction

In a multi-layer information-theoretic network (Last and Maimon, 1999), each extracted rule is assigned a connection weight expressing the mutual information between the rule condition (a conjunction of input values) and the rule consequence (a target value). The weight is positive if the conditional probability of a target attribute value, given the input values, is higher than its unconditional probability and negative otherwise. A weight close to zero means that the target attribute value is almost independent of the input values. Thus, each positive connection weight can be interpreted as an *information content* of a corresponding rule of the form "*if condition, then target value (is more likely)*". Accordingly, a negative weight refers to a rule of the form "*if condition, then* ***not*** *target value" (target value is less likely)*".

The most informative rules are found by ranking the information-theoretic connection weights in descending order. Both the rules having the highest positive and the lowest negative weights are of a potential interest to a user. Due to the disjunctive structure of the information-theoretic network, the sum of connection weights assigned to all the rules is equal to the estimated mutual information between a set of input attributes and a target attribute (see Table 33 above).

The information-theoretic network constructed from the original data (see sub-section 5.2 above) contains 1,783 connections with non-zero information-theoretic weights, each representing a disjunctive association rule. Most of these rules are not particularly interesting, since their weights are quite negligible (very close to zero). Like in other datasets, we would like to concentrate on the highest positive and the lowest negative connection weights only. The problem is that the target attribute in this database (Diagnosis) has 36 possible values, which makes listing all the rules in the descending order of their weights hardly meaningful. Therefore, we have decided to group together all rules having the same target value (diagnosis) and then represent them in the descending order of information-theoretic weights. Thus, we can *characterize* each cause of death.

In Table 77 below, we are showing the positive rules for the most common natural cause of death – the ischaemic heart disease. Since all the rules in this table have the same consequence (diagnosis), only the conditions of each rule are included. Thus, association rule no. 358, shown in the first line, reads:

If Age is between 61 and 69 and Gender is male then Diagnosis is ischaemic heart disease

The rules in Table 7 represent the characteristics of the population under a high risk of heart disease. The conditions of all the rules include males in the age of 61 and higher. Some rules are more specific. Thus, according to the Rules no. 1202 and 1231, males between 80 and 85 are more endangered by a heart disease during the months January – August. The winter months (January – April) seem more dangerous for males of 75 – 80 (Rule no. 978).

Table 2 shows the characteristics of those, who are *less likely* to die from a heart disease (though the likelihood is greater than zero). The rule in the first line is:

If Age is between 61 and 69, Gender is female, and Month is between January and April, then Diagnosis is ***not*** *ischaemic heart disease*

In this population group, we have mostly females, aged 47 to 69. Males between 39 and 47 are also under a lower risk. According to the Rule no. 759, the winter months are safer for women between 61 and 69.

Tables 9 and 10 represent the rules related to the unnatural cause, which, unfortunately, is the most common in Israel – motor-vehicle traffic accidents. The high-risk population groups include children (age: 4 – 17) and males between 17 and 28. September to November, happen to be more dangerous for young males on the road (maybe, because the first rains start during this period). In Table 7, we find people who drive less and thus are more subject to natural causes of death: males and females, aged 61 and higher. The winter months (January – April) prove to be particularly safe for them.

Rule No.	Rule Condition	Weight
358	Age is between 61 and 69 and Gender is male	0.00387
1202	Age is between 80 and 85 and Gender is male and Month is between January and April	0.00371
387	Age is between 69 and 72 and Gender is male	0.00329
479	Age is between 85 and 88 and Gender is male	0.00297
978	Age is between 75 and 80 and Gender is male and Month is between January and April	0.00233
1231	Age is between 80 and 85 and Gender is male and Month is between May and August	0.00224

Table 7. Ischaemic Heart Disease: Highest Positive Rule Weights.

Rule No.	Rule Condition	Weight
759	Age is between 61 and 69 and Gender is female and Month is between January and April	-0.00119
329	Age is between 57 and 61 and Gender is female	-0.00127
208	Age is between 39 and 47 and Gender is male	-0.00132
300	Age is between 47 and 57 and Gender is female	-0.00189

Table 8. Ischaemic Heart Disease: Lowest Negative Rule Weights.

Rule No.	Rule Condition	Weight
62	Age is between 4 and 17	0.00489
121	Age is between 23 and 28 and Gender is male	0.00458
556	Age is between 17 and 23 and Gender is male and Month is between September and November	0.00458

Table 9. Motor Vehicle Traffic Accidents: Highest Positive Rule Weights.

Rule No.	Rule Condition	Weight
522	Age is between 85 and 88 and Gender is female	-0.00020
992	Age is between 75 and 80 and Gender is male and Month is between January and April	-0.00020
1216	Age is between 80 and 85 and Gender is male and Month is between January and April	-0.00021
431	Age is between 69 and 72 and Gender is female	-0.00024
463	Age is between 72 and 75 and Gender is female	-0.00027
400	Age is between 69 and 72 and Gender is male	-0.00028
492	Age is between 85 and 88 and Gender is male	-0.00028
1327	Age is between 80 and 85 and Gender is female and Month is between January and April	-0.00028
371	Age is between 61 and 69 and Gender is male	-0.00051

Table 10. Motor Vehicle Traffic Accidents: Lowest Negative Rule Weights.

8.5.5 Data Reliability

In (Last and Kandel, 1999a) and (Maimon et al. 1999), we use the following definition of data reliability, based on the Computational Theory of Perception:

Definition. *Degree of Reliability of an attribute A in a tuple k is defined on a unit interval [0,1] as the degree of certainty that the value of attribute A stored in a tuple k is correct from the user's point of view.*

Our method of calculating data reliability (Maimon et al. 1999) can be applied to a target attribute in an information-theoretic network by measuring the distance between predicted and actual target values. The distance is zero, when the predicted (by the network) and the actual value are the same. In this case, the reliability is equal to one. On the other hand, when the probability of the actual value is much lower than the probability of the predicted value, the reliability becomes close to zero. The exact shape of the reliability function is determined by a user-specific approach to reliability of lowly probable values.

After calculating the predicted diagnosis in every record by using the Information-Fuzzy Network (IFN), the Mortality database has been extended to a fuzzy relational database (see Zemankova and Kandel, 1984) by adding a new, fuzzy attribute: the reliability degree of the recorded diagnosis. We are interested in identifying data errors by applying the *selection* operator of the fuzzy relational algebra (Klir and Yuan, 1995) to the extended database. In Table below, we are listing the records retrieved by the query "What are the records with reliability degree less than 0.1%?"

Though we could not check the actual correctness of these "suspicious" records, they certainly represent rather exceptional cases from the medical viewpoint. Thus, suicide and homicide are quite rare causes of death for people of age 85 and higher (records no. 4341 and 9083). Congenital anomalies are much unexpected for the old (records no. 15897 and no. 25324). Death of a 69-year old woman, caused by pregnancy is also hard to explain (record no. 14330). On the other hand, records no. 28328, 28723, 31260, 32966, and 33120 include quite uncommon diseases for the newborn (age = 0 years).

Record No.	Age	Gender	Month of Death	Recorded Diagnosis	Predicted Diagnosis
4341	85	Man	10	Suicide and Self-inflicted injuries	Ischaemic heart disease
9083	89	Man	2	Homicide	Ischaemic heart disease
9371	92	Woman	3	Congenital Anomalies	Ischaemic heart disease
10149	86	Woman	8	Diseases of the Muscoloskeletal System	Ischaemic heart disease
11847	77	Man	3	Diseases of the Genital Organs	Ischaemic heart disease
14330	69	Woman	11	Pregnancy etc.	Ischaemic heart disease
15807	64	Woman	8	Congenital Anomalies	Ischaemic heart disease
17961	77	Man	1	Diseases of the Genital Organs	Ischaemic heart disease
24060	79	Man	3	Diseases of the Genital Organs	Ischaemic heart disease
24676	71	Woman	7	Other Endocrine Diseases	Ischaemic heart disease

25324	89	Man	2	Congenital Anomalies	Ischaemic heart disease
25356	71	Man	10	Diseases of the Genital Organs	Ischaemic heart disease
28328	0	Woman	5	Diseases of Blood	Prenatal period
28723	0	Woman	9	Cerebrovascular disease	Prenatal period
30339	87	Woman	7	Diseases of the Muscoloskeletal System	Ischaemic heart disease
31260	0	Man	5	Mental Disorders	Prenatal period
32966	0	Woman	12	Non-Malignant Neoplasms	Prenatal period
33120	0	Woman	11	Diseases of the Urinary System	Prenatal period

Table 11. Low Reliability Records (Reliability < 0.1%).

8.6 Evaluation of the Discovered Knowledge

Following are the main results achieved, with respect to the project objectives, and the actions to be taken:

- *Data Cleaning.* The automated data cleaning procedure has revealed outliers in most attributes of the database (see sub-section 4.3 above). The outlying values have been explained by rare categories and missing / inaccurate information. We have "rectified" the data by correcting these values. Since the number of records containing outliers is low, the effect on the results of the data mining process has not been significant. Still, some of the results can be used to improve the quality of data in the original database (the Register of Deaths).
- *Dimensionality Reduction.* Traditionally, the mortality data has been analyzed with respect to age, gender, and ethnic origin. To the best of our knowledge, no attempt has been made to study the seasonal patterns in the causes of death. Our results suggest that time of year is a more important factor than place of birth and/or ethnic origin and it deserves a deeper analysis.
- *Discretization of Continuous Features.* This has been a by-product of using the information-theoretic network (IFN). The intervals of age,

calculated by the algorithm, can be used for defining age groups in different types of data analysis.

- *Rule Extraction.* Rules defining high-risk and low-risk groups (w.r.t. specific causes) have been extracted and scored by the information-theoretic network. These rules can be used for determining priorities in the health care budget. They may be also valuable for insurance companies and other commercial institutions.
- *Data Quality.* Most unreliable records in the database (see Table above) contain lowly probable information. This information should be checked by medical experts and possibly compared to the manual source. This comparison can lead to correcting the data in the original database.

8.7 Using the Discovered Knowledge

The Ministry of Health has not implemented the actions recommended on the achieved results yet. Our results have been based on the data of only one year (1993). Though the Ministry of Health representatives have considered most results as interesting and valuable, a comprehensive analysis of multi-year datasets is certainly required. Unfortunately, the complete data of other years has not been available during the time of the project. We believe that the data mining techniques used in this project are applicable to larger amounts of diagnoses data.

8.8 Conclusions

In this chapter, we have applied the process of knowledge discovery to a dataset of 33,134 mortality records. A significant amount of data preparation has been performed. The data mining methods applied have been based on the information-theoretic approach to data mining. The process has resulted in selection and scoring of the most important input attributes, discretization of continuous features, rule extraction, and calculation of data reliability. The main strengths of the information-theoretic methods, used for mining this dataset, include applicability to attributes of mixed nature, built-in dimensionality reduction, extraction of complex association rules, robustness to noisy data, and high scalability. All these features are especially important for knowledge discovery in medical databases that are characterized by heterogeneous structure, highly noisy data, and large number of records.

In the future, other techniques may be applied to the same type of data, including temporal data mining, rule reduction, and use of expert medical knowledge in the discovery process.

Acknowledgements

We thank Prof. Gabi Barabash, Director General of the Israel Ministry of Health, and his staff, for providing data and information, used in this research.

References

Blij, H.J. and Murphy, A.B. 1998. *Human Geography: Culture, Society, and Space*, 6th ed. Wiley

Cover, T. M. 1991. *Elements of Information Theory.* Wiley

Fayyad, U., Piatetsky-Shapiro, G. and Smyth, P. 1996. From Data Mining to Knowledge Discovery: An Overview. In: *Advances in Knowledge Discovery and Data Mining*, Fayyad, U. et al. (eds), AAAI/MIT Press, 1-30

Klir G. J. and Yuan, B. 1995. *Fuzzy Sets and Fuzzy Logic: Theory and Applications.* Prentice-Hall

Last M. and Kandel, A. 1999a. Automated Perceptions in Data Mining, invited paper. In: *1999 IEEE International Fuzzy Systems Conference Proceedings*, IEEE Press, Part I, 190 - 197

Last M. and Kandel, A. 1999b. Automated Detection of Outliers in Real-World Data. Submitted to publication.

Last M. and Maimon, O. 1999. An Information-Theoretic Approach to Data Mining. Submitted to publication.

Maimon, O., Kandel, A., and Last, M. 1999. Information-Theoretic Fuzzy Approach to Knowledge Discovery in Databases. In: *Advances in Soft Computing - Engineering Design and Manufacturing*, Roy, R. et al. (eds), Springer-Verlag

Pyle, D. 1999. *Data Preparation for Data Mining.* Morgan Kaufmann

Zemankova-Leech M. and Kandel, A. 1984. *Fuzzy Relational Databases - a Key to Expert Systems.* Verlag TUV

9 Consistent and Complete Data and "Expert" Mining in Medicine

Boris Kovalerchuk[1], **Evgenii Vityaev**[2] **and James F. Ruiz**[3]

[1]Department of Computer Science
Central Washington University
Ellensburg, WA, 98926-7520, U.S.A.
borisk@tahoma.cwu.edu
[2]Institute of Mathematics
Russian Academy of Sciences
Novosibirsk 630090, Russia
vityaev@math.nsc.ru
[3]Department of Radiology
Woman's Hospital
Baton Rouge, LA 70895-9009, U.S.A.
mdjr@womans.com

The ultimate purpose of many medical data mining systems is to create formalized knowledge for a computer-aided diagnostic system, which can in turn, provide a second diagnostic opinion. Such systems should be consistent and complete as much as possible. The system is consistent if it is free of contradictions (between rules in a computer-aided diagnostic system, rules used by an experienced medical expert and a database of pathologically confirmed cases). The system is complete if it is able to cover (classify) all (or largest possible number of) combinations of the used attributes. A method for discovering a consistent and complete set of diagnostic rules is presented in this chapter. Advantages of the method are shown for development of a breast cancer computer-aided diagnostic system

9.1 Introduction

Stages. Knowledge discovery is a complex multistage process. These stages include initial understanding the problem domain, understanding and preparation of data. Data mining, evaluation, and use of discovered knowledge follow the first three stages. In this chapter, knowledge discovery stages for two methods (BEM and MMDR)are presented. These methods belong to the promising class of complete and consistent data mining methods. Such methods produce **consistent knowledge**, i.e., **knowledge free of contradictions** (between rules in a computer-aided diagnostic system, rules used by an experienced medical expert and a database of pathologically confirmed cases). Similarly complete methods produce complete knowledge systems (models), i.e., models which classify all (or largest possible number of) combinations of the used attributes.

Data mining paradigms. Several modern approaches for knowledge discovery are known in the medical field. Neural networks, nearest neighbor methods, discriminant analysis, cluster analysis, linear programming, and genetic algorithms are among the most common knowledge discovery tools used in medicine.

These approaches are associated with different **learning paradigms**, which involve four major components:

- Representation of background and associated knowledge,
- Learning mechanism,
- Representation of learned knowledge, and
- Forecast performer.

Representation of background and associated knowledge sets a framework for representing **prior knowledge**. A **learning mechanism** produces new (learned) knowledge and identifies parameters for the forecast performer using prior knowledge. **Representation of learned knowledge** sets a framework for use of this knowledge including forecast and diagnosis. A **forecast performer** serves as a final product, generating a forecast from learned knowledge.

Figure 1 shows the interaction of these components of a learning paradigm. The training data and other available knowledge are embedded into some form of knowledge representation. The learning mechanism (method/algorithm) uses available information to produce a forecast performer and possibly a separate entity, **learned knowledge**, which can be **communicated to medical experts.**

The most controversial problem is the relation between a **forecast performer** and **learned knowledge**. The learned knowledge can exist in different forms. The widely accepted position is that the learning mechanism of a data mining system produces knowledge only if that knowledge can be put in a human-understandable form (Fu, 1999).

Some DM paradigms (such as neural networks) do not generate learned knowledge as a separate human-understandable entity. A forecast performer (trained neural network) contains this knowledge implicitly, but cryptically, coded as a large number of weights.

This knowledge should be decoded and communicated into the terms of the problem to be solved. Fu (1999) noted "Lack of comprehension causes concern about the credibility of the result when neural networks are applied to risky domains, such as **patient care**". As noted in many recent publications, obtaining **comprehensible learned knowledge** is one of the important and promising directions in data mining (e.g. (Muggleton, 1999; Graven and Shavlik, 1997)).

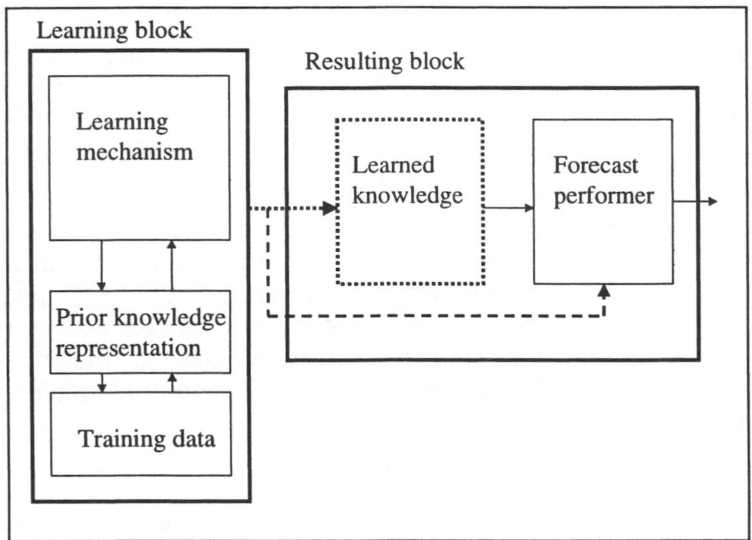

Figure 1. Learning paradigm.

This consideration shows the importance of knowledge representation to obtain decodable understandable knowledge and a understandable forecast performer. Five major forms of knowledge representation are listed below (Langley and Simon, 1995):

1. A multilayer network of units (**neural network paradigm**).

2. Specific cases applied to new situations by matching with new cases (**instance-based learning paradigm**).
3. Binary features used as the conditions and actions of rules (**genetic algorithms paradigm**).
4. Decision trees and propositional If-Then rules (**rule induction paradigm**).
5. Rules in first-order logic form (Horn clauses as in the Prolog language) (**analytic learning paradigm**).
6. A mixture of the previous representations (**hybrid paradigm**).

As it was already discussed, neural network learning identifies the forecast performer, but does not produce knowledge in a form understandable by humans.. The rule induction and analytical learning paradigms produce learned knowledge in the form of understandable if-then rules and the forecast performer is a derivative of these forms of knowledge. Therefore, this chapter concentrates on rule induction and analytical learning paradigms.

The next important component of each of leaning paradigms is a **learning mechanism**. These mechanisms include specific and general formal and informal steps. These steps are challenging for many reasons. Currently, the **least formalized steps** are reformulating the actual problem as a learning problem and identifying an effective knowledge representation.

It has become increasingly evident that effective **knowledge representation** is an important problem for the success of data mining. Close inspection of **successful projects** suggests that much of the power comes not from the specific induction method, but from proper formulation of the problems and from crafting the representation to make learning tractable (Langley and Simon, 1995). Thus, the **conceptual challenges** in data mining are:

- proper formulation of the problems and
- crafting the knowledge representation to make learning meaningful and tractable.

Munakata (1999) and Mitchell (1999) point out several especially promising and challenging tasks in current data mining:

1.enhancement of **background and associated knowledge** using

- incorporation of more comprehensible, non-oversimplified, **real-world types of data**,

- human-computer interaction for **extracting background knowledge**,

2. enhancement of **learning mechanism** using

   -interactive human **guided data mining** and

   -optimization of decisions, rather than prediction.

3. **hybrid systems** for taking advantage of different methods of data mining.

4. Learning from multiple databases and Web based systems.

Traditionally, the knowledge representation process in medical diagnosis includes two major steps:

extracting about a dozen diagnostic features from data or images and

representing a few hundred data units using the extracted features.

Data mining in fields outside of medicine tend to use larger databases and discover larger sets of rules using these techniques. However, mammography archives at hospitals around the world contain millions of mammograms and biopsy results. Currently, the American College of Radiology (ACR) supports the National Mammography Database (NMD) Project (http://www.eskimo.com/~briteoo/nmd) with a unified set of features (BI-RADS, 1998).

Several universities and hospitals have developed mammography image bases that are available on the Internet. Such efforts provide the opportunity for large-scale data mining and knowledge discovery in medicine. Data mining experience in business applications have shown that a large database can be a source of useful rules, but the useful rules may be accompanied by a larger set of irrelevant or incorrect rules. A great deal of time may be required for experts to select only non-trivial rules. This chapter addresses the problem by offering a method of rule extraction consistent with expert judgement using approaches listed above (1.2) **interactive extracting background knowledge** and (2.1) **human guided data mining**. These two new approaches in data mining recall well-known problems of more traditional expert systems (Giarratano and Riley, 1994).

"Expert mining" paradigm: data mining versus "expert mining". Traditional medical expert systems rely on knowledge extracted in the form of If-Then **diagnostic rules** extracted from **medical experts**. Systems based on Machine Learning technique rely on an available **database** for discovering diagnostic rules. These two sets of rules may contradict each other. A medical expert may not trust rules, as they may contradict his/her existing rules and experience.

Also, a medical expert may have questionable or incorrect rules while the data/image base may have questionable or incorrect records. Moreover, data mining discovery may not necessarily take the form of If-Then rules and these rules may need to be decoded before they are compared to expert rules. This makes the design of computer-aided diagnostic system extremely complex and raises two additional complex tasks:

(1) Identify contradictions between expert diagnostic rules and knowledge discovered by data mining mechanisms and

(2) eliminate contradictions between expert rules and machine discovered rules.

If the first task is solved, the second task can be approached by cleaning the records in the database, adding more features, using more sophisticated rule extraction methods and testing the competence of a medical expert.

This chapter concentrates on the **extraction of rules** from an expert (**"expert mining"**) and from a collection of data **(data mining).** Subsequently, an attempt must be made to **identify contradictions.** If rule extraction is performed without this purpose in mind, it is difficult to recognize a contradiction.

In addition, rules generated by an expert and data-driven rules maybe incomplete as they may cover only a small fraction of possible feature combinations. This may make it impossible to confirm that rules are consistent with an available database. Additional new cases or features can make the contradiction apparent. Therefore, the major problem here is **discovering sufficient, complete, and comparable sets of expert rules and data-driven rules**. Such completeness is critical for comparison. For example, suppose that expert and data-driven rules cover only 3% of possible feature combinations (cases). If it is found that there are no contradictions between these rules, there is still plenty of room for contradiction in the remaining 97% of the cases.

Discovering complete set of regularities. If data mining method X discovers an incomplete set of rules, R(X), then rules R(X) do not produce an output (forecast) for some inputs. If two data mining methods, X and Y, produce incomplete sets of rules R(X) and R(Y) then it would be difficult to compare them if their domains overlap in only a small percentage of their rules.

Similarly, an expert mining method, E, can produce a set of rules R(E) with very few overlapping rules from R(X) and R(Y). Again, this creates a problem in comparing the performances of R(X) and R(Y) with R(E). Therefore, completeness is a very valuable property of any data mining method. The Boolean Expert Mining method (BEM) described below is complete. If an expert has a judgement about a particular type of patient symptom or symptom complex then appropriate rules can be extracted by BEM.

The problem is to find a method, W, such that R(W)=R(X)UR(Y) for any X and Y, i.e., this method, W, will be the most general for a given data set. The MMDR is a complete method for relational data in this sense. Below we present more formally what it means for W to be the most general method available. Often, data are limited such that a complete set of rules can not be extracted.

Similarly, if an expert does not know answers to enough questions, rules can not be extracted from him. Assume that data are complete enough. How can it be guaranteed that a complete set of rules will be extracted by some method? If data are not sufficient, then MMDR utilizes the available data and attempts to keep statistical significance within an appropriate range. The MMDR will deliver a forecast for a maximum number of cases. Therefore, this method attempts to maximize the domain of the rules.

In other words, the **"expert mining" method** called BEM (Boolean Expert Mining) extracts a complete set of rules from and expert and the **data mining method** called MMDR (Machine Method for Discovering Regularities) extracts a complete set of rules from data. For MMDR and BEM, this has been proved in (Vityaev, 1992; Kovalerchuk et al. 1996).

Thus, the first goal of this chapter is to present methods for discovering complete sets of expert rules and data-driven rules. This objective presents us with an exponential, non-tractable problem of extracting diagnostic rules.

A brute-force method may require asking the expert thousands of questions. This is a well-known problem for expert system development (Kovalerchuk, Vityaev, 1999). For example, for 11 binary diagnostic features of clustered calcifications found in mammograms, there are (2^{11}=2,048) feature combinations, each representing a unique case. A brute-force method would require questioning a radiologist on each of these 2,048 combinations.

A related problem is that experts may find it difficult or impossible to articulate confidently the **large number of interactions** between features.

Dhar amd Stein (1997) pointer out that If a problem is "**decomposable**" (the interactions among variables are limited) and experts can articulate their decision process, a rule-based approach may scale well. An effective mechanism for decomposition based monotonicity is presented below.

Creating a consistent rule base includes the following steps:

1. Finding data-driven **rules not** discovered by asking an expert.
2. Analysis of these new rules by an expert using available proven cases. A list of these cases from the database can be presented to an expert. The expert can check:

2.1 Is a new rule discovered because of **misleading cases**? The rule may be rejected and training data can be extended.

2.2 Does the rule **confirm** existing expert knowledge? Perhaps the rule is not sufficiently transparent for the expert. The expert may find that the rule is consistent with his/her previous experience, but he/she would like more evidence. The rule can increase the confidence of his/her practice.

2.3 Does the rule **identify new** relationships, which were not previously known to the expert? The expert can find that the rule is promising.

3. Finding rules which are **contradictory** to the experts knowledge or understanding. There are two possibilities:

   3.1. The rule was discovered using misleading cases. The rule must be rejected and training data must be extended.

   3.2. The expert can admit that his/her ideas have no real ground. The system improves expert experience.

9.2 Understanding the Data

9.2.1 Collection of Initial Data: Monotone Boolean Function Approach

Data mining has a serious drawback. If data are scarce then data mining methods cannot produce useful regularities (models). An expert is a valuable source of **"artificial data"** and regularities for situations where an **explicit set of data** either does not exist or is **insufficient**.

For instance, an expert can say that the case with attributes <2,3,1,6,0,0> belongs to the class of benign cases. This "artificial case" can be added to training data. An efficient mechanism for **constructing "artificial data"** is one of the major goals of this chapter. The actual training data, "artificial data" and known regularities constitute **background knowledge**.

The idea of the approach under consideration is to develop:

1. the procedure of questioning (interviewing) an expert to obtain known regularities and additional "artificial data", and

2. the procedure of extracting new knowledge from "artificial data", known regularities and actual training data.

The idea of extracting knowledge by interviewing an expert is originated in traditional medical expert systems. The serious drawback of traditional knowledge-based (expert) systems is the slowness of the interviewing process for changing circumstances. This includes the extraction of artificial data, regularities, models, diagnostic rules and dynamic correction of them.

Next, an expert can learn from artificial data, already trained "artificial experts" and human experts. This learning is called **"expert mining,"** an umbrella term for extracting data and knowledge from "experts". An example of expert mining is extracting understandable rules from a learned neural network which serves as an artificial expert (Shavlik, 1994).

This chapter presents a method to "mine" data and regularities from an expert and significantly speed up this process. The method is based on the mathematical tools **of monotone Boolean functions (MBF)** (Kovalerchuk et al. 1996).

The essence of the property of **monotonicity** for this application is that:

> If an expert believes that property T is true for example x and attributes of example y are stronger than attributes of x, then property T is also true for example y.

Here the phrase *attributes are stronger* refers to the property that values of each attributes of x are larger than the corresponding values of y. Informally, larger is interpreted as "better" or "stronger." Sometimes to be consistent with this idea, the coding of attributes should be changed.

The **slowness of learning** associated with traditional expert systems, means that experts would be asked more questions than is practical when extracting rules and "artificial data". Thus, traditional experts take too much time for real systems with a large number of attributes. The new efficient approach is to represent the questioning procedure (interviewing) as a restoration of a monotone Boolean function interactively with an "oracle" (expert).

In the experiment below, the number actual questions needed for complete search was decreased to 60% of the total number of possible questions. This was accomplished for a small number of attributes (five attributes), using the method based on monotone Boolean functions.

The difference becomes increasingly significant as the number of attributes increases. Thus, full restoration of either one of the two functions f_1 and f_2 (considered below) with 11 arguments without any optimization of the interview process would have required up to 2^{11} or 2048 calls (membership inquiries) to an expert. However, an optimal dialogue (i.e. a minimal number of questions) for restoring each of these functions would require at most 924 questions:

$$\binom{11}{5}+\binom{11}{6} = 2\,x\,462 = 924,$$

This follows from the Hansel lemma (equation (1) below) (Hansel, 1963, Kovalerchuk at al. 1996), under the assumption of monotonicity of these functions. (To the best of our knowledge, Hansel's original paper has not been translated into English. There are numerous references to it in the non-English literature. See equation (1) below).

This new value, 924 questions, is 2.36 times smaller than the previous upper limit of 2048 calls. However, this upper limit of 924 questions can be reduced even further by using monotonicity and the **hierarchy** imbedded within the structured sequence of questions and answers. In one of the tasks, the maximum number of questions needed to restore the monotone Boolean function was reduced first to 72 questions and further reduced to 46 questions.

In fact, subsequently only about 40 questions were required for the two **nested** functions, i.e., about 20 questions per function. This number should be compared with the full search requiring 2^{11} or 2048 questions. Therefore, this procedure allowed us to ask about **100 times fewer questions** without relaxing the requirement of complete restoration of the functions.

The formal definitions of concepts from the theory of monotone Boolean functions used to obtain these results are presented in section 2.2.1.

1	Develop a hierarchy of Monotone Boolean functions
2	Interactively restore each function in the hierarchy
3	Combine functions into a complete diagnostic function
4	Present the complete function as a set of simple diagnostic rules: *If A and B and C…and F Then Z*

Figure 2. Major steps for extraction of expert diagnostic rules.

Figure 2 presents the major steps of extraction of rules from an expert using this mathematical technique. Figure 3 details the sequence of actions taken to accomplish step 2, i.e., restoring each of the monotone Boolean functions with a minimal sequence of questions to the expert. The last block (2.5) in figure 3 provides for interviewing an expert with a **minimal dynamic sequence of questions**. This sequence is based on the fundamental Hansel lemma (Hansel, 1966; Kovalerchuk at al. 1996) and the property of **monotonicity.**

Table 1 shows the general idea of these steps. It represents a complete interactive session. A minimal dynamic sequence of questions means that the minimum of the Shannon Function is reached, i.e., the **minimum number of questions required to restore the most complex monotone Boolean function of n arguments**.

This sequence is not a sequence written in advance. It depends on each answer of an expert. Each subsequent question is defined **dynamically** by the previous answer and in this way, the number of total questions is minimized.

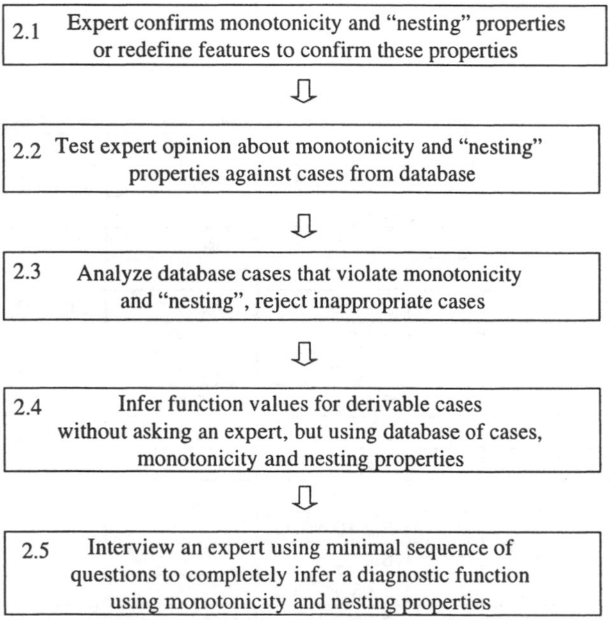

2.1 Expert confirms monotonicity and "nesting" properties or redefine features to confirm these properties

⇩

2.2 Test expert opinion about monotonicity and "nesting" properties against cases from database

⇩

2.3 Analyze database cases that violate monotonicity and "nesting", reject inappropriate cases

⇩

2.4 Infer function values for derivable cases without asking an expert, but using database of cases, monotonicity and nesting properties

⇩

2.5 Interview an expert using minimal sequence of questions to completely infer a diagnostic function using monotonicity and nesting properties

Figure 3. Iteratively restoring functions in hierarchy.

Columns 2, 3 and 4 in table 1 present values of the three functions f_1, f_2 and ψ of five arguments chosen for this example. These functions represent regularities that should be discovered by interviewing an expert. Column 5 & 6 indicate the chain/case # for those cases that are derived as extensions of the primary vector in column 1.

These extensions are based on the property of monotonicity and so no questions are posed to the expert. Column 5 is for extending values of functions from 1 to 1 and column 6 is for extending them from 0 to 0. In other words, if f(x)=1 then column 5 helps to find y such that f(y)=1.

Similarly, column 6 works for f(x)=0 by helping to find y such that f(y)=0. Assume that each of these functions has it's own target variable. Thus, the first question to the expert in column 2 is: "Does the sequence (01100) represent a case with the target attribute equal to 1 for f_1?"

Columns 3 and 4 represent expert's answers for functions f_2 and ψ. Here $(01100)=(x_1, x_2, x_3, x_4, x_5)$. If the answer is "yes" (1), then the next question will be about the target value for the case (01010). If the answer is "No" (0), then the next question will be about the target value for (11100).

This sequence of questions is not accidental. As mentioned above, it is inferred from the Hansel lemma. An asterisk is used to indicate that the result was obtained directly from the expert.

1	2	3	4	5	6	7	8
Vector	F_1	f_2	ψ	Monotone extension case #		Chain #	Case #
				$1 \rightarrow 1$	$0 \rightarrow 0$		
(01100)	1*	1*	1*	1.2;6.3;7.3	7.1;8.1	Chain 1	1.1
(11100)	1	1	1	6.4;7.4	5.1;3.1		1.2
(01010)	1*	0*	1*	2.2;6.3;8.3	6.1;8.1	Chain 2	2.1
(11010)	1	1*	1	6.4;8.4	3.1;6.1		2.2
(11000)	1*	1*	1*	3.2	8.1;9.1	Chain 3	3.1
(11001)	1	1	1	7.4;8.4	8.2;9.2		3.2
(10010)	1*	0*	1*	4.2;9.3	6.1;9.1	Chain 4	4.1
(10110)	1	1*	1	6.4;9.4	6.2;5.1		4.2
(10100)	1*	1*	1*	5.2	7.1;9.1	Chain 5	5.1
(10101)	1	1	1	7.4;9.4	7.2;9.2		5.2
(00010)	0*	0	0*	6.2;10.3	10.1	Chain 6	6.1
(00110)	1*	1*	0*	6.3;10.4	7.1		6.2
(01110)	1	1	1	6.4;10.5			6.3
(11110)	1	1	1	10.6			6.4
(00100)	1*	1*	0*	7.2;10.4	10.1	Chain 7	7.1
(00101)	1	1	0*	7.3;10.4	10.2		7.2
(01101)	1	1	1*	7.4;10.5	8.2;10.2		7.3
(11101)	1	1	1	5.6			7.4
(01000)	0*	0	1*	8.2	10.1	Chain 8	8.1
(01001)	1*	1*	1	8.3	10.2		8.2

(01011)	1	1	1	8.4	10.3		8.3
(11011)	1	1	1	10.6	9.3		8.4
(10000)	0*	0	1*	9.2	10.1	Chain 9	9.1
(10001)	1*	1*	1	9.3	10.2		9.2
(10011)	1	1	1	9.4	10.3		9.3
(10111)	1	1	1	10.6	10.4		9.4
(00000)	0	0	0	10.2		Chain 10	10.1
(00001)	1*	0*	0	10.3			10.2
(00011)	1	1*	0	10.4			10.3
(00111)	1	1	1	10.5			10.4
(01111)	1	1	1	10.6			10.5
(11111)	1	1	1				10.6
Total Calls	**13**	**13**	**12**				

Table 1. Dynamic sequence used to interview an expert.

For instance, the binary vector ((01100) could represent five binary attributes, such as positive for the disease (1) and negative for the disease (0) for the last five-year observations of a patient. These attributes could also be months, weeks, minutes, or any other time interval.

Suppose for case #1.1 an expert gave the answer $f_1(01100)=0$. This 0 value could be extended in column 2 for case #7.1 (00100) and case #8.1 (01000) as there is more evidence in support of $f_1=0$. These cases are listed in column 6 in the row for case #1.1. There is no need to ask an expert about cases #7.1 and #8.1. Monotonicity is working for them.

On the other hand, the negative answer $f_1(01100)=0$ can not be extended for $f_1(11100)$ as there is more evidence in support of $f_1=1$. An expert should be asked about $f_1(11100)$ value.

If the answer is negative, i.e., $f_1(11100)=0$, then this value can be extended for cases #5.1 and # 3.1. Similar to case #1.1 these cases are listed in column 6 for case #1.2.

Because of monotonicity, the value of f_1 for cases #5.1 and #3.1 will also be 0. In other words, the values in column 2 for f_1 are derived by **up-down sliding** in table 1 according to the following five steps:

Step 1.

Action: Begin with the first case #1.1, (01100). Ask the expert about the value of $f_1(01100)$.

Result: Here the expert reported that $f_1(01100)=1$.

Step 2.

Action: Write the value for case #1.1 under column 2.

Here a "1^*" is recorded next to vector (01100). Recall that an asterisk denotes an answer directly provided by the expert. The case of having the true value corresponds to column 5. (If the reply was false (0), then "0^*" is written in column 2. The case of having a false value corresponds to column 6.)

Step 3.

Action: Based on the response of true by the expert in step 1, check column 5 or 6 respectively to extend the given value. Here column 5 is checked as the response given for case #1.1 is true.

Result: Extend the response to the cases listed. Here cases #1.2, #6.3, and #7.3 are defined as 1. Therefore, in column 2 for cases #1.2, #6.3, and #7.3 the values of the function f1 must be (1). Note that no asterisk is used because these are extended values.

Step 4. (Iterate until finished).

Action: Go to the next vector (called sliding down), here case #1.2. Check whether the value of f_1 has already been derived. If the value of f_1 is not fixed (i.e., it is empty), repeat steps 1-3, above for this new vector. If f_1 is not empty (i.e., it has been already derived), then apply step 3 and slide down to the next vector. Here cases #6.4 and #7.4 are extended and then one moves to case #2.1. Note, that if the value has not yet been fixed, then it will be denoted by $f_1(x)=e$ (e for empty).

Result: Values of the function are extended. Here since for case #1.2 $f_1(11100)\ )\neq e$, the values of the function for the cases #6.4 and #7.4 are extended without asking an expert.

Here the total number of cases with an asterisk (*) in column 1 is equal to 13. For columns 3 and 4, the number of asterisks is 13 and 12, respectively. These numbers show that 13 questions are needed to restore each of f_1 and f_2 and 12 questions are needed to restore ψ as functions of five variables.

As we have already mentioned, this is only 37.5% of 32 total possible questions and 60% of the potential maximum of 20 questions generated by Hansel lemma. Table 2 shows this result more specifically.

Search methods	f_1, f_2	f_2	Decreasing coefficient	
			f_1, f_2	ψ
Non-optimized search (upper limit)	32	32	1	1
Optimal search (upper limit)	20	20	1.6	1.6
Optimal search (actual performance)	13	12	2.5	2.67

Table 2. Comparison of search results for five attributes.

The next step is obtaining learned rules from table 1. In order to construct rules, one needs to concentrate on the information contained in columns 2, 3 and 4 of table 1.

One needs to take the first vector marked with "1*" in each one of the chains and construct a conjunction of non-zero components. For instance, for the vector (01010) in chain 2, the corresponding conjunction is x_2x_4. Based on these conjunctions, column 4 in table 1 and the steps listed below, the following function $\psi(x_1,x_2,x_3,x_4,x_5)$ was obtained:

$$\psi(x)=x_1x_2 \vee x_2x_3 \vee x_2x_4 \vee x_1x_3 \vee x_1x_4 \vee x_2x_3x_4 \vee x_2x_3x_5 \vee x_2 \vee x_1 \vee x_3x_4x_5.$$

Steps:

1. Find all the **lower units** for all chains as elementary functions.
2. Exclude the redundant terms (conjunctions) from the end formula.

Let us explain the concept of lower unit with an example. In chain 6 of table 1 the case #6.2 is a maximal lower unit, because f_1 for this case is equal to 1 and the prior case, #6.1, has an f_1 value equal to 0. Similarly, the case #6.1 will be referred to as an **upper zero**.

The Boolean function $\psi(x)$ can be simplified to $\psi(x)=x_2 \vee x_1 \vee x_3x_4x_5$.

Similarly, the target functions $f_1(x)$ and $f_2(x)$ can be obtained from columns (2 and 3) in table 1 as follows:

$$f_1(x)= x_2x_3 \vee x_2x_4 \vee x_1x_2 \vee x_1x_4 \vee x_1x_3 \vee x_3x_4 \vee x_3 \vee x_2x_5 \vee x_1x_5 \vee x_5,$$

$$f_2(x)= x_2x_3 \vee x_1x_2x_4 \vee x_1x_2 \vee x_1x_3x_4 \vee x_1x_3 \vee x_3x_4 \vee x_3 \vee x_2x_5 \vee x_1x_5 \vee x_4x_5.$$

Hansel chains. This sequence of questions is not accidental. As mentioned above, it is inferred from the Hansel lemma to get a minimal number of questions in the process of restoring a **complete rule**. Here by complete rule we mean restoring a function for all possible inputs.

Below the general steps of the algorithm for chain construction are considered. All 32 possible cases with five binary attributes (x_1, x_2, x_3, x_4, x_5) are presented in column 1 in table 1. They have been grouped according to the Hansel lemma.

These groups are called Hansel chains. The sequence of chains begins from the shortest length chain #1 -- (01100) and (11100). This chain consists only of two ordered cases (vectors), (01100) < (11100) for five binary attributes. Then largest chain #10 consists of 6 ordered cases:

(00000) < (00001) <(00011) < (00111) < (01111) < (11111).

To construct chains presented in table 1 (with five dimensions like x_1, x_2, x_3, x_4, x_5) a sequential process is used, which starts with a single attribute and builds to all five attributes. A standard mathematical notation is used. For example, we will consider all five-dimensional vectors as points in 5-dimensional binary "cube",

$E_5 =\{0,1\}x\{0,1\}x\{0,1\}x\{0,1\}x\{0,1\}$.

First, all 1-dimensional chains (in $E_1=\{0,1\}$) are generated. Each step of chain generation consists of using current i–dimensional chains to generate (i+1) dimensional chains. Generating of chains for the next dimension (i+1) is four–step **"clone-grow-cut-add"** process. An i-dimensional chain is "cloned" by adding zero to all vectors in the chain. For example, the 1-dimensional chain:

(0) < (1)

clones to its two-dimensional copy:

(00) < (01).

Next we **grow** additional chains by changing the cloned zero to 1.

For example cloned chain 1 from above grows to chain 2:

Chain 1: (00) < (01)

Chain 2: (10) < (11).

Next we **cut** the head case, the largest vector (11), from chain 2 and **add** it as the head of chain 1 producing two Hansel 2-dimencional chains:

New chain 1: (00) < (01) <(11) and

New chain 2: (10).

This process continues through the fifth dimension for $<x_1, x_2, x_3, x_4, x_5>$. Table 1 presents result of this process. The chains are numbered from 1 to 10 in column 7 and each case number corresponds to its chain number, e.g., #1.2 means the second case in the first chain. Asterisks in columns 2, 3 and 4 mark answers obtained from an expert.

The remaining answers for **the same chain** in column 2 are automatically obtained using monotonicity. The value $f_1(01100)=1$ for case #1.1 is extended for cases #1.2, #6.3 and #7.3 in this way. Hansel chains are derived independently of the particular applied problem, they depend only on the number of attributes (five in this case).

9.2.2 Preparation and Construction of the Data and Rules Using MBF

9.2.2.1 Basic Definitions and Results

In this section, the formal definitions of concepts from theory of monotone Boolean functions (MBF) are presented. These concepts are used for construction of an optimal algorithm of interviewing an expert. An optimal interviewing process contains the smallest number of questions asked to obtain "artificial cases" sufficient to restore the diagnostic rules. Let E_n be the set of all binary vectors of length n. Let x and y be two such vectors.

Then, the **vector** $x = (x_1,x_2,x_3,\ldots,x_n)$ **precedes** the vector $(y_1,y_2,y_3,\ldots,y_n)$ (denoted as: $x \geq y$) if and only if the following is true for **all** i=1,…,n:

$$x_i \geq y_i$$

A Boolean function f(x) is **monotone** if for any vectors x, y $\in E_n$, the relation $f(x) \geq f(y)$ follows from the fact that $x \geq y$. Let M_n be the set of all monotone Boolean functions defined on n variables.

A binary vector x of length n is said to be an **upper zero** of a function $f(x) \in M_n$, if f(x) = 0 and, for any vector y such that $y \geq x$, we have f(y)=1.

Also, the term **level** represents the number of units (i.e., the number of the "1" elements) in the vector x and is denoted by U(x).

An upper zero x of a function f is said to be the **maximal upper zero** if

$$U(x) \geq U(y)$$

for any upper zero y of the function f (Kovalerchuk and Lavkov, 1984). We define the concepts of **lower unit** and **minimal lower unit** similarly. A binary vector x of length n is said to be a **lower unit** of a function $f(x) \in M_n$, if f(x) = 1 and, for any vector y from E_n such that $y \geq x$, we obtain f(y) = 0. A lower unit x of a function f is said to be the **minimal lower unit** if

$$U(y) \geq U(x)$$

for any lower unit y of the function f. The **number** of **monotone Boolean functions** of n variables, ψ(n), is given by:

$$\psi(n) = 2^{\binom{n}{\lfloor n/2 \rfloor}(1+\varepsilon(n))}$$

where

$0 < \varepsilon(n) < c(\log n)/n$

and c is a constant (see (Alekseev, 1988; Kleitman, 1969)). Thus, the number of monotone Boolean functions grows exponentially with n.

Let a monotone Boolean function f be defined by using a certain operator A_f (also called an **oracle**) which takes a vector $x = (x_1,x_2,x_3,...,x_n)$ and returns the value of f(x). Let **F** = {F} be the set of all **algorithms** which can solve the above problem and let φ(F, f) be the number of accesses to the operator A_f required to generate f(x) and completely restore a monotone function $f \in M_n$.

The **Shannon function** φ(*n*) (Korobkov, 1965) is defined as:

$$\varphi(n) = \min_{F \in \mathbf{F}} \max_{f \in M_n} \varphi(F, f)$$

Next consider the problem of finding all the maximal upper zeros (lower units) of an arbitrary function f∈Mn by accessing the operator Af. This set of Boolean vectors identifies a monotone Boolean function completely f.

It is shown in (Hansel, 1966) that for this problem the following relation is true (known as Hansel's lemma):

$$\varphi(n) = \binom{n}{\lfloor n/2 \rfloor} + \binom{n}{\lfloor n/2 \rfloor + 1} \quad (1)$$

Here $\lfloor n/2 \rfloor$ is the closest integer number to *n*/2, which is no greater than *n*/2 (floor function).

In terms of machine learning, the set of all maximal upper zeros represents the **border elements** of the negative patterns. In an analogous manner, set of all minimal lower units to represent the border of positive patterns. In this way, a monotone Boolean functionrepresents two **compact patterns**.

Restoration algorithms for monotone Boolean functions, which use Hansel's lemma are optimal in terms of the Shannon function. That is, they minimize the maximum time requirements of any possible restoration algorithm. This lemma is one of the final results of the long-term efforts in monotone Boolean functions started by Dedekind (1897).

9.2.2.2 Algorithm for Restoring a Monotone Boolean Function

Next the algorithm **RESTORE is presented**, for the interactive restoration of a monotone Boolean function, and two procedures **GENERATE** and **EXPAND**, for manipulation of chains.

ALGORITHM "RESTORE" $f(x_1,x_2,...,x_n)$

Input: Dimension n of the binary space and access to an oracle A_f.

Output: A monotone Boolean function restored after a minimal number (according to formula (1)) of calls to the oracle A_f.

Method:

1. Construction of Hansel chains (see section 2.2.3 below).
2. Restoration of a monotone Boolean function starting from chains of minimal length and finishing with chains of maximal length.

This ensures that the number of calls to the oracle A_f is no more than the limit presented in formula (1).

Set I=1; {initialization}
DO WHILE (function $f(x)$ is not entirely restored)
Step 1: Use procedure GENERATE to generate element a_i; which is a binary vector.
Step 2: Call oracle A_f to retrieve the value of $f(a_i)$;
Step 3: Use procedure EXPAND to deduce the values of other elements in Hansel chains (i.e., sequences of examples in E_n) by using the value of $f(a_i)$, the structure of element a_i and the monotonicity property of monotonicity.
Step 4: Set $i \rightarrow i$+1;
RETURN

Table 3. Procedure RESTORE.

PROCEDURE "GENERATE": Generate i-th element a_i to be classified by the oracle A_f.

Input: The dimension n of the binary space.
Output: The next element to send for classification by the oracle A_f.
Method: Begin with the minimal Hansel chain and proceed to maximal Hansel chains.

IF i=1 THEN {where i is the index of the current element} Step 1.1: Retrieve all Hansel chains of minimal length; Step 1.2: Randomly choose the first chain C_1 among the chains retrieved in step 1.1; Step 1.3: Set the first element a_1 as the minimal element of chain C_1; ELSE Set k=1 {where k is the index number of a Hansel chain}; DO WHILE (NOT all Hansel chains are tested) Step 2.1: Find the largest element a_i of chain C_k, which still has no $f(a_i)$ value; Step 2.2: If step 2.1 did not return an element a_i then randomly select the next Hansel Chain C_{k+1} of the same length l as the one of the current chain C_k; Step 2.3: Find the least element a_i from chain C_{k+1}, which still has no $f(a_i)$ value; Step 2.4: If Step 2.3 did not return an element a_i, then randomly choose chain C_{k+1} of the next available length $(l+1)$; Step 2.5: Set $k \leftarrow k+1$;

Table 4. Procedure GENERATE.

PROCEDURE "EXPAND": Assign values of $f(x)$ for $x \leq a_i$ or $x \geq a_i$ in chains of the given length l and in chains of the next length $l+2$. According to the Hansel lemma if for n the first chain has an even length then all other chains for this n will be even. A similar result holds for odd lengths.

Input. The $f(a_i)$ value.
Output. n extended set of elements with known $f(x)$ values.
Method: The method is based on monotone properties:

if $x \geq a_i$ and $f(a_i)$=1, then $f(x)$=1; and

if $a_i \geq x$ and $f(a_i)$=0, then $f(x)$=0.

Step 1.	Obtain x such that $x \geq a_i$ or $x \geq a_i$ and x is in a chain of the lengths l or l+2.
Step 2.	If $f(a_i)$=1, then for all x such that $x \geq a_i$ set $f(x)$=1;
	If $f(a_i)$=0, then for all x such that $a_i \geq x$ set $f(x)$=0;
Step 3:	Store the $f(x)$ values which were obtained in step 2;

Table 5. Procedure EXPAND.

9.2.2.3 Construction of Hansel Chains

Several steps in the previous algorithms deal with Hansel chains. Next we describe how to construct all Hansel chains for a given space E_n of dimension n. First, we give a formal definition of a general chain. A **chain** is a sequence of binary vectors a_1, a_2 ,...a_i, a_{i+1},..., $a_{,i}$ such that a_{i+1} is obtained from a_i by changing a "0" element to a "1". That is, there is an index k such that $a_{i,k}$ = 0, $a_{i+1,k}$ = 1 and for any $t \neq k$, the following is true

$a_{i,t}=a_{i+1,t}$. For instance, the following list of three vectors is a chain <01000, 01100, 01110>. To construct all Hansel chains, we will use an iterative procedure as follows. Let $E_n=\{0,1\}^n$ be the n-dimensional binary cube. All chains for E_n are constructed from chains for E_{n-1}. Therefore, we begin the construction for E_n by starting with E_1 and iteratively proceeding to E_n.

Chains for E_1.

For E_1 there is only a single (trivial) chain and it is <(0), (1)>.

Chains for E_2.

First we consider E_1 and add at the beginning of each one of its chains the element (0). Thus, we obtain the set {00, 01}. This set is called E_2^{min}. In addition, by changing the first "0" to "1" in E_2^{min}, we construct the set E_2^{max} = {10, 11}. To simplify notation, we will usually omit "( )" for vectors as (10) and (11). Both E_2^{min} and E_2^{max} are isomorphic to E_1, clearly,

$$E_2 = E_2^{min} \cup E_2^{max}.$$

However, they are not Hansel chains. To obtain Hansel chains we need to modify them as follows: Adjust the chain <00, 01> by adding the maximum element (11) from the chain <10, 11>. That is, obtain a new chain <00, 01, 11>. Then we need to remove element (11) from the chain <10, 11>. Thus, we obtain the two new chains: <00, 01, 11> and <10>. These chains are the **Hansel chains** for E_2. That is E_2 = {<00, 01, 11>, <10>}.

Chains for E_3.

The Hansel chains for E_3 are constructed in a manner similar to the chains for E_2. First, we double (clone) and adjust (grow) the Hansel chains of E_2 to obtain E_3^{min} and E_3^{max}. The following relation is also true:

$$E_3 = E_3^{min} \cup E_3^{max},$$

where

E_3^{min} = {<000, 001, 011>, <010>}

and

E_3^{max} = {<100, 101, 111>, <110>}.

We then proceed with the same chain modification as for E_2. That is, first we choose two isomorphic chains. At first, let it be two maximal length chains

<000, 001, 011> and <100, 101, 111>.

We add the maximal element (111) from <100, 101, 111> to <000, 001, 011> and drop it from <100, 101, 111>. In this way, we obtain the two new chains:

<000, 001, 011, 111> and <100, 101>.

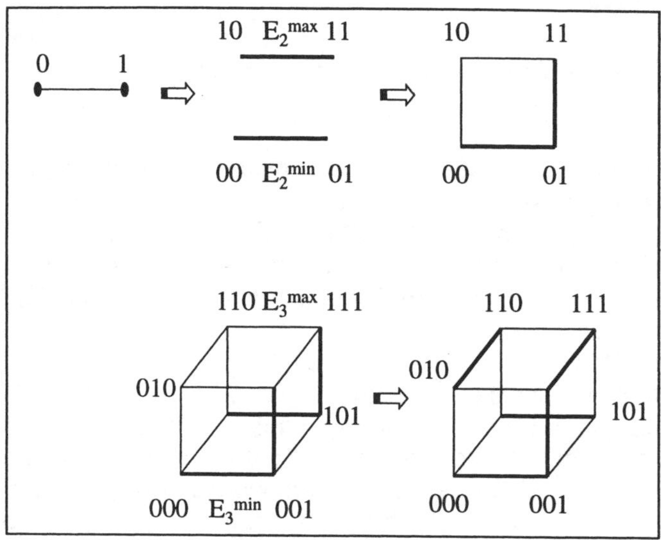

Figure 4. Construction of Hansel chains for E3.

Next, this procedure is repeated for the rest of the isomorphic chains <010> and <110>. In this simple case we will have just one new chain <010, 110> (note that the second chain will be empty). Therefore, E_3 consists of the three Hansel chains

<010, 110>, <100, 101> and <000, 001, 011, 111>.

In a similar manner, one can construct the Hansel chains for E_4, E_5 and so on. Note that the Hansel chains of E_{n-1} can be obtained recursively from the Hansel chains of E_1, E_2,...,E_{n-2}. Figure 4 depicts the above issues for the E_1, E_2 and E_3 spaces.

9.3 Preparation of the Data

9.3.1 Problem Outline

Below we discuss the application of above described methods for medical diagnosis using features extracted from mammograms. In the U.S., breast cancer is the most common female cancer (Wingo et a1. 1995). The most effective tool in the battle against breast cancer is screening mammography. However, it has been found that intra- and inter-observer variability in mammographic interpretation is significant (up to 25%) (Elmore et al. 1994). Additionally, several retrospective analyses have found error rates ranglng from 20% to 43%. These data clearly demonstrate the need to improve the reliability of mammographic interpretation.

The problem of identifying cases suspicious for breast cancer using mammographic information about clustered calcifications is considered. Examples of mammographic images with clustered calcifications are shown in figures 6-8. Calcifications are seen in most mammograms and commonly indicate the presence of benign fibrocystic change. However, certain features can indicate the presence of malignancy. Figures 5-7 illustrate the broad spectrum of appearances that might be present within a mammogram. Figure 5 shows calcifications that are irregular in size and shape. These are biopsy proven malignant type calcifications.

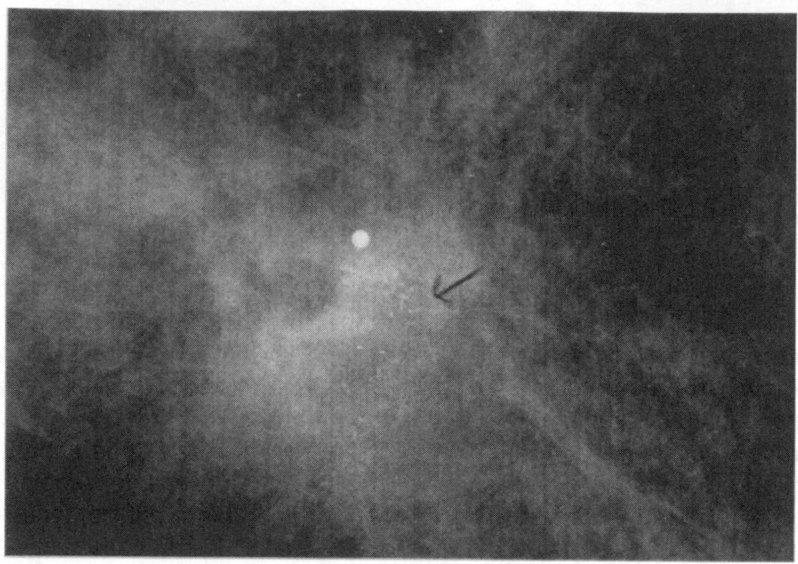

Figure 5. Clustered calcifications produced by breast cancer. Calcifications display irregular contours and vary in size and shape.

Figure 6 presents a cluster of calcifications within a low-density ill-defined mass. Again, these calcifications vary in size, shape and density suggesting that a cancer has produced them. Finally, Figure 7 is an example of a carcinoma, which has produced a high-density nodule with irregular spiculated margins. While there are calcifications in the area of this cancer, the calcifications are all nearly spherical in shape and quite in uniform in their density. This high degree of regularity suggests a benign origin. At biopsy, the nodule proved to be a cancer while the calcifications were associated with a benign fibrocystic change. There is promising Computer-Aided diagnostic research aimed to improve the situation (Shetrn, 1996; SCAR, 1998; TIWDM, 1996, 1998; CAR, 1996).

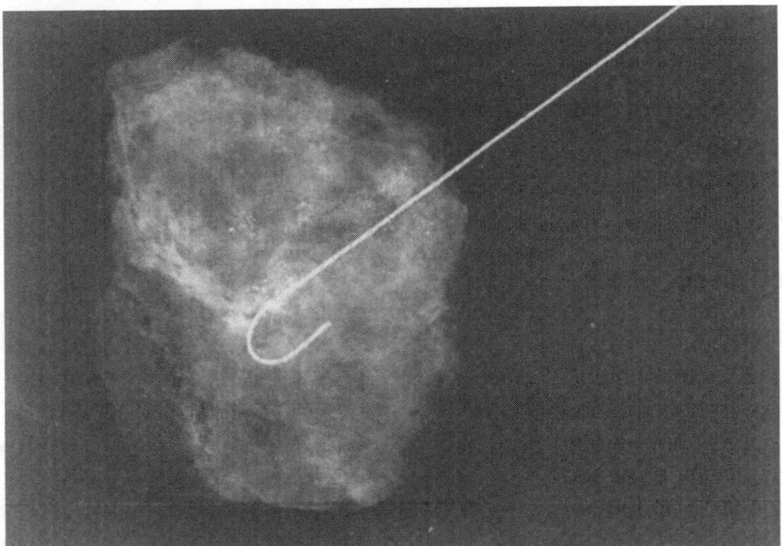

Figure 6. Low density, ill defined mass and associated calcifications.

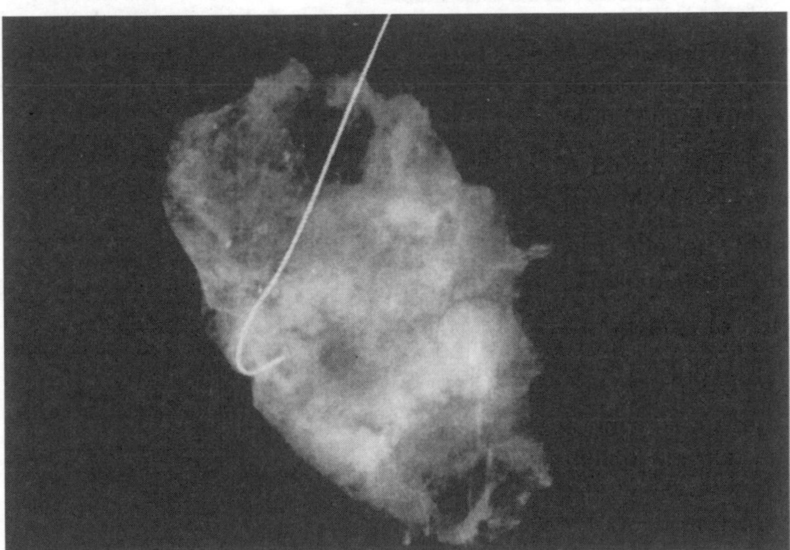

Figure 7. Carcinoma producing mass with spiculated margins and associated benign calcifications.

9.3.2 Hierarchical Approach

The interview of a radiologist to extract ("mine") breast cancer diagnostic rules is managed using an original method described in the previous section. One can ask a radiologist to evaluate a particular case when a number of features take on a set of specific values. A typical query will have the following format:

> "If feature 1 has value V_1, feature 2 has value V_2,..., feature n has value V_n, then should biopsy be recommended or not?
>
> Or, does the above setting of values correspond to a case suspicious of cancer or not?"

Each set of values (V_1, V_2, ...,V_n) represent a possible clinical case. It is practically impossible to ask a radiologist to generate diagnoses for thousands of possible cases. **A hierarchical approach combined with the use of the property of monotonicity makes the problem manageable.**

A hierarchy of medically interpretable features was constructed from a very generalized level to a less generalized level. This hierarchy follows from the definition of the 11 medically oriented binary attributes. The medical expert indicated that the original 11 binary attributes w_1, w_2, w_3, y_1, y_2, y_3, y_4, y_5, x_3, x_4, x_5 could be organized in terms of a hierarchy with development of two new generalized attributes x_1 and x_2:

Level 1 (5 attributes)	Level 2 (all 11 attributes)
x_1	w_1, w_2, w_3
x_2	y_1, y_2, y_3, y_4, y_5
x_3	x_3
x_4	x_4
x_5	x_5,

Five binary features x_1, x_2, x_3, x_4, and x_5 are considered on level 1.

A new generalized feature,

x_1 -- "Amount and volume of calcifications"

with grades (0 - "benign" and 1 - "cancer") was introduced based on features:

w_1—number of calcifications/cm^3,

w_2--volume of calcification, cm^3 and

w_3--total number of calcifications.

Variable x_1 is viewed as a function $x_1=\nu(w_1,w_2,w_3)$ to be identified. Similarly a new feature

x_2—"Shape and density of calcification"

with grades: (1) for "marked" and (0) for "minimal" or, equivalently (1)-"cancer" and (0)-"benign" generalizes features:

y_1 -- "Irregularity in shape of individual calcifications"

y_2 -- "Variation in shape of calcifications"

y_3 -- "Variation in size of calcifications"

y_4 -- "Variation in density of calcifications"

y_5 -- "Density of calcifications".

Variable x_2 is viewed as a function $x_2=\psi(y_1, y_2, y_3, y_4, y_5)$ to be identified for cancer diagnosis. The described structure is presented in fig. 9.

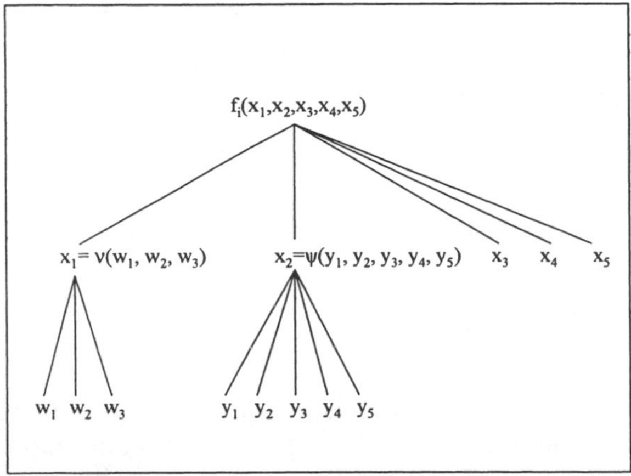

Figure 8. Task decomposition.

A similar structure was produced for a decision regarding biopsy. The expert was requested to review both the structure and answers for the questions:

"Can function f_1 be assumed the same for both problems?

"Can function f_2 be assumed the same for both problems?

The expert indicated that these two functions ν and ψ should be common to both problems: (P1) recommendation biopsy and (P2) cancer diagnosis. Therefore, the following relation is true regarding the f_i (for i = 1, 2) and the two φ, and ψ functions:

$$f_i(x_1,x_2,x_3,x_4,x_5) = f_i(\nu(w_1,w_2,w_3),\ \psi(y_1,y_2,y_3,y_4,y_5),\ x_3,x_4,x_5),\ i = 1,2.$$

Further levels of hierarchy can be developed for better describing the problem. For example, y_1 ("irregularity in shape of individual calcifications") may be found in 3 grades: "mild" (or t_1), "moderate" (or t_2) and "marked" (or t_3). Next observe that it is possible to change (i.e., generalize) the operations used in the function $\psi(y_1,y_2,..,y_5)$. For instance, we may have mentioned function ψ as follows: $\psi(y_1,y_2,..,y_5) = y_1 \& y_2 \vee y_3 \& y_4 \& y_5$, where & and $\vee$ are the binary, logical operations for "AND" and "OR", respectively. Then, & and $\vee$ can be substituted for one of their multivalued logic analogs, for example, $x \& y = \min(x,y)$ and $x \vee y = \max(x,y)$ as in fuzzy logic (see, for example in (Kovalerchuk and Talianski, 1992)). This decomposition is presented in fig. 4.

Assume that x_1 is the number and the volume occupied by calcifications, in a binary setting, as follows: (0-"against cancer", 1-"for cancer"). Similarly, let:

x_2--{shape and density of calcifications}, with values: 0-"benign", 1-"cancer"

x_3--{ductal orientation}, with values: 0-"benign", 1-"cancer"

x_4--{comparison with previous examination}, with values: 0-"benign",1-"cancer"

x_5--{associated findings}, with values: 0-"benign",1-"cancer".

9.3.3 Monotonicity

To understand how monotonicity is applied in the breast cancer problem, consider the evaluation of calcifications in a mammogram. Given the above definitions we can represent clinical cases in terms of binary vectors with five generalized features as: (x_1,x_2,x_3,x_4,x_5). Next consider the two clinical cases that are represented by the two binary sequences: (10110) and (10100). If one is given that a radiologist correctly diagnosed (10100) as a malignancy, then, by utilizing the property of monotonicity, we can also conclude that the clinical case (10110) should also be a malignancy.

This conclusion is based on the **systematic coding of all features "suggestive for cancer" as 1**. Observe that (10100) has two indications for cancer:

x_3=1 (ductal orientation having value of 1; suggesting cancer) and

x_1=1 (amount and volume of calcifications with value 1 indicating cancer).

In the second clinical case we have these two observations for cancer and also $x_4=1$ (a comparison with previous examinations suggesting cancer). In the same manner if (01010) is not considered suspicious for cancer, then the case (00000) should also not be considered suspicious. This is true because in the second case we have less evidence indicating the presence of cancer. The above considerations are the essence of how our algorithms function. They can combine logical analysis of data with monotonicity and generalize accordingly. In this way, the weaknesses of the brute-force methods can be avoided.

It is assumed that if the radiologist believes that the case is malignant, then he/she will recommend a biopsy. More formally, these two sub-problems are defined as follows:

The Clinical Management Sub-Problem (P1): One and only one of the following two disjoint outcomes is possible:

1) "Biopsy is necessary", or:

2) "Biopsy is not necessary".

The Diagnosis Sub-Problem (P2): Similarly as above, one and only one of two following disjoint outcomes is possible. That is, a given case is:

1) "Suspicious for malignancy", or:

2) "Not suspicious for malignancy".

The goal here is to extract the way the system operates in the form of two discriminant Boolean functions f_2 and f_1:

1. Function f_1 returns true (1) value if the decision is "biopsy is necessary", false (0) otherwise.
2. Function f_2 returns true (1) value if the decision is "suspicious for malignancy", false (0) otherwise.

The first function is related to the first sub-problem, while the second function is related to the second sub-problem. There is an important relation between these two sub-problems P1 and P2 and functions $f_1(\alpha)$, $f_2(\alpha)$. The problems are **nested,** i.e., if the case is suggestive of cancer ($f_2(\alpha)=1$) then biopsy should be recommended ($f_1(\alpha)=1$) for this case, therefore, $f_2(\alpha)=1 \Rightarrow f_1(\alpha)=1$. Also if biopsy is not recommended ($f_1(\alpha)=0$) then the case is not suggestive of cancer ($f_2(\alpha)=0$), therefore $f_1(\alpha)=0 \Rightarrow f_2(\alpha)=0$. The last two statements are equivalent to $f_2(\alpha) \geq f_1(\alpha)$ and $f_1(\alpha) \leq f_2(\alpha)$, respectively for case α. Let $E^+_{n,1}$, is a set of α sequences from E_n, such that $f_1(\alpha)=1$ (biopsy positive cases). Similarly, $E^+_{n,2}$ is a set of α sequences from E_n, such that $f_2(\alpha)=1$ (cancer positive cases). Observe, that the **nested property** formally means that $E^+_{n2} \subseteq E^+_{n1}$ (for all cases suggestive of cancer, biopsy should be recommended) and $f_2(\alpha) \geq f_1(\alpha)$ for all $\in E_n$.

The previous two interrelated sub-problems P1 and P2 can be formulated as a **restoration problem of two nested monotone Boolean functions** f_1 and f_2. A medical expert was presented with the ideas of monotonicity and nested functions as above and he felt comfortable with the idea of using nested monotone Boolean functions. Moreover, dialogue that followed confirmed the validity of this assumption. Similarly, the function $x_2=\psi(y_1, y_2, y_3, y_4, y_5)$ for x_2 ("Shape and density of calcification") was confirmed to be a monotone Boolean function.

A Boolean function is a compact presentation of a set of diagnostic rules. A Boolean discriminant function can be presented in the form of a set of logical "IF-THEN" rules, but it is not necessary that these rules stand for a single tree as in the decision tree method. A Boolean function can produce a diagnostic discriminant function, which cannot be produced by the decision tree method. For example, the **Biopsy** Sub-Problem is stated:

$$f_1(x)=x_2x_4 \vee x_1x_2 \vee x_1x_4 \vee x_3 \vee x_5 \qquad (2)$$

This formula is read as follows

IF (x_2 AND x_4) OR (x_1 AND x_2) OR (x_1 AND x_4) OR (x_3) OR (x_5)

THEN Biopsy is recommended

In medical terms this translates as:

IF (shape and density of calcifications suggests cancer AND comparison with previous examination suggests cancer) OR (the number and the volume occupied by calcifications suggests cancer AND shape and density of calcifications suggests cancer) OR (the number and the volume occupied by calcifications suggests cancer AND comparison with previous examination suggests cancer) OR (ductal orientation suggests cancer) OR (associated findings suggests cancer)

THEN Biopsy is recommended.

As was already mentioned in section 2, full restoration of either one of the functions f_1 and f_2 with 11 arguments without any optimization of the interview process would have required up to 2048 calls to the medical expert. Note that practically all studies in breast cancer computer-aided diagnostic systems derive diagnostic rules using significantly less than 1,000 cases (Gurney, 1994). Using the Hansel lemma restoring a monotone Boolean would require at most 924 calls to a medical expert. However, this upper limit of 924 calls can be reduced further. The hierarchy presented in fig. 9 reduces the maximum number of questions needed to restore Monotone Boolean functions of 11 binary variables to 72 questions (non-deterministic questioning) and to 46 using Hansel lemma. The actual number of questions asked was about 40, including both nested functions (cancer and biopsy) (i.e., about 20 questions per function).

9.3.4 Rules "Mined" from Expert

Examples of Extracted Diagnostic Rules. *Below examples of rules discovered using technique described in previous sections are presented.*
EXPERT RULE (ER1):

IF NUMBER of calcifications per cm^2 (w_1) is large

AND TOTAL number of calcifications (w_3) is large

AND irregularity in SHAPE of individual calcifications is marked

THEN suspicious for malignancy

EXPERT RULE 2 (ER2):

IF NUMBER of calcifications per cm^2 (w1) large

AND TOTAL number of calcifications is large (w_3)

AND variation in SIZE of calcifications (y_3) is marked

AND VARIATION in Density of calcifications (y_4) is marked

AND DENSITY of calcification (y_5) is marked

THEN *suspicious for malignancy.*

EXPERT RULE 3 (ER3):

IF (SHAPE and density of calcifications are positive for cancer

AND Comparison with previous examination is positive for cancer)

OR (the number and the VOLUME occupied by calcifications are positive for cancer

AND SHAPE and density of calcifications are positive for cancer)

OR (the number and the VOLUME occupied by calcifications are positive for cancer AND comparison with previous examination is positive for cancer)

OR (DUCTAL orientation is positive for cancer OR associated FINDINGS are positive for cancer)

THEN *Biopsy is recommended.*

In addition, some other rules were extracted. Below these rules are presented briefly in formal notation. MAL stands for suspicious for malignancy.

IF $w_2\&y_1$ THEN MAL

IF $w_2\&y_2$ THEN MAL

IF $w_2\&y\&_3\&y_4\&y_5$ THEN MAL

IF $w_1\&w_3\&y_2$ THEN MAL

IF $w_1\&w_3\&x_5$ THEN MAL

9.3.5 Rule Extraction through Monotone Boolean Functions

Boolean expressions were obtained for shape and density of calcification (see figure 8 for data structure) from the information depicted in table 1 (columns 1 and 4) with the following steps:

(i) Find all the maximal lower units for all chains as elementary conjunctions;

(ii) Exclude the redundant terms (conjunctions) from the end formula. See expression (3) below. Thus, from table 1 (columns 1 and 4) the following formula was obtained

$x_2=\psi(y_1, y_2, y_3, y_4, y_5) =y_1y_2y_2y_3\vee y_2y_4\vee y_1y_3\vee y_1y_4\vee y_2y_3y_4\vee y_2y_3y_5\vee y_2\vee y_1\vee y_3y_4y_5$

and then we simplified it to $y_2\vee y_1\vee y_3y_4y_5$. As above, from columns 2 and 3 in table 1 we obtained the initial components of the target functions of x_1, x_2, x_3, x_4, x_5 for the biopsy sub-problem as follows:

$$f_1(x) = x_2x_3\vee x_2x_4\vee x_1x_2\vee x_1x_4\vee x_1x_3\vee x_3x_4\vee x_3\vee x_2x_5\vee x_1x_5\vee x_5,$$

and for the cancer sub-problem to be defined as:

$$f_2(x) = x_2x_3\vee x_1x_2x_4\vee x_1x_2\vee x_1x_3x_4\vee x_1x_3\vee x_3x_4\vee x_3\vee x_2x_5\vee x_1x_5\vee x_4x_5.$$

The simplification of these disjunctive normal form (DNF) expressions allowed us to exclude redundant conjunctions and produce DNFs. For instance, in x_2 the term y_1y_4 is not necessary, because y_1 covers it.

Using this technique we extracted 16 rules for the diagnostic class "suspicious for malignancy" and 13 rules for the class "biopsy" (see formulas (6) and (7) for mathematical representation).

All of these rules are obtained from formula (6) presented below. Similarly, for the second sub-problem (highly suspicious for cancer) the function that we found was:

$$f_2(x) = x_1x_2 \vee x_3 \vee (x_2 \vee x_1 \vee x_4)x_5 \tag{3}$$

Regarding the second level of the hierarchy (which recall has 11 binary features) we interactively constructed the following functions (interpretation of the features is presented below):

$$x_1 = \nu(w_1, w_2, w_3) = w_2 \vee w_1w_3 \tag{4}$$

and

$$x_2 = \psi(y_1, y_2, y_3, y_4, y_5) = y_1 \vee y_2 \vee y_3y_4y_5 \tag{5}$$

By combining the functions in (2)-(5) the formulas of all 11 features for **biopsy** are obtained:

$$f_1(x) = (y_2 \vee y_1 \vee y_3y_4y_5)x_4 \vee (w_2 \vee w_1w_3)(y_2 \vee y_1 \vee y_3y_4y_5) \vee (w_2 \vee w_1w_3)x_4 \vee x_3 \vee x_5 \tag{6}$$

and for suspicious for **cancer**:

$$f_2(x) = x_1x_2 \vee x_3 \vee (x_2 \vee x_1 \vee x_4)x_5 = (w_2 \vee w_1w_3)(y_1 \vee y_2 \vee y_3y_4y_5) \vee x_3 \vee (y_1 \vee y_2 \vee y_3y_4y_5)$$
$$\vee (w_2 \vee w_1w_3 \vee x_4) \tag{7}$$

9.4 Data Mining

9.4.1 Relational Data Mining Method

A machine learning method called Machine Methods for Discovering Regularities (MMDR) (Vityaev et al. 1992;1993; 1998; Kovalerchuk and Vityaev, 1998; 1999; 2000) can be applied for the discovery of diagnostic rules for breast cancer diagnosis. The method expresses patterns as **relations** in first order logic and assigns probabilities to rules generated by composing patterns.

Learning systems based on first-order representations have been successfully applied to many problems in chemistry, physics, medicine, finance and other fields (Kovalerchuk et al, 1984; 1992; 1997; 1998; Kovalerchuk, Ruiz and Vityaev, 1997;1998;1999; Vityaev et al. 1992; 1993; 1998). As any technique based on logic rules, this technique allows one to obtain **human-readable forecasting rules** that are (Mitchell, 1997)

interpretable in medical language and it provides a presumptive diagnosis. A medical specialist can evaluate the correctness of the presumptive diagnosis as well as a diagnostic rule.

The critical issue in applying data-driven forecasting systems is generalization. MMDR and related “Discovery” software systems (Vityaev et al, 1992;1993;1998) generalize data through “law-like” logical probabilistic rules. Conceptually, **law-like rules** came from the philosophy of science. These rules attempt to mathematically capture the essential features of **scientific laws:** (1) high level of generalization; (2) simplicity (Occam’s razor); and, (3) refutability. The first feature -- generalization -- means that any other regularity covering the same events would be less general, i.e., applicable only to a subset of events covered by the law-like regularity. The second feature – simplicity--reflects the fact that a law-like rule is shorter than other rules. The law-like rule (R1) is more refutable than another rule (R2) if there are more testing examples which refute (R1) than (R2), but the examples fail to refute (R1).

Formally, an IF-THEN rule C is presented as

$$A_1\& \ldots \& A_k \Rightarrow A_0,$$

where the IF-part, $A_1\&\ldots\&A_k$, consists of true/false logical statements $A_1,\ldots,A_k$, and the THEN-part consists of a single logical statement A_0. Statements A_i are some given refutable statements or their negations, which are also refutable. Rule C allows one to generate sub-rules with a truncated IF-part, e.g. $A_1\&A_2 \Rightarrow A_0$, $A_1\&A_2\&A_3 \Rightarrow A_0$ and so on. It is known that a sub-rule is logically stronger than the rule used to construct the sub-rule. Thus, if some rule and its sub-rule C’ classify correctly the same set of examples, then the sub-rule is preferred. In general, there are three reasons to prefer the sub-rule:

1. The sub-rule is more general (logically stronger and describes the same set of events).
2. The sub-rule is simpler then the rule, because it consists of fewer statements in the IF-part.
3. Sub-rule is better testable (more refutable) then the rule, because the larger set of possible examples may falsify it (the IF-part of the sub-rule is less restrictive).

Thus, if a rule covers the set of examples then one can test that no one of its sub-rules also covers the same set of examples. Otherwise, this sub-rule or maybe some of its sub-rules will be preferred, because this sub-rule is simpler, more general and more refutable. In **deterministic case**, a **“law-like” rule** can be defined (for some set of examples) as a rule without sub-rules covering this set of examples. In other words, “law-like” rule is the rule, which is true for some set of examples, but no one of its sub-rule is true for this data.

If examples contain noise, which is typical in medical field, the probabilistic characteristics of the expressions are used instead of crisp (true/false) values. The conditional probability of the rule is used in the MMDR method as this charateristic. For rule C, its conditional probability Prob(C) = $Prob(A_0/A_1\&...\&A_k)$ is defined, assuming that $Prob(A_1\&...\&A_k) > 0$. Similarly conditional probabilities $Prob(A_0/ A_{i1}\&...\&A_{ih})$ are defined for sub-rules C_i, such as $A_{i1}\& ...\&A_{ih} \Rightarrow A_0$., assuming that $Prob(A_{i1}\&...\&A_{ih}) > 0$.

Conditional probability, Prob(C) = $Prob(A_0/A_1\&...\&A_k)$, is used for estimating forecasting power of the rule to predict A_0. In addition, the conditional probability is a major tool for defining **non-deterministic (probabilistic) law-like rules (regularities)** (Vityaev E et al. 1998;1992).

The rule is a **probabilistic "law-like" rule** iff all of its **sub-rules** have a statistically significant **lower conditional probability** than the rule. Another definition of "law-like" rules can be given in terms of generalization. The **rule is "law-like" iff it can not be generalized without producing a** statistically significant reduction in **its conditional probability.** "Law-like" rules defined in this way hold all three listed above properties (properties of scientific laws), i.e., these rules are (1) general from a logical perspective, (2) simple, and (3) refutable. Section 5 presents some breast cancer diagnostic rules extracted using this approach.

The "Discovery" software searches all chains C_1 , C_2 , ..., C_{m-1}, C_m of nested "law-like" subrules, where C_1 is a subrule of rule C_2 , $C_1 = sub(C_2)$, C_2 is a subrule of rule C_3, $C_2 = sub(C_3)$ and finally C_{m-1} is a subrule of rule C_m, $C_{m-1} = sub(C_m)$. Also

$$Prob(C_1) < Prob(C_2), \dots , Prob(C_{m-1}) < Prob(C_m).$$

There is a **theorem** (completeness theorem, Vityaev, 1992) that **all rules, which have a maximum value of conditional probability, can be found at the end of such chains**. The algorithm stops generating new rules when they become too complex (i.e., statistically insignificant for the data) even if the rules are highly accurate on training data. The Fisher statistical criterion is used in this algorithm for testing statistical significance. The obvious other stop criterion is time limitation.

Theoretical advantages of MMDR generalization are presented in (Vityaev et al. 1992;1993;1998, Kovalerchuk and Vityaev, 2000). This approach has some similarity with the hint approach (Abu-Mostafa, 1990). We use mathematical formalisms of first-order logic rules described in (Russel and Norvig, 1995; Halpern, 1990; Krantz et al. 1971; 1989; 1990). Note that a class of general propositional and first-order logic rules, covered by MMDR is wider than a class of decision trees (Mitchell, 1997).

Figure 9 describes the steps of MMDR. In the first step we select and/or generate a class of logical rules suitable for a particular task. The next step is learning the particular first-order logic rules using available training data. Then we test first-order logic rules on training data using Fisher statistical criterion.

After that statistically significant rules are selected and Occam's razor principle is applied: the simplest hypothesis (rule) that fits the data is preferred (Mitchell, 1997). The last step is creating interval and threshold forecasts using selected logical rules: IF A(x,y,...,z) THEN B(x,y,...,z).

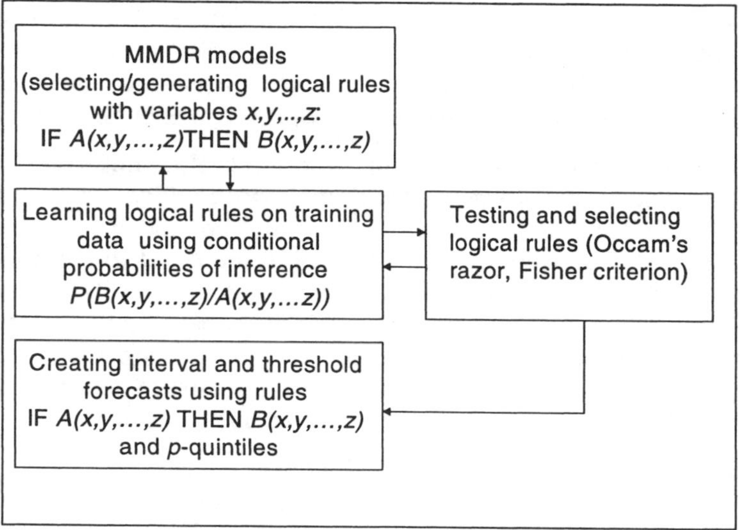

Figure 9. Flow diagram for MMDR: steps and technique applied.

9.4.2 Mining Diagnostic Rules from Breast Cancer Data

The next task is the discovery of rules from data. This study was accomplished using an extended set of features. A set of features listed in section 3.2 was extended with two features:

- *Le Gal type and*

- *Density of parenchyma*

with three diagnostic classes:

1. "malignant"

2. "high risk of malignancy" and

3. "benign".

Several dozen diagnostic rules were extractred with statistical significant on the 0.01, 0.05 and 0.1 levels (F-criterion).

These rules are based on 156 cases (73 malignant, 77 benign, 2 highly suspicious and 4 with mixed diagnosis). In the Round-Robin test the rules diagnosed 134 cases and refused to diagnose 22 cases.

The total accuracy of diagnosis is 86%. Incorrect diagnoses were obtained in 19 cases (14% of diagnosed cases). The false-negative rate was 5.2% (7 malignant cases were diagnosed as benign) and the false-positive rate was 8.9% (12 benign cases were diagnosed as malignant). Some of the rules are shown in table 6. This table resents examples of discovered rules with their statistical significance.

Diagnostic rule	F-criterion for features		Total significance of F-criterion			Accuracy of diagnosis for test cases (%)
			0.01	0.05	0.1	
IF NUMber of calcifications per cm^2 is between 10 and 20 AND VOLume > 5 cm^3 THEN Malignant	NUM VOL	0.003 0.004	+ +	+ +	+ +	93.3
IF TOTal number of calcifications >30 AND VOLume > 5 cm^3 AND DENsity of calcifications is moderate THEN Malignant	TOT VOL DEN	0.023 0.012 0.033	- - -	+ + +	+ + +	100.0
IF VARiation in shape of calcifications is marked AND NUMber of calcifications is between 10 and 20 AND IRRegularity in shape of calcifications is moderate THEN Malignant	VAR NUM IRR	0.004 0.004 0.025	+ + -	+ + +	+ + +	100.0
IF variation in SIZE of calcifications is moderate AND Variation in SHAPE of calcifications is mild AND IRRegularity in shape of calcifications is mild THEN Benign	SIZE SHAPE IRR	0.015 0.011 0.088	- - -	+ + -	+ + +	92.86

Table 6. Examples of extracted diagnostic rules.

Figure 10 presents results for another selection criterion: level of conditional probability of rules. Three groups of rules marked MMDR1, MMDR2 and MMDR3 with levels 0.7, 0.85 and 0.95 are used in this figure. A higher level of conditional probability decreases the number of rules and diagnosed patients, but increases accuracy of diagnosis.

Group MMDR1 contains extracted 44 statistically significant rules for 0.05 level of F –criterion with a conditional probability no less than 0.70. Group MMDR2 consists of 30 rules with a conditional probability no less than 0.85 and 18 rules with a conditional probability no less than 0.95 form MMDR3. The total accuracy of diagnosis is 82%. The false negative rate is 6.5% (9 malignant cases were diagnosed as benign) and the false positive rate was 11.9% (16 benign cases were diagnosed as malignant).

The most reliable 30 rules delivered a total accuracy of 90%, and the 18 most reliable rules performed with 96.6% accuracy with only 3 false positive cases (3.4%).

Neural Network ("Brainmaker", California Scientific Software) software had given 100% accuracy on training data, but for the Round-Robin test, the total accuracy fell to 66%.

The main reason for this low accuracy is that Neural Networks (NN) do not evaluate the statistical significance of the perfect performance (100%) on training data. Poor results (76% on training data test) were also obtained with Linear Discriminant Analysis ("SIGAMD" software, StatDialogue software, Moscow).

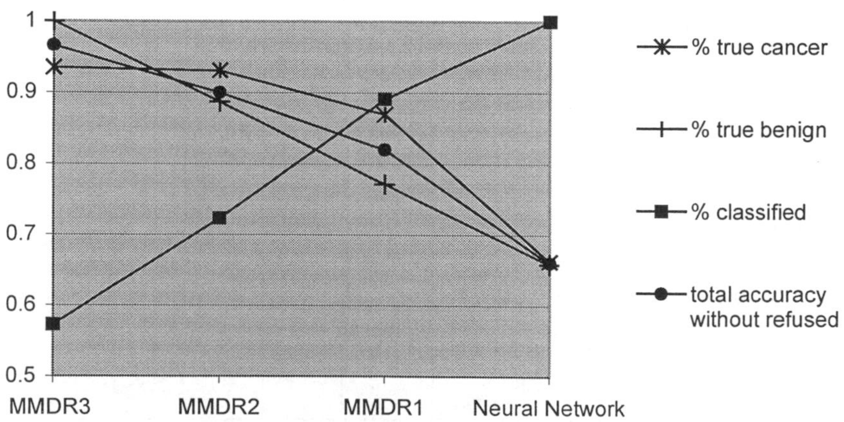

Figure 10. Performance of methods (Round-Robin test).

The Decision Tree approach ("SIPINA" software, Université Lumière, Lyon, France) performed with accuracy of 76%-82% on training data. This is worse than what we obtained for the MMDR method with the much more difficult Round-Robin test (fig. 10). The very important false-negative rate was 3-8 cases (MMDR), 8-9 cases (Decision Tree), 19 cases (Linear Discriminant Analysis) and 26 cases (NN).

In these experiments, rule-based methods (MMDR and decision trees) outperformed other methods. Note also that only MMDR and decision trees produce diagnostic rules. These rules make a computer-aided diagnostic decision process visible, transparent to radiologists. With these methods radiologists can control and evaluate the decision making process.

Linear discriminant analysis gives an equation, which separates benign and malignant classes. For example,

$$0.0670x_1-0.9653x_2+\ldots$$

represents a case. How would one interpret a weighted number of calcifications/cm^2 ($0.0670x_1$) plus a weighted volume (cm^3), i.e., $0.9653x_2$? There is no direct medical sense in this arithmetic.

9.5 Evaluation of Discovered Knowledge

Below we compare some rules extracted from 156 cases using data mining algorithms and by interviewing the radiologist.

From the database the rule DBR1 was extracted:

> **IF** NUMber of calcifications per cm^2 (w_1) is between 10 and 20
>
> AND VOLume (w_2)>5 cm^3
>
> **THEN** Malignant

The closest expert rule is ER1:

> **IF** NUMber of calcifications per cm^2 (w_1) large
>
> AND TOTal number of calcifications (w_3) is large AND
>
> irregularity in SHAPE of individual calcifications (y_1) is marked
>
> **THEN** Malignant

There is no rule DBR1 among the expert rules, but this rule is statistically significant (0.01, F-criterion). Rule DBR1 should be tested by the radiologist and included in diagnostic knowledge base after his verification. The same verification procedure should be done for ER1.

This rule should be analyzed against database of real cases. The analysis may lead to conclusion that the database is not sufficient and rule DB1 should be extracted from the extended database. Also, the radiologist can conclude that the feature set is not sufficient to incorporate rule DBR1 in to his knowledge base. This kind of analysis is not possible for Linear Discriminant analysis or Neural Networks. We also use fuzzy logic to clarify the meaning of such concepts as "Total number of calcifications (w_3) is *large*". The reliability of the expert radiologist against 30 actual cases was tested. The radiologist classified these cases into three categories:

1. "High probability of Cancer, Biopsy is necessary" (or CB).
2. "Low probability of cancer, probably Benign but Biopsy/short term follow-up is necessary" (or BB).
3. "Benign, biopsy is not necessary" (or BO).

These cases were selected from screening cases recalled for magnification views of calcifications. For the CB and BB cases, pathology reports of biopsies confirmed the diagnosis while a two-year follow-up had been used to confirm the benign status of BO.

The expert's diagnosis was in full agreement with his extracted diagnostic rules for 18 cases and for 12 cases he asked for more information than that given in the extracted rule. When he was interviewed he answered that he had cases with the same combination of 11 features but with different diagnosis. This suggests that we need to extend the feature set and the rule set to adequately cover complicated cases. Restoration of Monotone Boolean functions allowed us to identify this need. This is one of the useful outputs from these functions.

The following rule DBR2 was extracted from the database

IF variation in SIZE of calcifications is moderate

AND variation in SHAPE of calcifications is mild

AND IRRegularity in shape of calcifications is mild

THEN Benign.

This rule is confirmed by the database of 156 actual cases using the Round-Robin test. We extracted from this database all cases for which this rule is applicable, i.e., cases where the variation in SIZE of calcifications is moderate; variation in SHAPE of calcifications is mild and IRRegularity in shape of calcifications is mild.

For 92.86% of these cases the rule is accurate. The expert also has a rule with these premises, but the expert rule includes two extra premises:

ductal orientation is not present and there are no associated findings (see formula (6)). This suggests that the database should be extended to determine which rule is correct.

Radiologists Comments regarding Rules extracted from Database.

DB RULE 1:

IF TOTAL number of calcifications >30

AND VOLUME >5 cm^3

AND DENSITY of calcifications is moderate

THEN Malignant.

F-criterion—significant for 0.05.

Accuracy of diagnosis for test cases --100%.

Radiologist's comment—This rule might have promise, but I would consider it risky.

DB RULE 2:

IF VARIATION in shape of calcifications is marked

AND NUMBER of calcifications is between 10 and 20

AND IRREGULARITY in shape of calcifications is moderate

THEN Malignant.

F-criterion—significant for 0.05.

Accuracy of diagnosis for test cases -- 100%.

Radiologist's comment—I would trust this rule.

DB RULE 3:

IF variation in SIZE of calcifications is moderate

AND variation in SHAPE of calcifications is mild

AND IRREGULARITY in shape of calcifications is mild

THEN Benign.

F-criterion—significant for 0.05.

Accuracy of diagnosis for test cases -- 92.86%.

Radiologist's comment—I would trust this rule.

9.6 Discussion

The study has demonstrated how consistent and complete data mining in medical diagnosis can acquire a set of logical diagnostic rules for computer-aided diagnostic systems. Consistency avoids contradiction between rules generated using data mining software, rules used by an experienced radiologist, and a database of pathologically confirmed cases.

Two major problems are identified: (1) to find contradiction between diagnostic rules and (2) to eliminate contradiction. Two complimentary intelligent techniques were applied for extraction of rules and recognition of their contradiction.

The first technique is based on discovering statistically significant logical diagnostic rules. The second technique is based on the restoration of a monotone Boolean function to generate a minimal dynamic sequence of questions to a medical expert.

The results of this mutual verification of expert and data-driven rules demonstrate feasibility of the approach for designing consistent breast cancer computer-aided diagnostic systems.

References

Abu-Mostafa, Y. 1990. Learning from hints in neural networks. Journal of complexity, 6:192-198

Alekseev, V. 1988. Monotone Boolean functions. In: Encyclopedia of Mathematics, Vol. 6. Kluwer Academic Publishers, 306-307

[BI-RADS], 1998. Breast Imaging Reporting and Data System. American College of Radiology, Reston, VA

Dedekind, 1897. Rueber Zerlegungen von Zahlen durch ihre grossten gemeinsamen Teiler, Festschrift Hoch. Braunschweig (in German), u.ges. Werke, 103-148

Dhar, V. and Stein, R. 1997. Intelligent Decision Support Methods. Prentice Hall, NJ

CAR'96, 1996. Computer Assisted Radiology. In: Proceedings of the International Symposium on Computer and Communication Systems for Image Guided Diagnosis and Therapy, Eds. Lemke HU, Vannier MW, Inamura K, Farman AG. Paris, France, June 26-29. Elsevier Science, 1996

Craven, M. and Shavlik, J. 1997. Understanding Time-Series Networks: A Case Study in Rule extraction. International Journal of Neural Systems (special issue on Noisy Time Series), 8 (4):374-384

Elmore, J., Wells, M., Carol, M., Lee, H., Howard, D. and Feinstein, A. 1994. Variability in radiologists' interpretation of mammograms. New England Journal of Medicine 331(22): 1493-1449

Fu, Li Min, 1999. Knowledge Discovery Based on Neural Networks. Communications of ACM 42 (11):47-50

Halpern, J.Y. 1990. An analysis of first-order logic of probability. Artificial Intelligence 46: 311-350

Hansel, G. 1966. Sur le nombre des fonctions Boolenes monotones den variables. C.R. Acad. Sci. Paris, 262(20):1088-1090 (in French)

Giarratano, J. and Riley, G. 1994. Expert systems: principles and programming. RWS, Boston

Gurney, J. 1994. Neural Networks at the crossroads: caution ahead. Radiology 193(1): 27-28.

Kleitman, D. 1969. On Dedekind's problem: The number of monotone Boolean functions. In: 5-th Proceedings of the American Mathematics Society 21:677-682

Korobkov, V. 1965. On monotone Boolean functions of algebraic logic. Problemy Cybernetiki 13:5-28. Nauka, Moscow (in Russian)

Kovalerchuk, B. and Lavkov, V. 1984. Retrieval of the maximum upper zero for minimizing the number of attributes in regression analysis. USSR Computational Mathematics and Mathematical Physics 24(4):170-175

Kovalerchuk, B. and Talianski, V. 1992. Comparison of empirical and computed fuzzy values of conjunction. Fuzzy Sets and Systems, 46: 49-53

Kovalerchuk, B., Triantaphyllou, E. and Vityaev, E. 1995. Monotone Boolean functions learning techniques integrated with user interaction. In: Proceedings of the Workshop "Learning from examples vs. programming by demonstration", 12-th International Conference on Machine Learning, Tahoe City. CA, 41-48

Kovalerchuk, B., Triantaphyllou, E., Despande, A. and Vityaev, E. 1996. Interactive Learning of Monotone Boolean Function. Information Sciences, 94 (1-4):87-118

Kovalerchuk, B., Triantaphyllou, E. and Ruiz, J. 1996. Monotonicity and logical analysis of data: a mechanism for evaluation of mammographic and clinical data. In: Kilcoyne RF, Lear JL, Rowberg AH Eds. Computer applications to assist radiology. Carlsbad, CA, Symposia Foundation, 191-196

Kovalerchuk, B., Triantaphyllou, E., Ruiz, J. and Clayton, J. 1997. Fuzzy Logic in Computer-Aided Breast Cancer Diagnosis. Analysis of Lobulation. Artificial Intelligence in Medicine 11:75-85

Kovalerchuk, B., Vityaev, E. and Ruiz, J.F. 1997. Design of consistent system for radiologists to support breast cancer diagnosis. In: Joint Conf. of Information Sciences (Duke University, NC, USA) 2: 118-121

Kovalerchuk, B., Conner, N., Ruiz, J. and Clayton, J. 1998. Fuzzy logic for formalization of breast imaging lexicon and feature extraction. In: 4th Intern. Workshop on Digital

Mammography, June 7-10, 1998, University of Nijmegen, Netherlands, http://www.azn.nl/rrng/xray/digmam/iwdm98/Abstracts/node51.html

Kovalerchuk, B. and Vityaev, E. 1998. Discovering Lawlike Regularities in Financial Time Series. Journal of Computational Intelligence in Finance, 6 (3):12-26.

Kovalerchuk B., Vityaev, E. 2000. Data Mining in Finance, Kluwer (in print)

Kovalerchuk, B., Ruiz, J., Vityaev, E. and Fisher, S. 1998. Prototype Internet consultation system for radiologists. Journal of Digital Imaging, 11(3): 22-26, Suppl

Kovalerchuk, B., Vityaev, E. and Ruiz, J. 1999. Consistent knowledge discovery in medical diagnosis. Special issue of the journal: IEEE Engineering in Medicine and Biology Magazine: "Medical Data Mining".

Krantz, D.H., Luce, R.D., Suppes, P. and Tversky, A. 1971; 1989; 1990; Foundations of Measurement V.1-3. Acad. Press, NY, London

Mitchell, T. 1997. Machine Learning. NY, McCraw Hill

Muggleton, S. 1999. Scientific Knowledge Discovery Using Inductive Logic Programming. Communications of ACM, 42 (11):43-46

Munakata, T. 1999. Knowledge Discovery. Communications of ACM, 42 (11):27-29

Russel, S., Norvig, P. 1995. Artificial Intelligence. A Modern Approach, Prentice Hall

SCAR'96. 1996. Proceedings of the Symposium for Computer Applications in Radiology. Eds. Kilcoyne RF, Lear JL, Rowberg AH Computer applications to assist radiology. Carlsbad, CA, Symposia Foundation

SCAR'98. 1998. Proceedings of the Symposium for Computer Applications in Radiology. Journal of Digital Imaging 11(3), Suppl

Shavlik, J.W. 1994. Combining symbolic and neural learning. Machine Learning, 14:321-331

Shtern, F. 1996. Novel digital technologies for improved control of breast cancer. In: CAR'96, Computer Assisted Radiology, Proceedings of the International Symposium on Computer and Communication Systems for Image Guided Diagnosis and Therapy, Lemke, H.U., Vannier, M.W., Elsevier, pp.357-361

TIWDM. 1996. Third International Workshop on Digital Mammography. University of Chicago, Chicago, IL, Abstracts, June 9-12, 1996

TIWDM. 1998. 4th Intern. Workshop on Digital Mammography, June 7-10, 1998. University of Nijmegen, Netherlands, 1998, http://www.azn.nl/rrng/xray/digmam/iwdm98/Abstracts/node51.html

Vityaev, E.E. 1992. Semantic approach to knowledge base development. Semantic probabilistic inference. Computational Systems, 146: 19-49, Novosibirsk (in Russian)

Vityaev, E.E. and Moskvitin, A.A. 1993. Introduction to discovery theory: Discovery software system. Computational Systems, 148: 117-163, Novosibirsk (in Russian)

Vityaev, E.E. and Logvinenko, A.D. 1998. Laws discovery on empirical systems. Axiom systems of measurement theory testing. Sociology: methodology, methods, mathematical models (Scientific journal of Russian Academy of Science) 10:97-121 (in Russian)

Wingo, P.A., Tong, T. and Bolden, S. 1995. Cancer statistics. Ca-A Cancer Journal for Clinicians, 45(1): 8-30.

10 A Medical Data Mining Application Based on Evolutionary Computation

Man Leung Wong[1], Wai Lam[2] and Kwong Sak Leung[3]

[1]Department of Information Systems
Lingnan University
Hong Kong, China
[2]Department of Systems Engineering and Engineering Management
The Chinese University of Hong Kong
Hong Kong, China
[3]Department of Computer Science and Engineering
The Chinese University of Hong Kong
Hong Kong, China

In this chapter, we will present data mining techniques for discovering knowledge from a Scoliosis database in the medical domain. Two kinds of knowledge, namely causal structures and rule knowledge, are learned. We employ Bayesian networks to represent causal structures. These networks are capable of depicting the causality relationships among the attributes. Rule knowledge captures interesting patterns and regularities in the database. We develop discovery methods based on Evolutionary Algorithms. Evolutionary Algorithms simulate the natural evolution to perform function optimization and machine learning. In particular, our approach for discovering causality relationships is based on Evolutionary Programming which learns Bayesian network structures. For rule learning, we apply Generic Genetic Programming to discover the rule knowledge. We have discovered new knowledge about the classification of Scoliosis and about the treatment. We demonstrate that the data mining process helps clinicians make decisions and enhance professional training.

10.1 Introduction

Data Mining, or sometimes referred as Knowledge Discovery in Database (KDD), can be defined as the nontrivial process of identifying valid, novel, potentially useful, and ultimately understandable patterns in data (Fayyad et al., 1996). The whole process of KDD consists of several steps. First, the problem domain should be analyzed to determine the objectives. Then, data is collected and an initial exploration is conducted to understand the data. The quality of data should be verified. Next, data preparation such as selection is made to extract relevant or target data set from the database. The data is preprocessed to remove noise and to handle missing data fields. Transformation may be performed to reduce the number of variables under consideration. A suitable data mining algorithm is employed on the prepared data. Finally the result of data mining is interpreted and evaluated. If the discovered knowledge is not satisfactory, these steps will be iterated. The discovered knowledge is then applied in decision making.

10.2 The Problem Domain

We will introduce our approaches for discovering knowledge from a Scoliosis database in the medical domain. Two different kinds of knowledge, namely causal structures and rule knowledge, are learned. Causal structures represented by Bayesian networks capture the causality relationships among the attributes. Rules capture interesting patterns and regularities in the database. We employ Evolutionary Algorithms for these discovery tasks. Evolutionary Algorithms simulate the natural evolution to perform function optimization and machine learning. In particular, our approach for discovering causality relationships is based on Evolutionary Programming which learns Bayesian network structures. For rule learning, we apply Generic Genetic Programming to discover the rule knowledge.

10.3 Understanding the Data

The medical database comes from the Orthopaedic Department of the Prince of Wales Hospital of Hong Kong. Scoliosis refers to the spinal deformation. A Scoliosis patient has one or several curves in his spine. Among them, the curves with severe deformations are identified as major curves. The database stores measurements on the patients, such as the number of curves, the curve locations, degrees and directions. It also records the maturity of the patient, the class of Scoliosis and the treatment.

The database contains 45 attributes including patient name, sex, date of birth, referral source, first visit date, age when menstruction start, associated anomalies, date of initial assessment, major curve degree on initial assessment, major curve rotation on initial assessment, truck shift on initial assessment, risser sign on initial assessment, the vertebra that the first curve started at, date of bracing start, major curve when bracing start, major curve rotation when bracing start, truck shift when bracing start, truck shift direction when bracing start, risser sign when bracking start, risser sign at surgery, joint laxity, whether vertebra L4 is titled, apex of first major curve, apex of second major curve, degree of first curve, degree of second curve, degree of third curve, degree of forth curve, scoliosis classification, treatment, etc.

There are 515 records and information for referral source, first visit date, and associated anomalies is missing in some records.

10.4 Data Preparation

According to the domain expert, 20 attributes, as shown in Table 1, are useful and extracted from the database in the preprocessing step. Some attributes are constructed from other attributes in the database. For example, **Age** is calculated from date of birth, **1stCurveT1** is derived from the vertebra that the first curve started at, **1stMCGreater** is obtained from degrees of the curves. Moreover, **1stMCDeg** and **2ndtMCDeg** are also derived from degrees of the curves.

Some records in the database contain too many missing fields, and thus they are deleted. Finally, the preprocessed database contains 500 records.

Name	Explanation	Possible Value
Sex	Sex	'M' or 'F'
Age	Age	Positive integer
Lax	Joint Laxity	Integer between 0 and 3
1stCurveT1	Whether 1st curve started at vertebra T1	Y or N
1stMCGreater	Whether the degree of 1st Major Curve is greater the 2nd Major Curve	Y or N
L4Tilt	Whether vertebra L4 is tilted	Y or N
1stMCDeg	Degree of 1st Major Curve	Positive integer
2ndtMCDeg	Degree of 2nd Major Curve	Positive integer
1stMCApex	Apex of 1st Major Curve	Any vertebra
2ndMCApex	Apex of 2nd Major Curve	Any vertebra
Deg1	Degree of 1st Curve	Positive integer
Deg2	Degree of 2nd Curve	Positive integer
Deg3	Degree of 3rd Curve	Positive integer
Deg4	Degree of 4th Curve	Positive integer
Class	Scoliosis Classification	K-I, K-II, K-III, K-V, TL, L
Mens	Age of Menstruation	Positive integer
TSI	Trunk Shift (in cm) when bracing start	Positive integer
TSIDir	Trunk Shift Direction when bracing start	Null, left or right
RI	Risser Sign when bracing start	Integer between 0 and 5
Treatment	Treatment	Observation, surgery or bracing

(Vertebras are coded with T1-T12 or L1-L5), (Trunk Shift measures the displacement of the curve), (Risser Sign measures the maturity of the patient)

Table 1. Attributes in the Scoliosis database.

10.5 Data Mining

10.5.1 Evolutionary Computation Background

Evolutionary Computation is a term to describe computational methods that simulate the natural evolution to perform function optimization and machine learning. A potential solution to the problem is encoded as an *individual.* An evolutionary algorithm maintains a group of individuals, called the *population,* to explore the search space. A *fitness function* evaluates the performance of each individual to measure how close it is to the solution. The search space is explored by evolving new individuals. The evolution is based on the Darwinian principle of evolution through natural selection: the fitter individual has a higher chance of survival, and tends to pass on its favorable traits to its offspring. A 'good' parent is assumed to be able to produce 'good' or even better offspring. Thus an individual with a higher score in the fitness function have a higher chance of undergoing evolution. Evolution is performed by changing the existing individuals. New individuals are generated by applying *genetic operators* that alter the underlying structure of individuals. This search technique is a 'weak' method. It is a general, domain independent method that does not require any domain-specific heuristic to guide the search. Examples of algorithms in evolutionary computation include Genetic Algorithm, Genetic Programming, Evolutionary Programming and Evolution Strategy. They mainly differ in the evolution models assumed, the evolutionary operators employed, the selection methods, and the fitness functions used.

10.5.1.1 Genetic Algorithm

Genetic Algorithms (GA) (Goldberg, 1989; Holland, 1992) is a search method for optimization. The goal of GA is to search for values for parameters $x_1, x_2, \ldots, x_n$ that optimizes a fitness function, $f(x_1, x_2, \ldots, x_n)$. The values of parameters are encoded as a fixed-length binary bit string, which becomes the *chromosome* of an individual. For example, if the parameters are real numbers, the binary value of these parameters can be concatenated to form the chromosome, as illustrated in 1. Each individual stores one chromosome. The binary bit string is called the *genotype* of the individual, while the parameter values encoded by the bit string is called the *phenotype* of the individual.

Parameter values: $x_1 = 7$, $x_2 = 5$, $x_3 = 1$

Binary values: $x_1 = 111$, $x_2 = 101$, $x_3 = 01$

Chromosome:

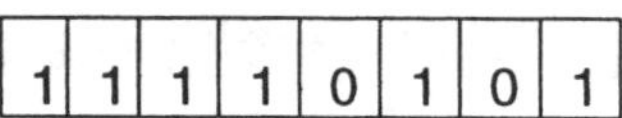

Figure 1. The chromosome in GA.

The algorithm of a simple GA is shown in Table 2. The algorithm begins with an initial population of individuals. The chromosomes of these individuals are randomly generated. Each individual is then evaluated by a fitness function to get a fitness value. The binary bits in the chromosome are decoded and the value of fitness function on this set of parameter values is calculated. Then a number of generations are iterated to evolve better individuals. In each generation, certain individuals are selected from the population of current generation as the parents. The selection is based on the Darwin's principle of survival of the fittest. The probability of an individual being selected is proportional to the fitness of the individual. This selection method is called fitness proportionate selection. The detail of selection methods is discussed in Section 5.1.5. Crossover is performed with a probability of p_c to recombine two parents. If crossover is not performed, then the children is just the same as the parents. The children will further undergo a mutation with a probability of p_m. The mutated children are put into the next generation of population. The generation is iterated until the termination criterion is met. An example of a termination criterion is that an individual can achieved a requirement of fitness value, or the maximum number of generation is exceeded.

Initialize the generation, t, to be 0.

Initialize a population of individual, Pop(t), with size popsize

Evaluate the fitness of all individual in Pop(t)

While the termination criteria is not satisfied

    Initialize Pop(t+1) as an empty set

    While size of Pop(t+1) < popsize

        Select two individuals, parent1 and parent2, from Pop'(t)

        Cross-over parent1 and parent2 to produce child1 and child2

        Mutate child1 and child2

        Evaluate the fitness of child1 and child2

        Put child1 and child2 into Pop(t+1)

    Increase the generation t by 1

Return the individual with the highest fitness value

Table 2. The Simple Genetic Algorithm.

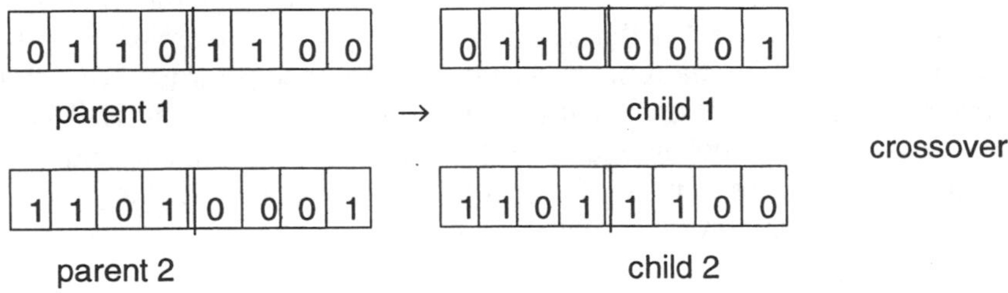

Figure 2. Crossover in GA. The crossover point is the 4th bit and the bits after it are exchanged.

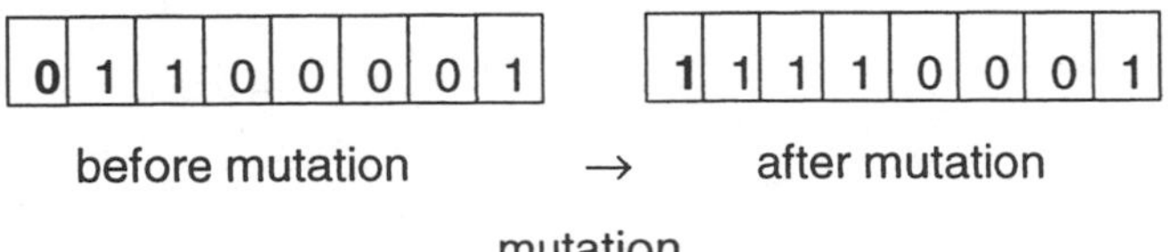

Figure 3. Mutation in GA. Mutation occurs at the 1st bit and the 4th bit.

Crossover exchanges the genetic materials in the chromosomes of two parents to produce two children. A random position in the bit string is chosen. The bits after this crossover point in the parental chromosomes are exchanged, as illustrated in Figure 2. This kind of crossover is called one point crossover. Mutation flips a bit from 0 to 1 or vice versa, as illustrated in Figure 3. Each bit has the same probability p_m of mutation. Mutation is a secondary operator that can restore lost genetic materials. For example, if all the individuals with 0 in the first bit are not selected as parents, then crossover only cannot re-generate a 0 at the first bit. However, mutation can re-introduce this lost 'gene' into the population.

10.5.1.2 Genetic Programming (GP)

Genetic Programming (GP) (Koza, 1992; 1994) is an extension of Genetic Algorithm. They mainly differ on the representation of chromosomes. The chromosome of GA is with fixed length. Each bit in the chromosome has its own meaning. The chromosome of GP is a tree consists of functions and terminals. The phenotype of the chromosome is a computer program, which when executed can solve the problem.

GP evolves a computer program in the language **L**isp. In **L**isp, all operations are executed by performing functions to arguments. A function call is represented as a list of the function and the arguments, enclosed by parentheses. The first element in the list is the function and the subsequent elements are the arguments. This kind of expression is called a S-expression. Every S-expression can be represented in a tree format. A function becomes a parent node and the arguments become the branches. For example, Figure 4 is the tree representing the S-expression **(+ 1 2 (IF (> TIME 10) 3 4))**. The function **IF** returns the second argument if the first argument is true, otherwise the third argument. The symbol **TIME** is a variable. The internal nodes of this tree are the functions and the leaf nodes are the terminals. This tree representation is the knowledge representation of chromosomes used in GP.

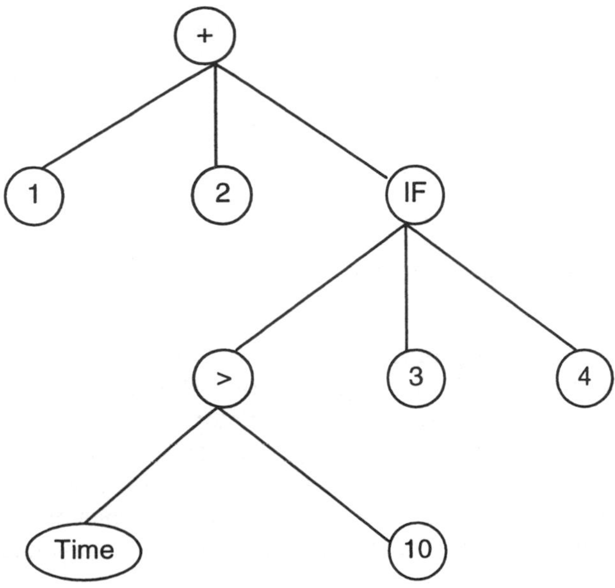

Figure 4. The tree representation of a S-expression.

Initialize the generation, t, to be 0.

Initialize a population of individual, Pop(t), with size popsize

While the termination criteria is not satisfied

    Evaluate the fitness of all individuals in Pop(t)

    Initialize Pop(t+1) as an empty set

    While size of Pop(t+1) < popsize

        Choose a genetic operation probabilistically

        If reproduction

            Select one individual based on fitness

            Copy the individual into Pop(t+1)

        If crossover

            Select two individuals based on fitness

            Perform crossover

            Insert the two offspring into Pop(t+1)

If mutation

Select one individual based on fitness

Perform mutation

Insert the offspring into Pop(t+1)

Increase the generation t by 1

Return the individual with the highest fitness value

Table 3. The Algorithm of Genetic Programming.

To apply GP to a problem, a set of functions *F* and a set of terminals *T* have to be defined. The algorithm of GP is very similar to GA. A set of initial individuals are created randomly from the function set and the terminal set. Each individual is evaluated by a fitness function. New individuals are evolved by genetic operators, including reproduction, crossover and mutation. The generation of evolutions repeated until the termination criterion is satisfied. The algorithm is sketched in Table 3.

To create an individual, a function is selected from *F* to be the root. A number of branches, which equals to the arity of this function, are created from the root. At each branch a symbol is selected from the set $F \cup T$. If a function is selected, the above process repeated recursively.

The genetic operators typically used in GP are reproduction, crossover and mutation. In reproduction, the parent is just copied unchanged to the new population. In crossover, two subtrees are selected from the trees of each parent. These subtrees are exchanged to produce two children, as shown in Figure 5. In mutation, a subtree is selected from the parental tree, and then replaced by a randomly generated subtree, as shown in Figure 6. The generation of the replacing subtree is the same as the generation of the initial population. Mutation is considered as less important in GP. It is because particular functions and terminals are not associated with fixed positions. It is rare for a function or terminal to disappear entirely from all the nodes of all individuals. Thus, mutation is not a necessary operation to restore the lost genetic materials.

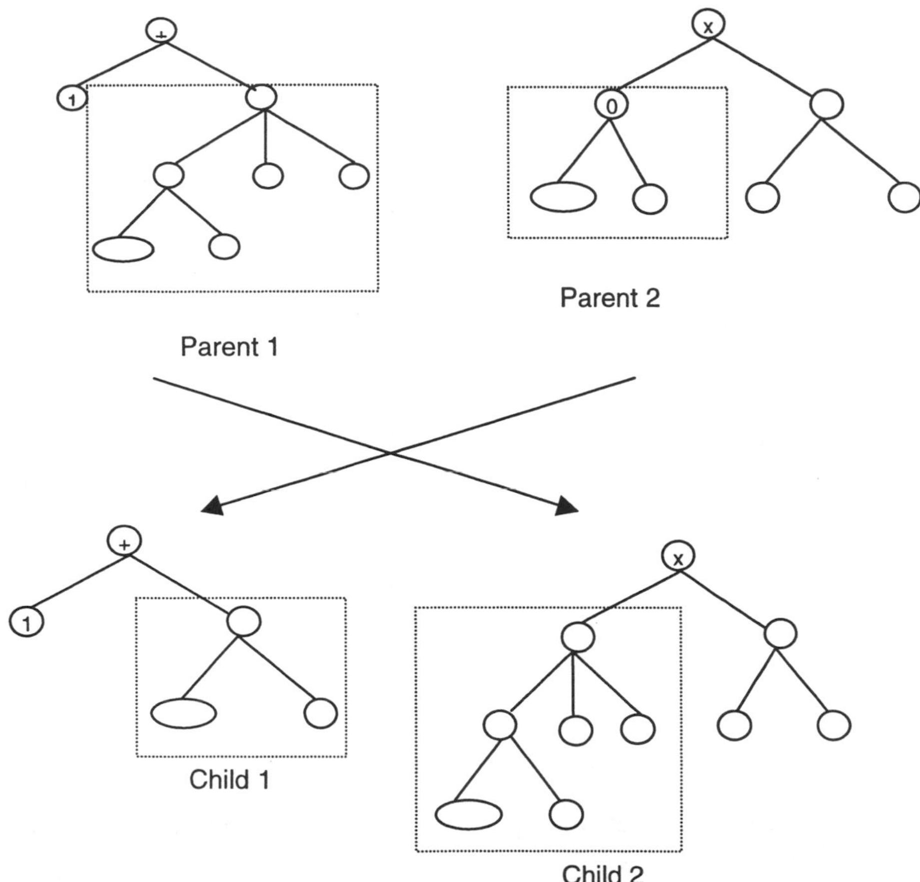

Figure 5. An example of crossover in GP. The selected subtree is enclosed by the dashed box.

10.5.1.3 Evolutionary Programming

Evolutionary Programming (EP) (Fogel et al. 1966; Fogel, 1994) emphasizes on the behavioral linkage between parents and their offspring, rather than seeking to emulate specific genetic operators as observed in nature. Different from GA, EP does not require any specific genotype in the individual. EP employs a model of evolution at a higher abstraction. Mutation is the only operator used for evolution.

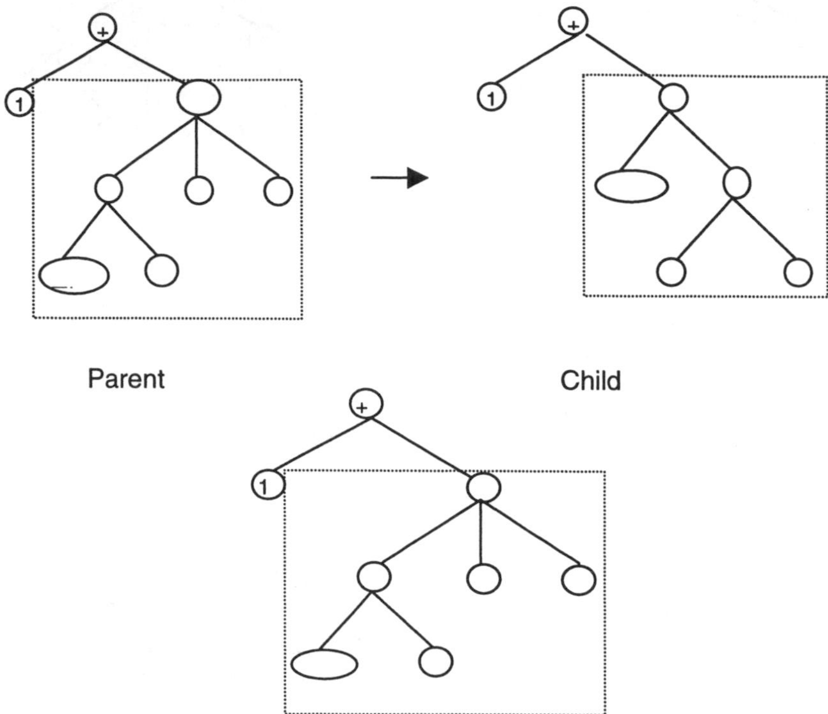

Figure 6. An example of mutation in GP. The selected subtree is enclosed by the dashed box.

A typical process of EP is outlined in Table 4. A set of individuals is randomly created to make up the initial population. Each individual is evaluated by the fitness function. Then each individual produces a child by mutation. There is a distribution of different types of mutation, ranging from minor to extreme. Minor modifications in the behavior of the offspring occur more frequently and substantial modifications occur more unlikely. The offspring is also evaluated by fitness function. Then tournaments are performed to select the individuals for the next generation. For each individual, a number of rivals are selected among the parents and offspring. The tournament score of the individual is the number of rivals with lower fitness scores than itself. Individuals with higher tournament scores are selected as the population of next generation. There is no requirement that the population size is held constant. The process is iterated until the termination criterion is satisfied.

Initialize the generation, t, to be 0.

Initialize a population of individual, Pop(t)

Evaluate the fitness of all individual in Pop(t)

While the termination criteria is not satisfied

  Produce one or more offspring from each individual by mutation

  Evaluate the fitness of each offspring

  Perform a tournament for each individual

  Put the individuals with high tournament scores into Pop(t+1)

  Increase the generation t by 1

Return the individual with the highest fitness value

Table 4. The Algorithm of Evolutionary Programming.

EP has two characteristics. First, there is no constraint on the representation. Mutation operator does not demand a particular genotype. The representation can follow from the problem. Second, mutations in EP attempt to preserve behavioral similarity between offspring and their parents. An offspring is generally similar to its parent at the behavioral level with slight variations. EP assumes that the distribution of potential offspring is under a normal distribution around the parent's behavior. Thus, the severity of mutations is according to a statistical distribution.

10.5.1.4 Evolution Strategy

Evolution Strategy (ES) (Rechenberg, 1973; Schwefel, 1981) is originally designed for real-valued function optimization. It emphasizes on the individual, i.e. the phenotype, to be the object to be optimized. Each parameter is represented as a object variable x_j. Each x_j is associated with a strategy variable σ_j, which controls the degree of mutation to x_j. The genotype of an individual is a vector of pair (x_j, σ_j).

There are various models of evolution strategy. In $(\mu + \lambda)$-ES, the population size is μ, and λ more individuals are evolved in each generation by recombination and mutation. Among these $(\mu + \lambda)$ individuals, only the best μ individuals are kept in the population. The selection is based on the score of an objective function *F*. The evolution terminates when the optimal set of values for all the objective values are found, or when the maximum number of generations is reached.

There are various methods of recombination, and can be classified as non-global and global. In non-global combination, two individuals are selected as parents. For non-global discrete recombination, the value of the pair (x_j,σ_j) of the offspring is selected randomly from one of the parents. For non-global intermediate recombination, the value of the pair (x_j,σ_j) of the offspring is set to the mean value of the two parents. On the other hand, in global recombination, a pair of individuals are selected for each pair of (x_j,σ_j). Thus if the individual contains L pairs of (x_j,σ_j). L pairs of parents are selected. For global discrete recombination, the value of each pair (x_j,σ_j) of the offspring is selected randomly from one of its parents. For global intermediate recombination, the value of each pair (x_j,σ_j) of the offspring is set to the mean value of its parents.

Mutation modifies the value of each x_j as well as each σ_j. According to the biological observation, offspring are similar to their parents and that smaller modifications occur more frequently than larger modifications. Thus the new value of x_j after mutation, x'_j, is equal

$$x'_j = x_j + N(0, \sigma_j)$$

where $N(0, \sigma_j)$ is a Gaussian random number with mean 0 and standard derivation σ_j. A mutation is regarded as successful if the mutated individual has a higher score on F than the parent. The ratio r is the ratio of successful mutations to all mutations. It is observed that the convergence rate is optimal if r equals to 1/5. Thus the new value of σ_j of each individual, σ'_j, is changed based on r:

$$\sigma'_j = \begin{cases} c_d\sigma_j & if \quad r < 1/5 \\ c_i\sigma_j & if \quad r > 1/5 \\ \sigma_j & if \quad r = 1/5 \end{cases}$$

where c_d and c_i are constants. If r is smaller than 1/5, σ is decreased by multiplying a constant $c_d < 1$, so as to generate offspring closer to the parents. If r is larger than 1/5, σ is increased by multiplying a constant $c_i >$ 1, so as to broaden the search.

ES and EP both use a statistical distribution of mutations. However, ES typically uses deterministic selection that the worst individuals are eliminated, while EP typically uses a stochastic tournament selection. EP is an abstraction of evolution at the level of *species* and thus no recombination is used because recombination does not occur between species. In contrast, ES is an abstraction of evolution at the level of individual behavior and hence recombination is reasonable.

10.5.1.5 Selection Methods

The classical method for selection of parents is the fitness proportionate selection (Holland, 1992), or called the 'roulette wheel' selection. The individuals in the population form a roulette wheel, where each individual has a slot sized in proportion to its fitness. The roulette wheel is turned to select the parent. Thus the probability of the i th individual being selected is $f_i / \sum_i f_i$, where f_i is the fitness of the i th individual. However, there is a deficiency in this selection method. In the early generations, a few individuals may have extraordinarily high fitness values. Fitness proportionate selection allocates a large number of offspring to these individuals, and cause premature convergence. At the later stages, the individuals may have very close fitness values. Fitness proportionate selection cannot differentiate the better individuals and allocates an almost equal number of offspring to all individuals.

Alternative selection methods have been proposed. In the rank selection method (Baker, 1985), the population is sorted according to the fitness. The probability of an individual being selected is proportional to its rank, with the better one getting a higher chance. For example, the probability for selecting an individual can be $(N + 1 - r_i) / \sum^{N}_{k=1} k$, where N is the population size and r_i is the rank of the individual. This selection method gives less emphasis on comparatively high-fitness individuals. On the other hands, it can distinguish individuals with a slightly difference in the fitness scores. In the tournament selection method, a group of individuals with size q are selected from the population. Among this group, the individual with the highest fitness value is selected. This selection method simulates the phenomenon that several individuals fight over the right of mating. However in these two methods, the probability of selection is not directly linked with the value of the objective function for optimization.

10.5.1.6 Data Mining using Evolutionary Computation

Data mining can be considered as an optimization problem, which tries to search for the most accurate information from all possible hypotheses. Since evolutionary computation is a robust and parallel search algorithm, it can be used in data mining to find interesting knowledge in noisy environment. Several systems have been built for learning concepts using evolutionary computation. GA can be used as the search algorithm by encoding a description of a concept into a bit string. However, the fixed-length chromosome in GA limited the representation of concept.

GABIL (De Jong et al. 1993) uses a flat string representation to encode classification rules in disjunctive normal form (DNF). It uses the Pittsburgh's approach (Smith, 1980; 1983) that a single individual contains all the necessary descriptions for a concept and corresponds to a set of rules. Each individual is a variable-length string representing a set of rules. Each rule has a fixed length and consists of one test for each feature. The system uses *k* bits for the *k* values of a nominal feature. For example, the bit string in Table 5 represents the rule "if (F1 = 1 or 2 or 3) and (F2 = 1) then (class = 0)". Adaptive GABIL can adaptively allow or prohibit certain genetic operations for certain individuals. Extra bits are introduced to control the uses of certain genetic operations. These bits are also parts of evolution in GA.

F1			F2				Class
1	1	1	1	0	0	0	0

Table 5. Bit string in GABIL.

GIL (Janikow, 1993) also used the Pittsburgh's approach. The bit string of an individual represents a rule in multiple-valued logic language VL_1. It utilizes 14 genetic operators, such as rules exchange, new event, rules drops, rule split, condition drop, condition introduce, reference change and etc. These operators perform generalization, specialization or other modifications to the individuals in the rule set level, the rule level and the condition level.

In REGAL (Giodana and Neri, 1995), each individual encodes a disjunct consists of a conjunctive formula. Each individual is only a partial solutions, and the whole population is a redundant set of these partial solutions. An individual encodes a concept represented in the first-order logic, which is a language with variables. Several good individuals co-exist in the population by the use of a selection operator called Universal Suffrage operator to select the parents. At each generation, a set of examples is selected. The individuals covering a selected example are collected into a set. This set corresponds to a roulette wheel and a spin is made to select a winning individual. The winning individual from the selected examples becomes the parents. A parallel model is designed to enhance the execution speed.

GP can perform data mining by learning a program for classification. An example is the approach developed by (Tackett, 1993). It uses a function set of (+,-,×,÷) and the conditional operator ≤, and a terminal set of all the 20 input features plus a random floating point constant. A program is evolved by GP. If the program returns a value larger than or equal to 0 given an input case, the input case is classified as a target. Otherwise it is classified as a non-target. Since the learned program is human understandable, knowledge can be obtained by examining the program. However, the program can be very complicated and difficult to interpret.

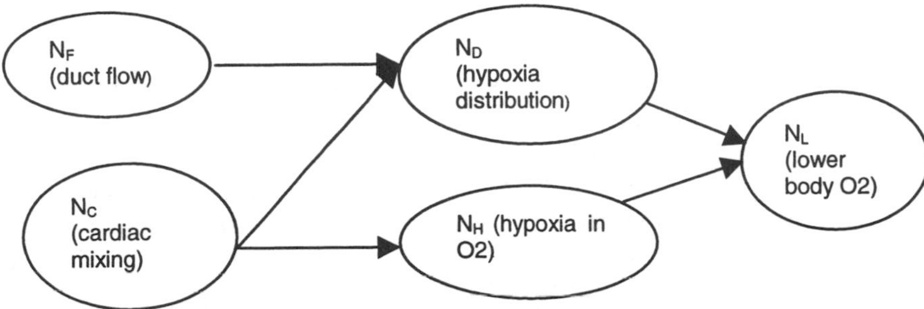

Figuare 7. A Bayesian Network Structure in a "Blue" Baby Domain.

10.5.2 Causal Structure Analysis

10.5.2.1 Bayesian Networks

The causal structure analysis mainly discovers a Bayesian network from the data. A Bayesian network is a formal knowledge representation supported by the well-developed Bayesian probability theory. A Bayesian network captures the conditional probabilities between attributes. It can be used to perform reasoning under uncertainty. A Bayesian network is a directed acyclic graph. Each node represents a domain variable, and each edge represents a dependency between two nodes. An edge from node *A* to node *B* can represent a causality, with *A* being the cause and *B* being the effect. The value of each variable should be discrete. Each node is associated with a set of parameters. Let N_i denote a node and Π_{Ni} denote the set of parents of N_i The parameters of N_i are conditional probability distributions in the form of $P(N_i | \Pi_{Ni})$with one distribution for each possible instance of Π_{Ni}. Figure 7 is an example Bayesian network structure modeling a medical domain concerned with "blue" baby diagnosis. This structure shows the causality relationships between the direction of duct flow, the degree of cardiac mixing, hypoxia distribution, hypoxia in O_2 and the degree of lower body O_2.

After the network is constructed, it can be used for conducting reasoning. A common and useful kind of reasoning is to perform probabilistic inferences. The process of inference is to use the evidence of some of the nodes that have observations to find the probability of some of the other nodes in the network. We calculate the posterior probability distribution of some other nodes given the observed nodes instantiated with some states. More details of Bayesian networks can be found in (Charniak, 1991; Heckerman and Wellman, 1995).

The main task of learning Bayesian network from data is to automatically find directed edges between the nodes, such that the network can best describe the causalities. Once the network structure is constructed, the conditional probabilities are calculated based on the data. The problem of Bayesian network learning is computationally intractable (Cooper, 1990). However, Bayesian network learning can be implemented by imposing limitations and assumptions. For instance, the algorithms of Chow and Liu (1968) and Rebane and Pearl (1989) can learn networks with tree structures, while the algorithms of Herskovits and Cooper (1990; 1992) and Bouckaert (1994) require the variables to have a total ordering. More general algorithms include Heckerman *et al.* (1995), Spirtes *et al.* (1993) and Singh and Valtorta (1993). More recently, Larranaga *et al.* (1996; 1996) have proposed algorithms for learning Bayesian networks using Genetic Algorithms.

10.5.2.2 The Learning Approach

The learning approach is based on Lam and Bacchus's work (1994; 1998) on employing the Minimum Description Length principle to evaluate a Bayesian network. Evolutionary Programming is employed to optimize this metric in order to search for the best network structure (Wong et al. 1999).

The *Minimum Description Length* (MDL) metric measures the *total description length* $D_t(B)$ of a network structure B. A better network has a smaller value on this metric. Let $N = \{N_1, \ldots, N_n\}$ denote the set of nodes in the network (and thus the set of variables, since each node represents a variable), and Π_{N_i} denote the set of parents of node N_i. The total description length of a network is the sum of description lengths of each node:

$$D_t(B) = \sum_{N_i \in N} D_t(N_i, \Pi_{N_i})$$

(1)

This length is based on two components, the *network description length D_n* and the *data description length D_d* :

$$D_t(N_i, \Pi_{N_i}) = D_n(N_i, \Pi_{N_i}) + D_d(N_i, \Pi_{N_i})$$

(2)

The formula for the network description length is:

$$D_n(N_i, \Pi_{N_i}) = k_i \log_2(n) + d(s_i - 1) \prod_{j \in \Pi_{N_i}} s_j$$

(3)

where k_i is the number of parents of variable N_i, s_i is the number of values N_i can take on, s_j is the number of values a particular variable in Π_{Ni} can take on, and d is the number of bits required to store a numerical value. This is the description length for encoding the network structure. The first part in the addition is the length for encoding the parents, while the second part is the length for encoding the probability parameters. This length can measure the simplicity of the network.

The formula for the data description length is:

$$D_d(N_i, \Pi_{N_i}) = \sum_{N_i \in \Pi_{N_i}} M(N_i, \Pi_{N_i}) \log_2 \frac{M(\Pi_{N_i})}{M(N_i, \Pi_{N_i})}$$

(4)

where $M(.)$ is the number of cases that match a particular instantiation in the database. This is the description length for encoding the data. A Huffman code is used to encode the data using the probability measure defined by the network. This length can measure the accuracy of the network.

10.5.2.3 Combining MDL and EP

We combine the MDL metric and EP for Bayesian network learning (Lam et al. 1998). The flowchart in Figure 8 shows the process. Each individual represents a network structure, which is a directed acyclic graph (DAG). A set of individuals is randomly created to make up the initial population.

Each graph is evaluated by the MDL metric described above. Then, each individual produces a child by performing a number of mutations. The child is also evaluated by the MDL metric. The next generation of population is selected among the parents and children by tournaments. Each DAG B is compared with q other randomly selected DAGs. The tournament score of B equals to the number of rivals that B can win, that is, the number of DAGs among those selected that have higher MDL scores than B. In our setting, the value of q is 5. One half of DAGs with the highest tournament scores are retained for the next generation. The process is repeated until the maximum number of generations is reached. The number of the maximum number of generations depends on the complexity of the network structure. If we expect a simple network, the maximum number of generations can be set to a lower value. The network with the lowest MDL score is output as the result.

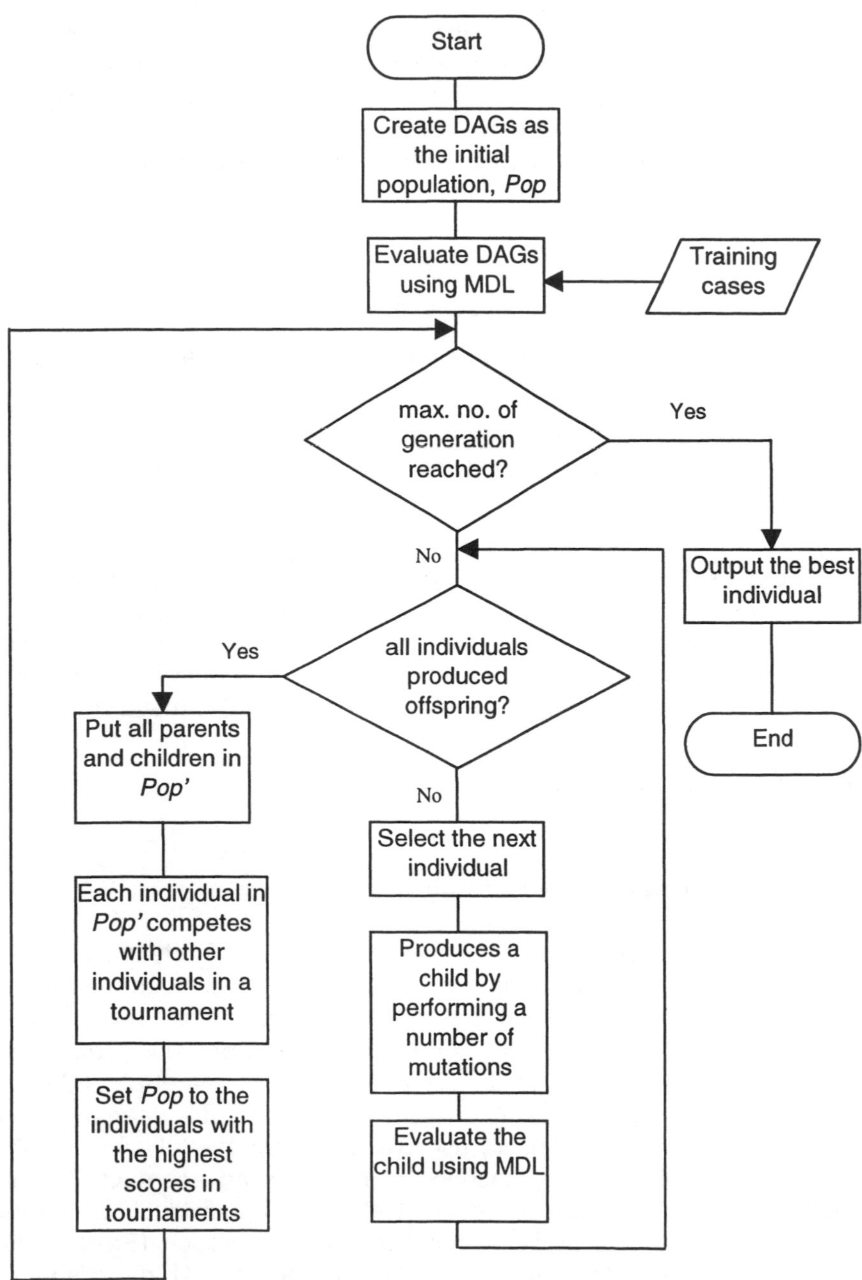

Figure 8. The flowchart of the Bayesian network learning process.

10.5.2.4 The Mutation Operators

Offspring in EP is produced by using a specific number of mutations. The probabilities of using 1, 2, 3, 4, 5 or 6 mutations are set to 0.2, 0.2, 0.2, 0.2, 0.1 and 0.1 respectively. The mutation operators modify the edges of the DAG. If a cyclic graph is formed after the mutation, edges in the cycles are removed to keep it acyclic. Our approach uses four mutation operators, with the same probabilities of being used:

1. Simple mutation randomly adds an edge between two nodes or randomly deletes an existing edge from the parent.
2. Reversion mutation randomly selects an existing edge and reverses its direction.
3. Move mutation randomly selects an existing edge. It moves the parent of the edge to another node, or moves the child of the edge to another node.
4. Knowledge-Guided mutation is similar to simple mutation, but the MDL scores of the edges guide the selection of the edge to be added or removed. The MDL metric of all possible edges in the network is computed before the learning algorithm starts. This mutation operator stochastically adds an edge with a small MDL metric to the parental network or deletes an existing edge with a large MDL metric.

10.5.3 Rule Learning

10.5.3.1 Rule Learning Background

Another kind of knowledge to be discovered are rules. A rule is a sentence of the form "if *antecedents*, then *consequent*". Rules are commonly used in expressing knowledge and are easily understood by human. Rule learning is the process of inducing rules from a set of training examples. Classical algorithms in this field include AQ15 (Michalski et al. 1986) and CN2 (Clark and Niblett, 1989). Previous works in rule learning using Evolutionary Computation mainly use GA (Goldberg 1989; Holland, 1992). There are two different approaches. In the Michigan approach (Holland and Reitman, 1978; Booker et al. 1989) each individual in the GA corresponds to a rule, while in the Pittsburgh approach (Smith, 1980; 1983) it corresponds to a *set* of rules. The system REGAL (Giordana and Neri, 1995) uses the Michigan approach and a distributed genetic algorithm to learn first-order logic concept descriptions. It uses a selection operator, called Universal Suffrage operator, to achieve the learning of multi-modal concepts. Another system GABIL (De Jong et al. 1993) uses the Pittsburgh approach. It can adaptively allow or prohibit certain genetic operations for certain individuals. GIL (Janikow, 1993) also uses the Pittsburgh's approach and utilizes 14 genetic operators. These operators perform generalization, specialization or other modifications to the individuals at the rule set level, the rule level and the condition level.

Our learning approach is based on Generic Genetic Programming (GGP) (Wong and Leung, 1992; 1997; Wong 1995), which is an extension to Genetic Programming (GP). It uses a grammar (Hopcroft and Ullman, 1979) to control the structures evolved in GP.

10.5.3.2 The Generic Genetic Programming Process

The flowchart in Figure 9 shows the process of using GGP for rule learning. A grammar is provided as a template for rules. The algorithm starts with an initial population of randomly created rules using the user-defined grammar. One individual corresponds to one rule. Each rule is evaluated by a fitness function. Then, individuals are selected stochastically to evolve offspring by the genetic operators. Rules with higher fitness scores have higher chances of being selected. The three genetic operators, crossover, mutation and dropping condition are presented in detail below. In each generation, the number of new individuals evolved equals to the population size. Thus at this stage, the number of individuals is doubled. All individuals participate in a token competition and a replacement step (Ngan et al. 1999), so as to eliminate similar rules and increase the diversity. One half of the individuals with the higher fitness scores after token competition are passed to the next generation.

To estimate the fitness scores of individuals a data set is used in GGP. The data set should be partitioned into a training set and a testing set. Only the training set is available for the learning process. After the maximum number of generations is reached, the discovered rules are further evaluated with the unseen testing set, so as to verify their accuracy and reject the rules that over-fit the training set. Our system uses 60% of the data for the training set and 40% for the testing set.

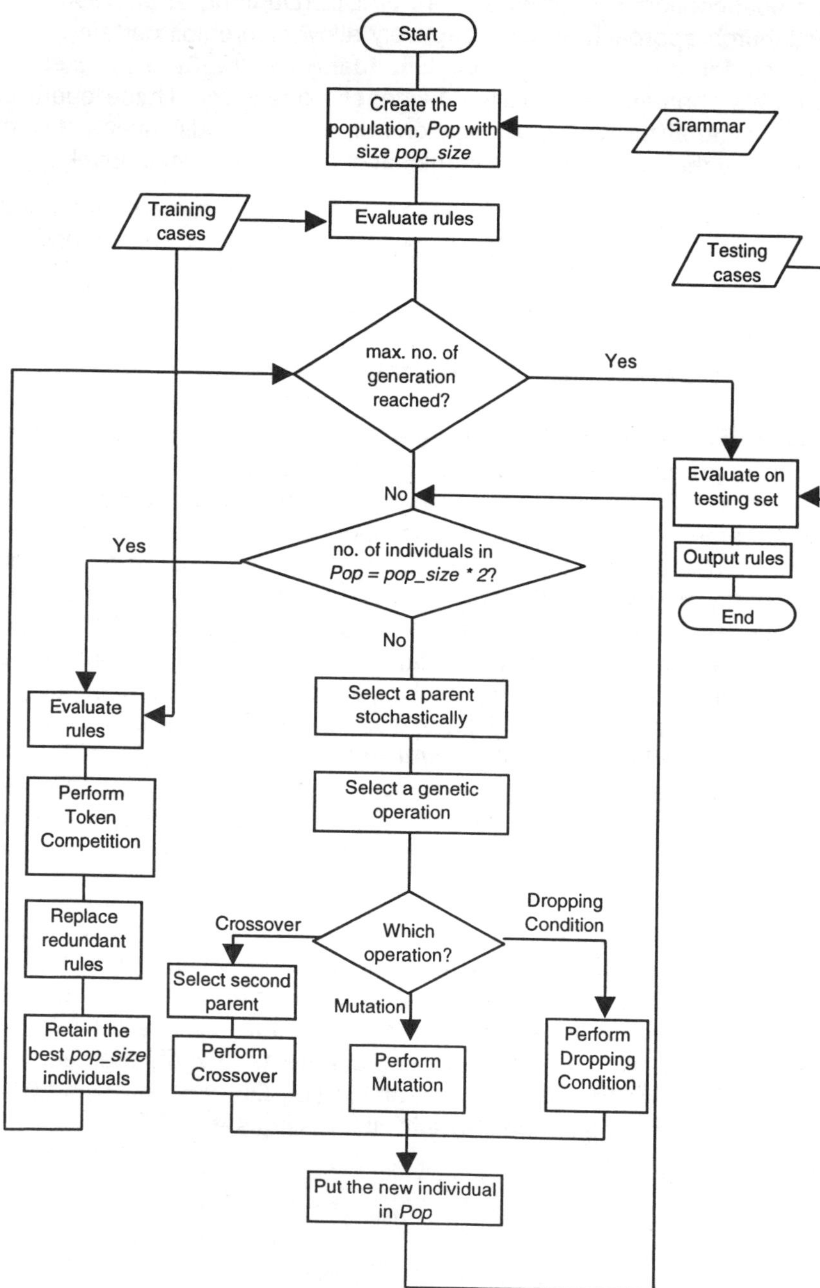

Figure 9. The flowchart of the Rule Learning process.

10.5.3.3 Grammar

The grammar specifies the rule structures to be evolved from GGP. The format of rules in each problem can be different. Thus for each problem, a specific grammar is written so that the format of the rules can best fit the domain. In general, the grammar specifies a rule is of the form "if *antecedents* then *consequent*". The antecedent part is a conjunction of attribute descriptors. The consequent part is an attribute descriptor as well. An attribute descriptor assigns a value to a nominal attribute, a range of values to a continuous attribute, or can be used to compare attribute values.

For example, consider a database with 4 attributes. We want to learn rules about **attr4**, which is Boolean. The attribute **attr1** is nominal and coded with 0, 1 or 2. The attribute **attr2** is continuous between 0-200. The domain of **attr3** is similar to **attr2** and we want the rule to compare them. An example of the context free grammar for rule learning in given in Table 6. The symbols in cursive are the *non-terminals* and the other symbols are the *terminals*. A production rule of the form $\alpha \rightarrow \beta$ specifies that the non-terminals α can be expanded to β. $\alpha \rightarrow \beta|\gamma$ denotes $\{\alpha \rightarrow \beta, \alpha \rightarrow \gamma\}$. The symbols **erc1**, **erc2**, **erc3** and **boolean_erc** in this grammar are ephemeral random constants (ERCs). Each ERC has it own range for instantiation: **erc1** is within {0,1,2}, **erc2** and **erc3** is between 0-200, **boolean_erc** can only be T or F. In this grammar the antecedent part consists of descriptors of all attributes. However a rule does not need specifications for *all* attributes. The symbol '**any**' is a generic descriptor that allows an attribute to be ignored in the rule. An attribute can be described either by its descriptor, or by '**any**' such that it can be disregarded in the antecedent.

The grammar is used to derive rules to make up the initial population. The *start symbol* is the first symbol of the first line of the grammar. From the start symbol, a complete derivation is performed. Table 5.3.3 is an example of how a rule is derived from the grammar. This grammar allows rules like:

- if attr1 = 0 and attr2 between 100 150 and attr3 $\neq$ 50, then attr4 = T.
- if attr1 = 1 and any and attr3 >= attr2, then attr4 = F.

- *Rule → i1f Antes, then Consq.*
- *Antes → Attr1 and Attr2 and Attr3*
- *Attr1 → any | Attr1_descriptor*
- *Attr2 → any | Attr2_descriptor*
- *Attr3 → any | Attr3_descriptor*
- *Attr1_descriptor → attr1 = erc1*
- *Attr2_descriptor → attr2 between erc2 erc2*
- *Attr3_descriptor → attr3 Comparator Attr3_term*
- *Comparator → = | ≠ | <= | >= | < | >*
- *Attr3_term → attr2 | erc3*
- *Consq → Attr4_descriptor*
- *Attr4_descriptor → attr4 = boolean_erc*

Table 6. An example grammar for rule learning.

Rule

if *Antes* , then *Consq.*

if *Attr1* and *Attr2* and *Attr3*, then *Consq.*

If *Attr1_descriptor* and *Attr2_descriptor* and *Attr3_descriptor*, then *Attr4_descriptor.*

If attr1 = erc1 and attr2 between erc2 erc2 and attr3 Comparator *Attr3_term*, then attr4 = boolean_erc.

If attr1 = erc1 and attr2 between erc2 erc2 and attr3 ≠ erc3 , then Attr4 = boolean_erc.

If attr1 = 0 and attr2 between 100 150 and attr3 ≠ 50, then attr4 = T.

Table 7. An example derivation of rules.

GGP provides a powerful knowledge representation and allows a great flexibility on the rule format. The representation of rules is not fixed but depends on the grammar. The descriptor is not restricted to compare attributes with values. Rather, the descriptors can be comparisons between attributes. Rules with other formats can be learned, provided that the suitable grammar is supplied. Moreover, rules with the user-desired structure can be learned because the user can specify the required rule format in the grammar.

10.5.3.4 Use of Causality Model and Temporal Order

The use of grammar can ensure syntactical correctness in the rule, but not semantical correctness. It is desirable to eliminate meaningless rules in the search process. This requires a certain degree of knowledge on the causality between the attributes. The causal structure analysis steps in our data mining module can provide this knowledge. The Bayesian network may provide an overview of the relationships among the attributes. For example, if we know that attribute *A* is not related to any other attributes, then we don't need to learn rules about *A*. If we know attribute *B* should depend on attributes *C* and *D*, then we can specify a rule format like 'if <attribute *C* descriptor> and <attribute *D* descriptor>, then <attribute *B* descriptor>'.

The temporal order among attributes can also provide knowledge to increase the learning efficiency. For example, in a medical domain, the rule "if treatment is plaster, then diagnosis is radius fracture" is inappropriate. This rule does not make sense, because an operation is taken based on the treatment, not the other way round. In general, an event that occurs later will not be a cause of an event occurred earlier! Thus, we can order the attributes according the temporal relationship. The grammar should be designed such that an attribute is not placed in the 'if' part if it occurs later then the attribute in the 'then' part. This temporal order can be represented easily using a grammar. Both causality model and temporal order may significantly reduce search space and prune meaningless rules.

10.5.3.5 Genetic Operators

The search space is explored by generating new rules using three genetic operators: crossover, mutation and a newly defined operator called dropping condition. A rule is composed of attribute descriptors. The genetic operators try to change the descriptors in order to search for better rules. Rank selection (Goldberg, 1989) method is being used to select the parents. The probabilities of using crossover, mutation and dropping condition in our system are 0.5, 0.4 and 0.1, respectively.

Crossover is a sexual operation that produces one child from two parents. One parent is designated as the primary parent and the other one as the secondary parent. A part of the primary parent is selected and replaced by another part from the secondary parent. Suppose that the following primary and secondary parents are selected:

If **attr1**=0 and **attr2** between 100 150 and **attr3≠50**, then **attr4**=T.

If **attr1**=1 and any and **attr3>=attr2**, then **attr4**=F.

The underlined parts are selected for crossover. The offspring will be

If **attr1**=0 and **attr2** between 100 150 and **attr3>=attr2**, then **attr4**=T.

The replaced part is selected randomly from the primary parent, hence genetic changes may occur either on the whole rule, on several descriptors, or on just one descriptor. The replacing part is also selected randomly, but under the constraint that the offspring produced must be valid according to the grammar. If a conjunction of descriptors is selected, it will be replaced by another conjunction of descriptors, but never by a single descriptor. If a descriptor is selected, then it can only be replaced by another descriptor of the same attribute. This can maintain the validity of the rule.

Mutation is an asexual operation. The genetic changes may occur on the whole rule, several descriptors, one descriptor, or the constants in the rule. A part in the parental rule is selected and replaced by a randomly generated part. The new part is generated by the same derivation mechanism using the same grammar. Similar to crossover, because the offspring have to be valid according to the grammar, a selected part can only mutate to another part with a compatible structure. For example, the parent

If **attr1**=0 and **attr2** between 100 150 and **attr3≠50**, then **attr4**=T.

May mutate to

If **attr1**=0 and **attr2** between 100 150 and attr3=40, then **attr4**=T.

Due to the probabilistic nature of GP, redundant constraints may be generated in the rule. For example, suppose that the actual knowledge is 'if $A<20$ then X=T'. We may learn rules like 'if $A<20$ and $B<20$ then X=T'. This rule is, of course, correct; but it does not completely represent the actual knowledge. Dropping condition is an operator designed to generalize the rules. The rule can be generalized if one descriptor in the antecedent part is dropped. Dropping condition selects randomly one attribute descriptor, and then turns it into 'any'. That particular attribute is no longer considered in the rule, hence the rule can be generalized.

Reproduction operator is not used in our approach. In conventional GP, an individual can exploit its genetic material through the use of the reproduction operator. Good individuals can reproduce themselves in the population and gradually dominate the population. However, in our system, we do not want a good rule to replicate itself. Rather, we need to diversify the population in order to find several good rules. Hence reproduction isnot used. Our system will only keep one copy for each good individual through token competition (Ngan et al. 1999).

10.6 Evaluation of the Discovered Knowledge

10.6.1 Evaluation of Causal Structure Analysis

We have used a population size of 50 and a maximum number of generations of 1000 to run in the causality and structure analysis. The execution time was 3 minutes on a Sun Ultra 1/140. The best Bayesian network structure learned is shown in Figure 10. The right part of the network shows that sex implies menstruation, and menstruation implies age, and age in turn implies **RI**. The network also shows that **TSIDir** can imply **TSI** because if TSI direction is null, **TSI** should be 0.

The main part of the network shows that **2ndMCDeg** can imply **2ndMCApex** and **1stMCGreater**. This is because if **2ndMCDeg** =0, the patient does not have the second major curve, and thus **2ndMCApex** must be null and the first major curve must be the greater curve. The value of **2ndMCDeg** also imply the degree of the second curve (**Deg2**), because if the patient has two major curves, most of the time the second major curve is the second curve. The value of **1stMCDeg** is affected by **1stMCGreater** and **Deg2**. When the degree of first major curve is greater than the second curve, most likely **1stMCDeg** is large. When **Deg2** is large, most likely the first major curve will be the second curve. The value of **1stMCDeg** can imply **Deg1** because when the value of **1stMCDeg** is small, the degree first curve is not large. **Deg2** can imply the value of **L4Tilt** and **Deg3**, while **Deg3** can imply **1stCurveT1**. If degree of the second curve is large, then usually L4 is tilt. If the patient does not have the second curve, then he will not have the third curve. Moreover, if he has at least three curves, then most of the time the deformation will start at the first vertebra T1. The network also shows that the value of **treatment** mainly depends on **1stMCDeg**. On the other hand, **Class** depends on **Deg2**.

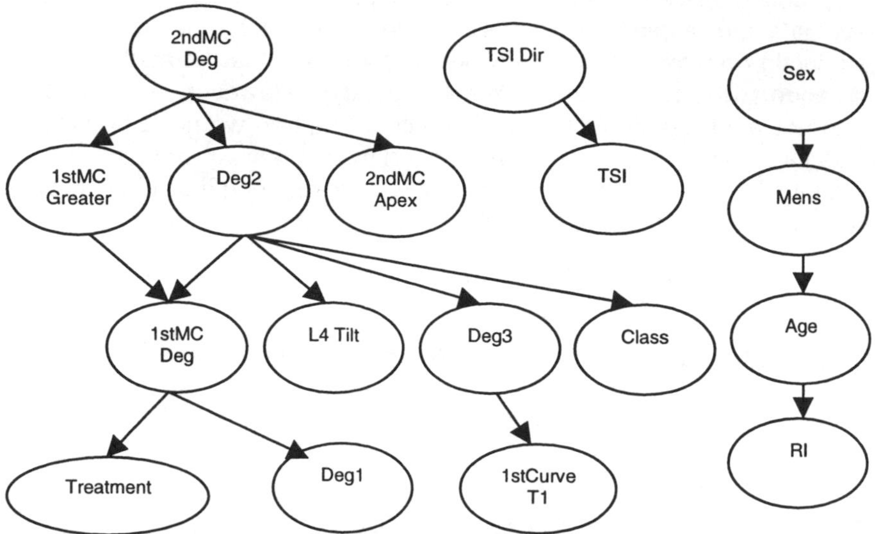

Figure 10: The best network structure for the Scoliosis database.

10.6.2 Evaluation of Rule Learning

The medical experts are interested to discover knowledge about classification of Scoliosis and treatment. Scoliosis can be classified as Kings, Thoracolumbar(TL) and Lumbar(L), while Kings can be further subdivided into K-I, II, III, IV and V. Treatment can be observation, surgery and bracing. The determinations of these two attributes are complicated. Although the induced Bayesian network provides valid and useful relationships, the domain expert is more interested in finding relationships between classification and the attributes **1stCurveT1**, **1stMCGreater**, **L4Tilt**, **1stMCDeg**, **2ndMCDeg**, **1stMCApex** and **2ndMCApex**, and relationships between treatment and age, laxity, degrees of the curves, maturity of the patient, displacement of the vertebra and the class of Scoliosis. This domain knowledge can be easily incorporated in the design of the rule grammar. There are two types of rules, one for classification of Scoliosis and the other for suggesting treatment. The grammar is outlined in Appendix A

Class	No. of Rules	cf			support			prob
		mean	max	min	mean	max	min	
King-I	5	94.84%	100%	90.48%	5.67%	10.73%	0.86%	28.33%
King-II	5	80.93%	100%	52.17%	6.61%	14.38%	1.07%	35.41%
King-III	4	23.58%	25.87%	16.90%	1.56%	2.58%	0.86%	7.94%
King-IV	2	24.38%	29.41%	19.35%	1.18%	1.29%	1.07%	2.79%
King-V	5	51.13%	62.50%	45.45%	0.97%	1.07%	0.86%	6.44%
TL	1	41.18%	41.18%	41.18%	1.50%	1.50%	1.50%	2.15%
L	3	54.04%	62.50%	45.45%	2.00%	2.79%	1.07%	4.51%

Table 8. Results of the rules for Scoliosis classification.

The population size used in the rule learning step is 100 and the maximum number of generations is 50. The execution time was about one hour on a Sun Ultra 1/140. The results of rule learning from this database are listed below.

1. Rules for Scoliosis classification.
   An example of this kind of rules is:

   If **1stMCGreater = N and 1stMCApex = T1-T8 and 2ndMCApex = L3-L4, then King-I. (cf=100%)**

   For each class of Scoliosis, a number of rules are mined. The results are summarized in Table 8. For King-I and II, the rules have high confidence and generally match with the knowledge of medical experts.However there is one unexpected rule for the classification of King-II. Under the conditions specified in the antecedents, our system found a rule with a confidence factor of 52% that classified to King-II. However, the domain expert suggests the class should be King-V! After an analysis on the database, we revealed that serious data errors existed in the current database and that some records contained an incorrect Scoliosis classification.
   For King-III and IV, the confidence of the rules discovered is just around 20%. According to the domain expert, one common characteristic for these two classes is that there is only one major curve or the second major curve is insignificant. However there is no rigid definition for a 'major curve' and the concept of 'insignificant' is fuzzy. These depend on the interpretation of doctors. Because of the

lack of this important information, the system cannot find accurate rules for these two classes. Another problem is that only a small number of patients in the database where classified to King-III or IV (see *prob* in Table 8). The database cannot provide a large number of cases for training. Similar problems also existed for King-V, TL and L. For the class King-V, TL and L, the system found rules with confidence around 40% to 60%. Nevertheless, the rules for TL and L show something different in comparison with the rules suggested by the clinicians. According to our rules, the classification always depends on the *first major curve*, while according to the domain expert, the classification depends on the *larger major curve*. After discussion with the domain expert, it is agreed that the existing rules are not defined clearly enough, and our rules are more accurate than them. Our rules provide hints to the clinicians to re-formulate their concepts.

2. Rules about treatment.

   An typical rule of this kind is:

   If age=2-12 and Deg1=20-26 and Deg2=24-47 and Deg3=27-52 and Deg4=0, then Bracing. (cf=100%)

   The results are summarized in Table 9. The rules for observation and bracing have very high confidence factors. However, the support is not high, showing that the rules only cover fragments of the cases. Our system prefers accurate rules to general rules. If the user prefers more general rules, the weights in the fitness function can be tuned. For surgery, no interesting rule was found because only 3.65% of the patients are treated with surgery.

Type	No. of Rules	*cf*			*Support*			*prob*
		mean	max	min	mean	max	min	
Observation	4	98.89%	100%	95.55%	3.49%	6.01%	1.07%	62.45%
Bracing	5	79.57%	100%	71.43%	1.03%	1.29%	0.86%	24.46%
Surgery	0	-	-	-	-	-	-	3.65%

Table 9. Results of the rules about treatment.

10.7 Using the Discovered Knowledge

This system is particularly suitable for the analysis of the real-life databases that cannot be described completely by just a few rules. Building a complete model for such a database is difficult and usually results in a complicated model. The system has been applied to a real-life medical Scoliosis database. The results can provide interesting knowledge as well as suggest refinements to the existing knowledge.

The biggest impact on the clinicians from the data mining analysis of the Scoliosis database is the fact that many rules set out in the clinical practice are not clearly defined. The usual clinical interpretation depends on the subjective experience. Data mining reveals quite a number of mismatches in the classification on the type of Kings curves. After a careful review by the senior surgeon, it appears that the database entries by junior surgeons may not be accurate and that the data mining rules discovered are in fact more accurate! The classification rules must therefore be quantified. The rules discovered can help in the training of younger doctors and act as an intelligent means to validate and evaluate the accuracy of the clinical database. An accurate and validated clinical database is very important for helping clinicians to make decisions, to assess and evaluate treatment strategies, to conduct clinical and related basic research, and to enhance teaching and professional training.

Furthermore, knowledge from domain experts can be very useful to data mining. The use of grammar allows the domain knowledge to be easily and effectively utilized. The grammar on one hand can prune the search space on meaningless rules while on the other hand can ensure that the output knowledge is in the user desired format.

10.8 Conclusions

We have presented a data mining application based on Evolutionary Computation. Two different kinds of knowledge, namely causal structures and rule knowledge, are discovered from a Scoliosis database. Causal structure analysis focuses on the general causality model between the *variables*. Bayesian network learning is adopted to learn the causal structure. The Bayesian network is easy to understand while it has a well-developed mathematical model.

On the other hand, rules capture the specific behavior between particular *values* of the variables. In many real-life situations, the available rules are general guidelines with many exceptional cases. The rule learning step aims at learning such kind of knowledge from data. Generic Genetic Programming is employed for the rule learning task. Token competition is used so as to learn as many rules as possible. Rules related to the classification of Scoliosis and treatment are discovered. It compares the confidence of the rule with the average probability and search for the patterns significantly deviated from the normal. Unexpected rules are also discovered and they lead to the discovery of errors in the database. For instance, we have discovered new knowledge about the classification of Scoliosis and about the treatment. We demonstrate that the data mining process helps clinicians make decisions and enhance professional training.

References

Baker, J. E. 1985. Adaptive selection methods for genetic algorithms. In Proceedings of an International Conference on Genetic Algorithms and Their Applications.

Booker, L., Goldberg, D. E. and Holland, J. H. 1989. Classifier systems and genetic algorithms. Artificial Intelligence, 40:235-282.

Bouckaert, R. R. 1994. Properties of belief networks learning algorithms. In Proceed ings of the Conference on Uncertainty in Artificial Intelligence, pages 102-109.

Charniak, E. 1991.Bayesian networks without tears. AI Magazine, 12(4):50-63.

Chow, C. K. and Liu, C. N. 1968. Approximating discrete probability distributions with dependence trees. IEEE Transactions on Information Theory, 14(3):462- 467.

Clark, P. and Niblett, T. 1989. The CN2 induction algorithm. Machine Learning, 3:261-283.

Cooper, G. F. 1990.The computational complexity of probabilistic inference using Bayesian belief networks. Artificial Intelligence, 42:393-405.

Cooper, G. F. and Herskovits, E. 1992. A Bayesian method for the induction of probabilistic networks from data. Machine Learning, 9:309-347.

De Jong, K. A., Spaers, W. M., and Gordon, D. F. 1993. Using genetic algorithms for concept learning. Machine Learning, 13:161-188.

Fayyad, U. M., Piatesky-Shapiro, G. and Smyth, P. Fall 1996. From data mining to knowledge discovery : An overview. AI Magazine, pages 37-54.

Fogel, D. B. 1994. An introduction to simulated evolutionary optimization. IEEE Transactions on Neural Network, 5:3-14.

Fogel, L., Owens, A. and Walsh, M. 1966. Artificial Intelligence through Simulated Evolution. New York: John Wiley and Sons.

Giordana, A. and Neri, F. 1995. Search-intensive concept induction. Evolutionary Computation, 3:375-416.

Goldberg, D. E. 1989. Genetic Algorithms in Search, Optimization and Machine Learning. Addison-Wesley.

Heckerman, D., Geiger, D., and Chickering, D. M. 1995. Learning Bayesian networks: The combination of knowledge and statistical data. Machine Learning, 20(3):197-243.

Heckerman, D. and Wellman, M. P. March 1995. Bayesian networks. Communications of the ACM, 38(3):27-30.

Herskovits, E. and Cooper, G. 1990. KUTATO: An entropy-driven system for construction of probabilistic expert systems from databases. Technical Report KSL-90-22, Knowledge Systems Laboratory, Medical Computer Science, Stanford University.

Holland, J. H. 1992. Adaptation in Natural and Artificial Systems. Bradford/MIT Press.

Holland, J. H. and Reitman, J. S. 1978. Cognitive systems based on adaptive algorithms. In D. A. Waterman and F. Hayes-Roth, editors, Pattern-Directed Inference Systems. Academic Press.

Hopcroft, J. E. and Ullman, J. D. 1979. Introduction to automata theory, languages, and computation. Reading, MA: Addison-Wesley.

Janikow, C. Z. 1993. A knowledge-intensive genetic algorithm for supervised learning. Machine Learning, 13:189-228.

Koza, J. R. 1992. Genetic Programming : on the programming of computers by means of natural selection. Bradford/MIT Press.

Koza, J. R. 1994. Genetic Programming II : automatic discovery of reusable programs. Bradford/MIT Press.

Lam, W. 1998. Bayesian network refinement via machine learning approach. IEEE Transactions on Pattern Analysis and Machine Intelligence, 20(3):240-251.

Lam, W. and Bacchus, F. 1994. Learning Bayesian belief networks - an approach based on the MDL principle. Computational Intelligence, 10(3):269-293.

Lam, W., Wong, M. L., Leung, K. S., and Ngan, P. S. 1998. Discovering probabilistic knowledge from databases using evolutionary computation and minimum description length principle. In Genetic Programming 1998: Proceedings of the Third Annual Conference, pages 786-794.

Larranaga, P., Kuijpers, C., Murga, R., and Yurramendi, Y. 1996. Learning Bayesian network structures by searching for the best ordering with genetic algorithms. IEEE Transactions on System, Man, and Cybernetics - Part A: Systems and Humans, 26(4):487-493.

Larranaga, P., Poza, M., Yurramendi, Y., Murga, R., and Kuijpers, C. 1996. Structure learning of Bayesian network by genetic algorithms: A performance analysis of control parameters. IEEE Transactions on Pattern Analysis and Machine Intelligence, 18(9):9.

Michalski, R. S., Mozetic, I., Hong, J., and Lavrac, N. 1986. The multi-purpose in cremental learning system AQ15 and its testing application to three medical domains. In Proceedings of the 5th National Conference on Artificial Intelligence, pages 1041-1045.

Ngan, P. S., Lam, W., Wong, M. L., Leung, K. S., and Cheng, J. C. Y. 1999. Medical data mining using evolutionary computation. Artificial Intelligence in Medicine, special issue of data mining in medicine, 16(1):73-96.

Rebane, G. and Pearl, J. 1989. The recovery of causal poly-trees from statistical data. In Uncertainty in Artificial Intelligence 3, pages 175-182. North-Holland, Amsterdam.

Rechenberg, I. 1973. Evolutionsstrategie: Optimierung technischer Systeme nach Prinzipien der biologischen Evolution (In English: Evolution Strategy: Optimization of technical systems by means of biological evolution). Stuttgart: Fromman-Holzboog.

Schwefel, H. P. 1981. Numerical Optimization of Computer Models. Chichester: Wiley.

Singh, M. and Valtorta, M. 1993. An algorithm for the construction of Bayesian network structures from data. In Proceedings of the Conference on Uncertainty in Artificial Intelligence, pages 259-265.

Smith, S. F. 1980. A Learning System based on Genetic Adaptive Algorithms. PhD thesis, University of Pittsburgh.

Smith, S. F. 1983. Flexible learning of problem solving heuristics through adaptive search. In Proceedings of the Eighth International Conference On Artificial Intelligence. Morgan Kaufmann.

Spirtes, P., Glymour, C., and Scheines, R. 1993. Causation, Prediction and Search. Springer-Verlag.

Tackett, W. A. 1993. Genetic programming for feature discovery and image discrimination. In Proceedings of the Fifth International Conference on Genetic Algorithms, pages 303-309.

Wong, M. L. 1995. Evolutionary program induction directed by logic grammars. PhD thesis, The Chinese University of Hong Kong.

Wong, M. L., Lam, W., and Leung, K. S. 1999. Using evolutionary computation and minimum description length principle for data mining of probabilistic knowledge. IEEE Transactions on Pattern Analysis and Machine Intelligence, 21(2):174-178.

Wong, M. L. and Leung, K. S. 1995. Inducing logic programs with genetic algorithms: The genetic logic programming system. IEEE Expert, 10(5):68-76.

Wong, M. L. and Leung, K. S. 1997. Evolutionary program induction directed by logic grammars. Evolutionary Computation, 5:143-180.

Appendix The Grammar for the Scoliosis Database

This grammar is not completely listed. The grammar for the other attribute descriptors is similar to the part of the grammar in lines 7-12.

1: *Rule* → *Rule1* | *Rule2*

2: *Rule1* → if *Antes1*, then *Consq1*.

3: *Rule2* → if *Antes2*, then *Consq2*.

4: *Antes1* → *1stCurveT1 1stMCGreater* and *L4Tilt* and *1stMCDeg* and *2ndMCDeg* and *1stMCApex* and *2ndMCApex*

5: *Antes2* → *Age* and *Lax* and *Deg1* and *Deg2* and *Deg3* and *Deg4* and *Mens* and *RI* and *TSI* and *ScoliosisType*

6: *Consq1* → *ScoliosisType_descriptor*

7: *1stMCGreater* → any | *1stMCGreater_descriptor*

8: *1stMCGreater_descriptor* → 1stMCGreater = boolean_const

9: *1stMCDeg* → any | *1stMCDeg_descriptor*

10: *1stMCDeg_descriptor* → 1stMCDeg between deg_const deg_const

11: *1stMCApex* → any | *1stMCApex_descriptor*

12: *1stMCApex_descriptor* → 1stMCApex between Apex_const Apex_const ...

---

11 Methods of Temporal Data Validation and Abstraction in High-Frequency Domains

Silvia Miksch[1], Andreas Seyfang[1], Werner Horn[2, 3], Christian Popow[4] and Franz Paky[5]

[1]Institute of Software Technology
Vienna University of Technology, Austria
{silvia, seyfang}@ifs.tuwien.ac.at, www.ifs.tuwien.ac.at/~{silvia, seyfang}
[2] Department of Medical Cybernetics and Artificial Intelligence
University of Vienna, Austria
werner@ai.univie.ac.at
[3] Austrian Research Institute for Artificial Intelligence
Vienna, Austria
[4] NICU, Department of Pediatrics
University of Vienna, Austria
popow@akh-wien.ac.at
[5] Department of Pediatrics
Hospital of Mödling, Austria
franz.paky@magnet.at

In medical domains, like Intensive Care Units both large amounts of on-line data and expert knowledge are available, but their automatic combination is hindered by practical concerns, like poor signal quality. In this chapter we present a set of methods to bridge this gap between erroneous high-frequency raw data and high-level symbolic representations. Interpretation of high-frequency data requires both time-oriented data validation and analysis resulting in high-level qualitative descriptions. The validation process consists of time-independent, time-point-, time-interval-, and trend-based methods to detect errors in the observed raw data as well as methods for its repair. The aim is to arrive at the most reliable data possible to obtain. The analysis abstracts different types of qualitative information concerning trends, values, and quality of the data. We developed various robust algorithms for both periodical and non-periodical curves to arrive at qualitative descriptions over time and to cope with artifacts in the data, which cannot possibly be detected in the previous validation steps.

11.1 Introduction

Most Intensive Care Units (ICUs) are well equipped with modern devices for patient monitoring. On-line recording of patient data and storage in computer-based patient records (CPR) and patient data management systems (PDMS) become common-place in today's ICUs. Currently, the medical staff is suffering from information overloading caused by too many channels of on-line recording and from a vast amount of false alarms due to simple alarming policies (Lawless, 1994).

On the one hand, during the last years, several sophisticated knowledge-based monitoring and therapy-planning systems have been introduced (Uckun, 1994). These systems concentrate on optimizing data analyses and interpretation, on applying different kinds of accessible knowledge and information to enrich the reasoning process, and on minimizing manual data input by improving the technical equipment at modern clinics and by accessing computer-based patient records. However, particular time-oriented data-analysis methods are needed to cope with data in high-frequency domains and to ensure proper operation in life-threatening situations.

On the other hand, the monitors available at the ICUs are equipped with alarming systems, which can only detect obvious errors. These alarming systems apply simple methods of range checking, which are obviously too simple to be useful in a complex medical setting. As a result, the medical staff has a burdensome time to distinguish dangerous situations from false alarms. So, the supporting monitoring and therapy-planning systems are ineffective without error-detection methods because of the quite poor quality of the data (Carlson et al., 1993).

Therefore, we are aiming to overcome the problem of information overload and to improve the quality of data by applying the following four strategies:
First, we propose data validation methods to arrive at reliable data. The importance of data validation has been neglected in the past—the data received from the monitors is more faulty than is often realized (Gardner et al., 1992). Intensive efforts to detect artifacts require the combination of all information available, cross-validating various data sources, inspecting and reasoning about data points over time, and looking at trends to get a

complete and consistent picture of the situation of the patient of the past and at present. In section we describe the methods for data validation and repair implemented in VIE-VENT, an open-loop knowledge-based monitoring and therapy planning system for artificially ventilated newborn infants (Miksch et al., 1993; 1996; Horn et al., 1997), which has been tested and evaluated in real clinical scenarios.

Second, data analysis methods are needed, which can handle time-oriented states and events, shifting contexts, and different expectations concerning the development of parameters. The process of this analysis is called *temporal data abstraction*. We describe the methods implemented in VIE-VENT and upcoming improvements in section . An advantage of using these qualitative descriptions is their unified usability and interchangeability in further reasoning processes, regardless of the origin of the described data.

Third, a lot of non-systematic errors, called noise, can be eliminated by the data validation methods. However, not all errors can be detected. Therefore, the temporal data abstraction methods should be made less sensitive to such errors and at the same time provide information about the estimated quality of the data. In section we describe the calculation of a reliability score as a byproduct of the validation as implemented in VIE-VENT and in section we describe our approach to utilize statistical measures for the reliability of the data in the abstraction process.

Fourth, periodic high-frequency data call for a method to reason over changes in the form of the oscillations—not only its frequency and amplitude—in an intuitive way. Descriptions in terms of frequency spectrums or function matrices as used by popular approaches in the field of signal processing are not compatible with the representation physician use when describing curves. In section 4.3 we describe our ongoing research on this topic.

In section 2 we describe the need for data validation and abstraction and describe the characteristics of the used data. We present our approaches to preprocessing data (time-oriented data validation) in section 3 and those to time-oriented data abstraction in section 4. The evaluation and benefits of our approach are discussed in section 5 and future work in section 6.

11.2 Motivation - The Characteristics of the Data

11.2.1 The Need for Time-Oriented Data Validation

In the following we will motivate the necessity of effective data validation illustrating our experiences with medical on-line data from ICUs.

We evaluated on-line data sets obtained from newborn infants with various respiratory diseases. The data were collected from the monitoring system of a neonatal Intensive Care Unit (NICU) once per second (16-28 hours of continuous data recording for each newborn infant). The data sets consist of measurements of continuously assessed quantitative data (e.g. transcutaneous partial pressure of oxygen ($P_{tc}O_2$), the pulse frequency (*PULS*) given from pulsoximetry), discontinuously assessed quantitative data (e.g. ventilator settings like *PIP*, *PEEP*, results of invasive blood-gas analyses like *pH*, P_aO_2 where *a* denotes a measurement from arterial blood), and continuously assessed qualitative data (e.g. clinical parameters like spontaneous breathing effort, chest wall extension).

Visualization and analysis of these data sets enabled a closer insight into the validity and the quality of the observed data, as well as the importance of secure and trustworthy data for further reasoning:

1. Small movements of the infant resulted in an unexpectedly high volume of data oscillation. This is specifically a problem of pulsoximetry. For example, small movements of the neonate result in sequences of unusable oxygen saturation (S_aO_2) measurements.
2. The measurements were frequently invalid caused by external events, which have to be performed regularly (e.g. calibration of transcutaneous sensors every three to four hours, scheduled endotracheal suctioning).
3. Continuously and discontinuously assessed measurements, which should reflect the same clinical context, frequently deviated from each other as a result of the individual situation of the patient or of variations in the environmental conditions under which the sensors operate.
4. Additional invalid measurements were caused by on-line transmission problems or were unexplainable.
5. Some errors occur because different people input data from in different environments and in different experimental settings.

Noisy and erroneous data is a serious problem—the data analysis and data mining methods should be made less sensitive to such non-systematic errors. In the machine learning literature the problem of noisy data has been expensively studied. On the one hand, when generating the rules from training data, the noise should be eliminated to make the rules more general and accurate. On the other hand, in some systems just the opposite is true: adding the noise to training data resulted in smaller misclassification of unseen examples ((Quinlan 1986) cited in (Cios, Pedrycz, & Swiniarski, 1998)). However, in our domain noise is seen as distracting from the real information and thus both data validation and abstraction must provide various methods to minimize the influence of noise on the outcome.

11.2.1.1 Related Work

Classical artifact-recognition methods mostly come from the field of statistical signal processing techniques and neural networks. Statistical signal processing, like Kalman filtering, is computationally expensive (Sittig & Factor, 1990). It puts much power in processing signals at a very low level, which may be unnecessary, if we know from high-level reasoning processes that the signal is useless. The same arguments hold for artificial neural networks (Sittig & Orr, 1992).

Error detection is inevitable in anesthesia monitoring (van der Aa, 1990) and post-operative care (Sukuvaara et al., 1992). The combination of range checks and validation and invalidation rules has been successfully applied by (Garfinkel et al., 1989) to eliminate false alarms and at least range checking facilities are standard for today's monitors in ICUs. However, commonly used systems produce numerous false alarms—or, if switched off—missing alarms (Lawless, 1994).

Most methods used today concentrate on numerical methods and do not take into account the clinical context. These methods are successful for particular problem characteristics—detecting values, which are not within certain ranges and trend values, which are physiologically implausible. But they cannot classify data as unreliable, because a large portion of reliability checking is dependent on the correct interpretation of the clinical context. Further, cross-checking of different parameters needs a very high, abstract level of reasoning. Such a reasoning gives insight into the reliability of measured data, both on a specific data point and on the trend over some selected time period.

Avoidance of wrong alarms, reliable monitoring, and effective therapy planning requires data validation procedures, which combine numerical methods with validation methods operating on derived qualitative time-oriented descriptions of state and grade values and various combinations thereof.

11.2.2 The Need for Deriving Temporal Abstractions

Beside the quality of data, monitoring and therapy planning in real-world environments involves numerous other data analysis problems:

1. Long-term monitoring requires the processing of a huge volume of data generated from several (monitoring) devices and individuals.
2. The available data occur at various observation frequencies (e.g. high or low frequency data), at various regularities (e.g. continuously or discontinuously sampled data), and are of various types (e.g. qualitative or quantitative data).
3. A time-oriented analysis process has to cope with a combination of all these data sources.
4. The underlying domain knowledge about the interactions of parameters is vague and incomplete.
5. The interpretation context is shifting depending on observed data.
6. The underlying expectations regarding the development of parameters are different according to the interpretation context and to the degrees of the parameters' abnormality.

11.2.2.1 Related Work

Traditional theories of data analysis (Avent & Charlton, 1990; Kay, 1993) mostly deal with well-defined problems. However, in many real-world cases the underlying structure-function models or the domain knowledge and models are poorly understood or not applicable because of their complexity and because knowledge is often incomplete or vague. Therefore, in the medical domain statistical analysis, control theory, or other techniques are often unusable, inappropriate or at least only partially applicable (Miksch et al., 1996; Horn et al., 1997).

To overcome the mentioned limitations, time-oriented analysis methods were proposed to derive qualitative values or patterns of the current and the past situation of a patient (e.g. transcutaneous partial pressure of carbon dioxide ($P_{tc}CO_2$) is *slightly below the target range*, or $P_{tc}CO_2$ is *increasing*). These data analysis methods are referred as *data-abstraction methods*, a term originally introduced by Clancey in his classical proposal on heuristic classification (Clancey, 1985). *Temporal* data abstraction represents an important subgroup where the processed data are temporal.

Atemporal data abstraction is substantially simpler than temporal abstraction, because time adds a new dimension and temporal dependencies dramatically increase the complexity of a problem.

An advantage of using such qualitative descriptions is their unified usability in the system model, regardless of their origin. Several significant and encouraging approaches have been developed in the past years.

Haimowitz et al. (1995) have developed the concept of trend templates ($TrenD_x$) to represent all the information available during an observation process. A trend template defines disorders as typical patterns of relevant parameters. These patterns consist of a partially ordered set of temporal intervals with uncertain end-points. Trend templates are used to detect trends in time-stamped data. The RÉSUMÉ project (Shahar & Musen, 1996) performs temporal abstraction of time-stamped data without predefined trends. The system is based on a knowledge-based temporal-abstraction method, which is decomposed into five sub-tasks: temporal context restriction, vertical temporal inference, horizontal temporal inference, temporal interpolation, and temporal pattern matching. Larizza et al. (1997) have developed methods to detect predefined courses in a time series. Complex abstraction allows to detect specific temporal relationships between intervals. The overall aim was to summarize the patient's behavior over a predefined time interval. Belazzi et al. (1999) utilize Bayesian techniques to extract overall trends from cyclic data in the field of diabetes. Keravnou (1997) focuses on the periodicity of events derived from the patient history.

All these approaches are dealing with low-frequency data. Therefore, the problems of oscillating data, frequently shifting contexts, and different context-specific expectations of the development of parameters are not covered.

In the field of NICUs, Hunter et al. (1999) developed a tool to detect significant events like probe changes in recorded data from monitors. The algorithm is based on joining temporal intervals until the error of the linear regression calculated from the raw data points within that window exceeds a particular threshold. Although our approach utilizing a *spread* (see section 4.1 and (Miksch et al., 1999)) differs significantly, its development was inspired by this.

11.3 Preprocessing: Time-Oriented Data Validation

The parts of the data abstraction methods described in section 4 are interwoven with the data validation process. First, the data validation process uses the numerical values of the parameters to arrive at reliable values which are transformed into unified qualitative descriptions by the data abstraction process. Second, it applies these derived qualitative descriptions to detect faulty measurements. The major aim of the data validation process is to detect faulty measurements or artifacts and finally to arrive at reliable measurements. An artifact is a situation where a measured variable does not reflect the clinical context.

We perform a two-step data validation process based on different temporal ontologies: first, a context-sensitive examination of the plausibility of input data and second, applying repair and adjustment methods for correcting wrong or ambiguous data. The final result is a classification of the input data as "correct", "wrong", "unknown", or "adjusted". A measurement is classified as "adjusted" if a "wrong" or "unknown" value is corrected by a repair or adjustment method. If a faulty measurement is recognized and no repair or adjustment method can be applied, the measurement is classified as "wrong". If no data for a measurement from the monitor is received and no value could be estimated, then the measurement is classified as "unknown". Otherwise it is classified as "correct". Not all methods mentioned below lead to a final classification. Some of them (like, the time-point-based functional dependencies) result in an intermediate and ambiguous classification of "some are wrong". This information is forwarded to and handled by the repair and adjustment module which provides strategies for repairing and adjusting not plausible or missing values based on the same temporal ontologies as the data validation module.

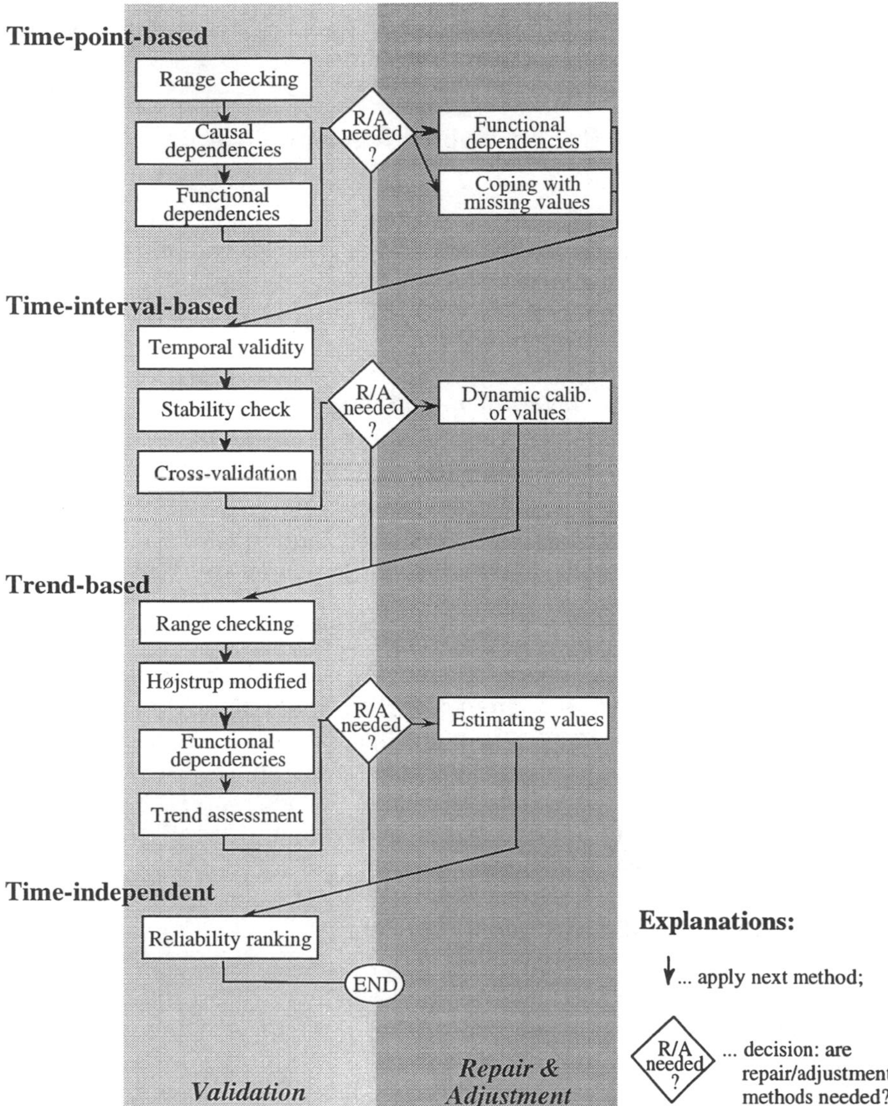

Figure 1. Overview and interaction of the components of the data validation and repair/adjustment modules. The left-hand side labels indicate the different temporal-based ontologies and the corresponding validation methods. On the right-hand side the possible repair or adjustment methods are mentioned.

We divide our methods into four types based on their underlying temporal ontologies: time-point-based, time-interval-based, trend-based, and time-independent validation and repair. Figure 1 gives an overview of the particular categories and their interactions. A detailed description of the whole process is given in (Horn et al., 1997).

11.3.1 Time-Point-Based Validation and Repair

The time-point-based category uses the value of a variable at a particular time point for the reasoning process. This concept can handle any kind of data. It benefits from the transparent and fast reasoning process but suffers from neglecting any information about the history of the observed parameters.

We distinguish the following validation and repair methods:

11.3.1.1 Validation: Range Checking

The range checking determines whether a quantitative value is within an acceptable range. It is simple but has shown very powerful to detect disconnections and missing measurements. Most modern ICU's equipment is able to perform range checks by itself.

We have enhanced this method by adding additional attributes, which define the clinical context (e.g. arterial, IPPV). There are look-up tables for all input parameters covering the plausible ranges. A parameter in the look-up table is specified by a parameter name, a list of attribute descriptors, an upper limit and a lower limit. For example, (CO_2, (arterial, IPPV), 10, 140), where "arterial" refers to the kind of blood gas analysis and IPPV to the mode of ventilation.

11.3.1.2 Validation: Causal Dependencies

Causal dependencies establish a relationship between different parameters. Qualitative values (e.g. *chest wall extension = small*) are related to numerical ranges of other parameters (e.g. *tidal volume < 5 ml/kg*). A causal dependency can be bidirectional—as shown in the example above—or unidirectional. In the bidirectional case we can only conclude that some of the parameters are wrong if the dependency is violated. The unidirectional case allows to invalidate a specific parameter. For example, S_aO_2 is invalidated if we cannot find a valid pulse (from pulsoximetry) or if we detect a substantial difference between the pulse and the heart rate from ECG (*HR*, measured in *beats/min*):

$$valid\,(PULS) = false \rightarrow valid\,(S_aO_2) = false \qquad (1)$$

$$|\,HR - PULS\,| > 8 \rightarrow valid\,(S_aO_2) = false \qquad (2)$$

Equation 2 can be used only if we have a valid *HR* and a valid *PULS*. In fact, such dependencies define an implicit ordering of parameters with respect to the application of validation procedures.

11.3.1.3 Validation and Repair: Functional Dependencies

Functional dependencies are useful for both numerical and qualitative parameters. Applying a functional dependency not only provides a mean for validating the parameters of the function, but also for repair of an invalid parameter.

Functional numerical dependencies are used to provide a value for a dependent parameter and to check inadequate data transmission for parameters where we know the exact functional relation.

Qualitative functional dependencies establish a relationship between derived qualitative values of different parameters. Due to the unified scheme for the qualitative values of all blood-gas measurements as shown in section it is easy to compare different measurements. For blood-gas measurements we expect that measures taken from different sites (arterial, venous, capillary, and transcutaneous) belong to the same qualitative data point region, or at least to the neighboring one. For example, we expect the same classification of the transcutaneous $P_{tc}CO_2$ and the invasive capillary P_cCO_2 measurements. If we detect, e.g. $P_{tc}CO_2$ is *substantially above the target range* and P_cCO_2 is *normal* we remember the ambiguity of the transcutaneous and the capillary carbon dioxide measurement. Which of the values is more plausible depends on the static reliability ranking discussed in section and the dynamic reliability score computed by each of the various validation methods. Later on in the validation process we will either invalidate one of the two measurements or repair it using dynamic calibration.

11.3.1.4 Repair: Coping with Missing Values

This method is applied if a value is marked as "unknown", "wrong", or "some are wrong" and if it could not be adjusted by any other method. There are two options to deal with missing values:

- *Simplified reasoning process.* This process uses only a few—most essential—parameters for further reasoning.
- *No solution.* When a critical situation has arisen in the past, no solution can be derived and the recommendations of appropriate treatments are delegated to the physicians.

Although not providing a solution might not seem to be a feature at first glance, for a system deployed in the medical domain it is vital to ensure that any output is based on solid grounds and that erroneous recommendations are strongly prohibited. The other advantage of a system "knowing its limits" is that operation is resumed immediately after input is valid again, without any need for an intervention by the user, as would be unavoidable for systems just "getting lost" in case of unexpected failure of input devices.

11.3.2 Time-Interval-Based Validation and Repair

The time-interval-based category of validation and repair deals with the values of different variables within a time interval.

We distinguish the following validation and repair methods:

11.3.2.1 Validation: Temporal Validity

Temporal validity sets the time interval during which a parameter is valid. We distinguish two kinds of temporal validity according to the regularities of the sampled data.

1. For *discontinuously* assessed data there are two possibilities for setting the valid time interval:

   (a) The user can specify the duration of validity for each entered datum. E.g., "P_aO_2 should be valid for the next 30 minutes".

   (b) For each parameter there is a predefined default maximum duration of validity.

   (c) A discontinuously assessed parameter value looses its validity, if one of the following conditions becomes true:

   (d) the time interval of the parameter's validity has elapsed,

   (e) a new value of the parameter is available, or

   (f) an external event (e.g. calibration of sensors) enforces to set the parameter invalid.

   The reliability score of a discontinuous parameter becomes smaller over time. For each parameter, a temporal validity interval is defined, which determines how long the time-interval-based repair method *dynamic calibration* (see below) can be active.

2. *Continuously* assessed data are handled in a different way: instead of valid time intervals we define *invalid* time intervals. The user can set a

parameter invalid explicitly, if specific external events take place (e.g. calibration of sensors, new application of sensors, disconnection).

11.3.2.2 Validation: Stability Check

After a period of invalidity of a parameter it is essential to enforce some (short) period of stability before the parameter is set back valid. This is specifically true for rapidly changing parameters like S_aO_2. The stability check defines allowed changes in the values of parameters. It compares the new value of a parameter with previously assessed values within a predefined time interval. This method is applicable for continuously assessed data only. We distinguish two situations:

1. Allowed changes of parameter values *without* a therapeutic action: The first value of a parameter, which is classified valid by all other validation methods becomes a candidate for stability testing. During time interval n we require, e.g.

$$\forall_{i,\, i=1,\dots,n}: |\, S_aO_2(t) - S_aO_2(t+i)\,| \leq \varepsilon \tag{3}$$

   For excellent stability of S_aO_2 we currently use $n = 120sec$ and $\varepsilon = 5\%$. The effect of the stability check is a delay in setting a parameter valid again. E.g., for S_aO_2 we will wait 120 seconds until the data values can be used again. If the stability check succeeds, we are able to reuse the values of the last 120 seconds. This results in a recalculation of the trends.

2. Allowed changes of parameter values *after* a therapeutic action: we expect a particular parameter to improve towards the normal range after a certain delay time. Besides the fact that therapeutic actions are not recommended in case the guiding parameters are invalid, a stability check as defined above is less useful. A larger ε for the direction of the desired improvement is used in this case.

11.3.2.3 Validation: Cross-Validation

Cross-validation of data from different sources is the time-interval-based utilization of qualitative functional dependencies described in section 3.1. Its specific use is the correlation of a parameter X which gives a quite exact measurement but is rarely available with a parameter Y which is inexact but available continuously. The basic assumption is that X behaves like Y.

As an example taken from ventilation management, X is an invasively measured blood gas and Y is a transcutaneous blood gas. If cross-validation detects a significant qualitative difference between, e.g. P_aCO_2 and $P_{tc}CO_2$ as described above, and both parameters are not invalidated by other methods, we apply dynamic calibration.

11.3.2.4 Repair: Dynamic Calibration

Dynamic calibration is a time-interval-based repair method, which repairs continuously assessed data values by applying a repair function which utilizes the difference between the discontinuously assessed data value X and the corresponding continuously assessed data value Y. This repair function adjusts the less reliable continuos value over a *temporal validity interval* to the reliable value of X. The resulting repaired value of Y receives a high reliability score which subsequently decreases over time. More details can be found in (Horn et al., 1997).

11.3.3 Trend-Based Validation and Repair

Trend-based validation analyzes the behavior of a variable during a time interval. A trend is a significant pattern in a sequence of time-ordered data. Therefore, the following methods can handle only continuously observed variables. They benefit from dynamically derived qualitative trend descriptions presented in section 4.4.

Based on physiological criteria, four kinds of trends of the time-stamped data samples can be discerned. They differ in the length of the sequence of data they use to calculate the trend. Further, they differ in the validity criteria for the determination of a valid trend. In monitoring more recent data are more important compared to older measurements. Thus we defined two criteria of validity to ensure that a trend is actually meaningful: (1) a certain minimum amount of valid measurements within the whole period, and (2) a certain amount of valid measurements during the last 20 percent of the time interval. These limits are defined by experts based on their clinical experience. They may easily be adapted to a specific clinical situation based on the frequency at which data arrives. Table 1 summarizes the trends and their criteria. For each kind of trend the actual growth rate and the derived qualitative trend category is determined as detailed in section 4.4.

kind of trend	sequence duration (minutes)	percentage of valid measurements for	
		whole sequence	last 20% of sequence
very short	1	50%	100%
short	10	40%	80%
medium	30	30%	60%
long	180	20%	40%

Table 1. Criteria of trend validity.

We distinguish the following validation and repair methods:

11.3.3.1 Validation: Range Check of the Growth Rate

A first basic check is the inspection of the growth rate. It is a sensible method for recognizing problems with the technical equipment, e.g. sensor loss. Range checks are applied on the very short-term trend and therefore react very fast.

11.3.3.2 Validation: Højstrup Method Modified

The modified Højstrup method recognizes growth rates, which are unacceptable after a certain amount of time. It recognizes implausible values by inspecting the temporal behavior of measurements. The temporal behavior is given as a function of measured values over time. Measurements are classified as implausible if the growth of this function is either too steep or the growth rate lies above a threshold and lasts for too long. The basic idea is given in (Højstrup, 1992). We have modified the algorithm to the needs of real-time monitoring in ICUs: the correlation function K is replaced by a measurement for the deviation of the last two points from the mean. We further may not assume a normal distribution of the differences. Therefore, the error threshold E is derived from knowledge about the maximum growth rate to accept and the desired rigidity of the system.

The algorithm is given in (Egghart, 1995; Horn et al., 1997). The main advantage of the method is the ability to select an area of growth between a value where it never signals an invalidity and a value where it immediately signals an invalidity. In between, the lower the growth rate the longer it will take to signal an invalidity.

11.3.3.3 Validation: Trend-Based Functional Dependencies

Trend-based functional dependencies model expectations on trends. They compare the behavior of two different parameters, which are related measurements within the same physiological context. For example, S_aO_2 and $P_{tc}O_2$ both give insight into the oxygenation of the patient. However, they react different in detail, but the global trend should be in parallel for both. We use the qualitative trend categories described in section 4.4 to compare the trends of such related parameters. The comparison is done using the short-term trend and the medium-term trend. If the trends differ by more than one category both measurements are marked as ambiguous.

A second usage of trend-based functional dependencies is to check whether the desired effect of a therapeutic action takes place. It is performed after a significant change of a parameter (ventilator setting), which controls the condition of the neonate. The method utilizes a specific delay time required to make a change in the ventilator setting visible in monitored parameters. For example, an increase of the inspired oxygen fraction F_iO_2 should cause an increase of the neonate's oxygen level O_2. This should be visible after a delay of 10 minutes in S_aO_2 and $P_{tc}O_2$.

The combination of inspecting trends of different parameters, which measure the same physiological context, with the inspection of trends after a therapeutic action gives a quite good insight into the validity of parameters. For example, if we find after an increase of FiO_2 that S_aO_2 is increasing, but $P_{tc}O_2$ is not, we can assume that $P_{tc}O_2$ giving invalid readings due to some other causes, like bad circulation.

11.3.3.4 Validation: Trend Assessment

The assessment of the parameter development examines the short-term trend. It compares two successive qualitative trend values of the parameter. An invalidity of the parameter is signaled if the trend categories are not the same or at least neighboring. The assessment procedure is applicable for the short-term trend only. The very-short-term trend reacts too rapidly to small oscillations of the values. The medium-term and the long-term trend are too insensitive.

The qualitative trend-categories are divided in an upper and a lower region by the normal region (see 4.4 for a detailed description of the process). According to these regions the ordering of the qualitative categories is defined as follows (compare figure 2):

- upper region: A1 - A2 - A3 - ZA - C
- lower region: B1 - B2 - B3 - ZB - D

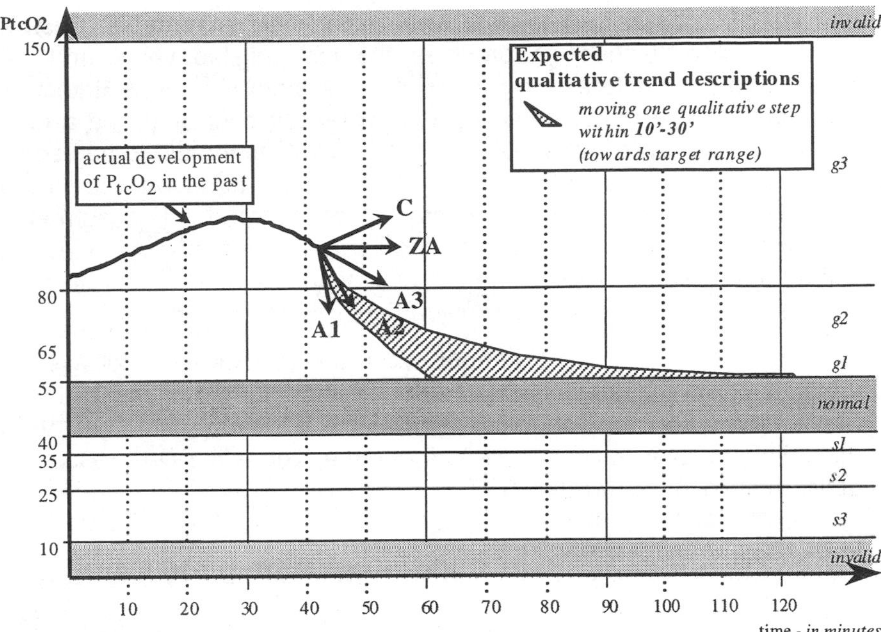

Figure 2. Trends defined in VIE-VENT. Values above the normal range can increase dangerously (C), stay constant (ZA), decrease too fast (A1), normal (A2), or too slow (A3).

The lower region is not shown in figure 2 but in figure 10 and in table 2.

The assessment procedure compares the previous qualitative short-term trend-category with the current one. If both belong to the same qualitative category or to a neighboring qualitative category then the parameter is validated as “correct”. Otherwise the parameter is classified as “wrong”.

The advantage of assessing qualitative trends is the ability to classify changes on a basis, which is better founded physiologically. For severe deviations from the target range we expect a return to the target range, which is fast initially and becomes slower and slower the nearer we approach the normal value. The trend-curve-fitting scheme and its resulting qualitative trend categories dynamically models this behavior.

11.3.3.5 Repair: Estimating Missing Values

During a monitoring process the position of a sensor has to be changed frequently and regularly. Therefore, the measurements are often missing. The implicit assumption of missing measurements during such a position change is that they will be steady keeping their previously observed values.

There are two possibilities to deal with missing measurements. First, a stepwise backward checking provides the last reliable value and we continue with this value as long as no other system change is detected. The reliability score of estimated values decreases over time and a user defined timeout prevents estimations based on values too old to be useful. Second, applying the growth rate of the short-term trend we estimate a "correct" value. A precondition is the stability of the trend. It is assumed to be true, if the medium-term and short-term qualitative trend-categories are identical. The trend-based estimation of a value is more accurate then simply using the last valid value, provided stability of the trend.

Estimating values is less problematic when the medical staff follows the general guideline that sensors should not be changed or calibrated during critical phases of the neonate. However, if we cannot get valid measurements over a longer period of time, the simplified reasoning process is applied (see section 3.1).

11.3.4 Time-Independent Validation: Reliability Ranking

This last category is based on time-independent reliability ranking of variables. From the medical and technical sampling point of view, there is a well-defined priority which measurement is more reliable than another, depending on different conditions.

This allows the definition of a reliability ranking scheme by the user. In case of contradicting parameter values which cannot be resolved by other methods, the more reliable one is selected according to the rating scheme.

Examples of reliability ranking of VIE-VENT are: arterial blood gases are more reliable than venous blood gases; invasive blood gases are more reliable than both transcutaneous blood gases and S_aO_2; S_aO_2 is more reliable than $P_{tc}O_2$. On the one hand these lists facilitate the data-validation task and on the other hand they also help the pruning of different and concurrent therapy recommendations.

11.4 Data Mining - Time-Oriented Data Abstraction

There are two fields of applications for the data abstracted from measuring devices in the clinical environment: Knowledge discovery and on-line monitoring.

Knowledge discovery retrospectively looks at recorded data to find significant patterns or to relate the raw data either to other information from the patient data management system or to rules in a knowledge base (Fayyad & Uthurusamy, 1996). On-line monitoring (a.k.a. intelligent alarming) tries to detect dangerous situations in real-time and to suggest countermeasures to assist the physician in the treatment process.

Both applications share most of their requirements concerning the data abstraction process. The main difference lies in the point of view on the data—retrospective vs. real-time. In retrospective analysis all information for the whole period of interest is available. So for each point in time the past, the present and the future are known. Opposed to this, in real-time analysis, only past and present are known. In the following we will explain the general approach first and discuss the special aspects of on-line monitoring at the end of each subsection if appropriate.

We distinguish three basic qualitative abstractions of a curve at a given position: *state*, *grade*, and *bends*. *State* (section 4.1) is the qualitative expression of the value itself, e.g. slightly high, normal, or extremely low. *Grade* (section 4.2) is the first deviation or slope of the curve, e.g. slightly increasing or stable. Since both state and grade are not only extracted for a single instant, but for a interval of time, the output of the abstraction process is not a series of point data, but a sequence of time intervals, during which a certain qualitative value stays stable.

Bend (section 4.3) abstraction transforms the curve from a series of data points to a sequel of bends with lines in between. This representation matches the intuitive or naive terms users often use when describing curves like “first it goes up, then it makes a bend down, and then up again”.

Trend curve fitting (section 4.4) is a method to abstract trends as utilized in section 3.3 from state and grade of a value.

In section 4.5 we show how *derived status information* can be produced by rules in a knowledge base using basic qualitative abstractions and information from the validation process.

11.4.1 State Abstraction

The state of a value is its classification according to a list of qualitative values and their borders, also called qualitative regions. E.g. the qualitative region of normal transcutaneously measured pressure of CO_2 ($P_{tc}CO_2$) might be from 35 to 49 mmHg during ventilation mode IPPV. Figure 3 shows an example from VIE-VENT, where we defined seven qualitative regions: *s1*, *s2*, and *s3*, for increased values, *normal* for values within the target range and *g1*, *g2*, and *g3*, for decreased values.

The transformation from quantitative to qualitative values has four advantages: First, qualitative information is easier to comprehend than an number. Second, uniform rating schemes provide convenient access to the data for rules applied on that data. Third, equal rating schemes for different parameters make them comparable, even if their numerical values are not, and independent of the origin of data. Fourth, the maintenance of a knowledge base or reasoning component is facilitated if the medical knowledge about value of a qualitative regions' limits changed.

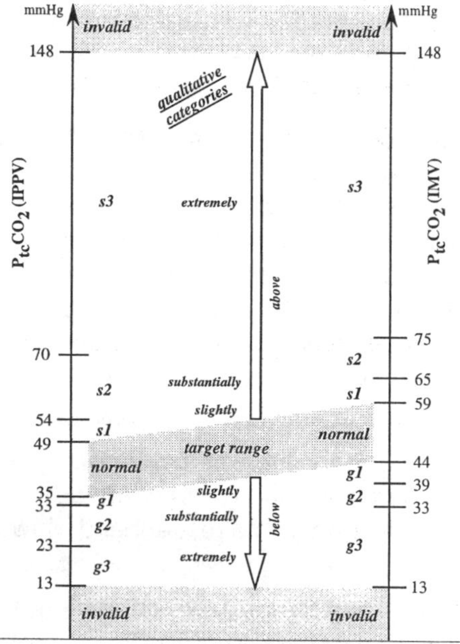

Figure 3. Qualitative regions of PtcCO2 in the context of IPPV and IMV.

Each set of qualitative regions is valid for a certain *context* only. The context is defined by the mode of ventilation—like in the above example—

by the diagnoses, or by constraints like acute problems or defects of the patient. Changes in context are derived automatically from the input data.

Although this transformation seems simple, it is not when the data is noisy like the signals obtained from monitors in the ICU environment.

Sophisticated data validation (as described in section 3) can contribute a lot to the quality of high-frequency data. Still many signals recorded in the medical domain exhibit more or less small random oscillations, which are hard to separate from meaningful changes in the curve.

If such a curve would be changed to a series of intervals, during which the qualitative value stays stable, and if the curve oscillates on the border between two qualitative regions, these intervals would be too small to be meaningful. In some cases the range of oscillation can be wider than the width of each qualitative region which leads to unusable output for most of the recording time.

There are two simple remedies to the problem: Averaging and thresholds. Both fail, if the quality of the signal or the range of oscillation changes dynamically as it is the case in the medical domain (e.g. small movements of the patient lead to short periods of random oscillations in the measured S_aO_2). To cope with such cases, we developed a method to abstract qualitative values from a statistical representation of the distribution of data points at each part of the curve called spread. It is explain third.

11.4.1.1 Averaging

The first approach—averaging—simply means that each measurement is replaced by the average of a certain number of data points in its surrounding. The approach is quite simple but the number of points involved in the calculation and the kind of averaging (mean, moving average, etc.) are very sensible parameters. Too much smoothing (e.g. averaging too many data points) hides meaningful peaks in the curve while moderate smoothing still fails to suppress more significant oscillations.

11.4.1.2 Thresholds

The second approach—thresholds—defeats errors by imposing a threshold when crossing the border between two qualitative regions. Thus, the qualitative value only changes, if the quantitative value exceeds the borders of the current qualitative region by a certain percentage of its width—the threshold. To avoid excessive postponement of changes in cases where the quantitative value crosses the border of a qualitative region but does not exceed the threshold, a timeout period is defined, after which smoothing is terminated by defining the qualitative value according to the current quantitative value, even if it is near a region's border. Figure 4 illustrates such a smoothing algorithm implemented in VIE-VENT. The ε-region corresponds to the threshold and the activated period reflects the time period until the timeout is reached. In the example in figure 4, the smoothing takes place from time point *t* until *t* + 7, called the smoothing period. More details are given in (Miksch et al., 1993).

The problem lies in finding the best values for threshold and timeout. If they are too big, every change in qualitative value is unnecessary postponed. If it is too small, it does not suppress all undesired oscillations. As with averaging good parameter settings might be found for curves of constant quality but no good solution can be found for dynamic changes in quality of measurement.

This algorithm was implemented in VIE-VENT (Miksch et al., 1993; 1996) but suffered from the inability to adjust the parameters in a way which fits the changing quality of the input.

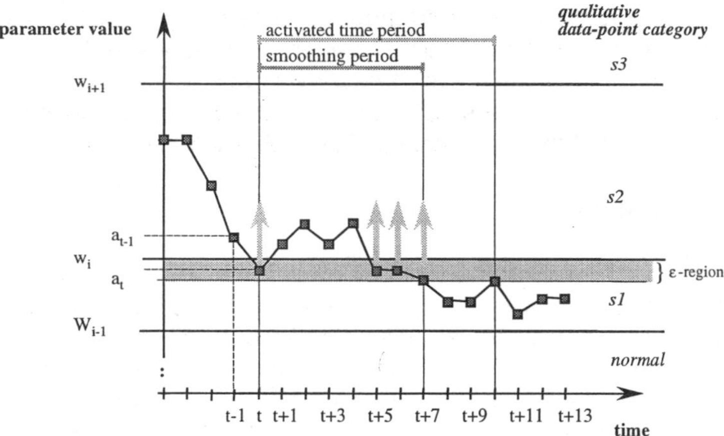

Figure 4. Smoothing of a curve oscillation on the border between two qualitative regions.

11.4.1.3 The Spread

To cope with these changing oscillations we developed a more complex representation of the curve, which we call the *spread* (Miksch et al., 1999). To calculate the spread, we slide a time window of constant width over the curve in small steps. For each position of the time window, we calculate a linear regression of the valid data points (i.e. not discarded by validation methods described in section 3) within the window. On the center of the line we plot the adapted standard error (s_a).

$$s_a = \frac{s}{\sqrt{N_{valid}}} \sqrt{N_{max}} \tag{4}$$

This is the standard deviation (s) of the linear regression divided by the square root of the number of valid data points involved in the calculation (N_{valid}) and multiplied by the square root of the maximum number of points possible in the interval (N_{max}).

Doing so we arrive at a vertical bar representing a statistically motivated estimation of the distribution of the data points in the time window. Connecting the ends of each bar with those of its neighbors yields a band (called *spread*), which vertically follows the average of the curve and the width of which shows the uncertainty involved in its calculation. The smaller the spread, the better the quality of the curve. Figure 5 shows the steps of the algorithm while figure 6 shows an example where the qualitative value is not influenced by a short peak which is not considered significant.

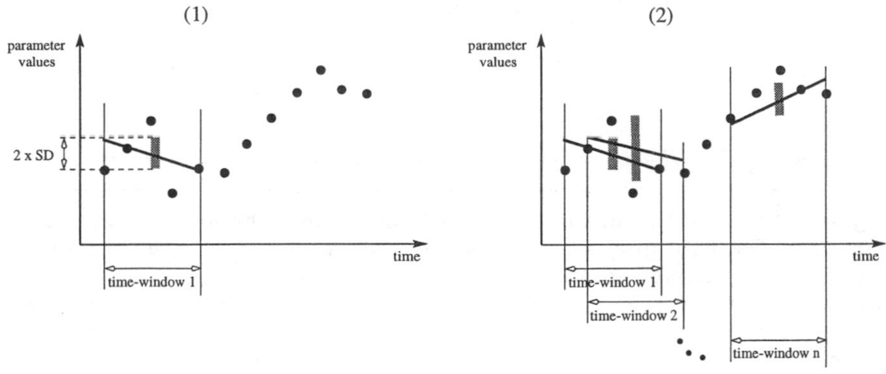

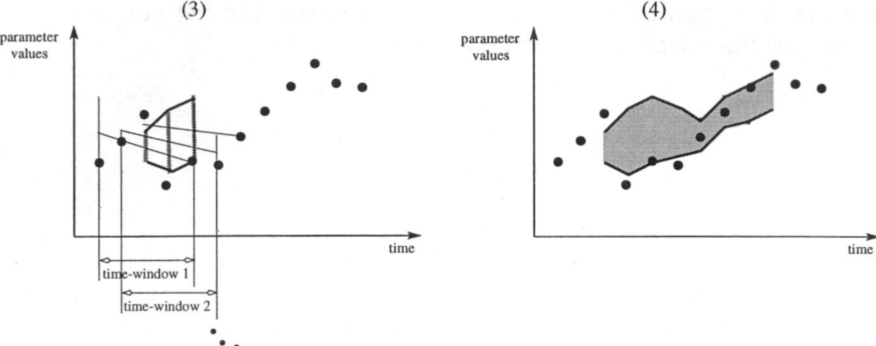

Figure 5. Calculation of the spread. For a given time-window (1) we calculate the linear regression line (long black line). On its center we plot the adapted standard error (equitation 4) up and down (gray vertical bar). This is repeated for all positions of the time-window (2). Connecting the ends of the bars (3) yields the spread (4). It represents the distribution of the data points based on statistical information.

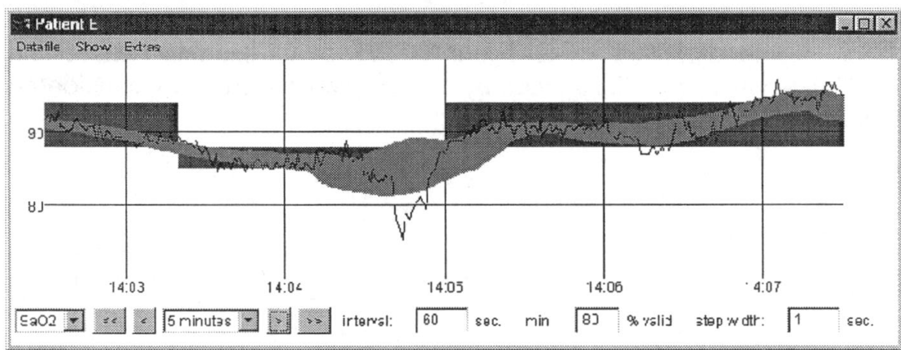

Figure 6. Practical example of the spread application. The thin line shows the raw data. The light gray area depicts the spread, the dark gray rectangles represent the derived temporal intervals of steady qualitative values. The lower part of the screen shot shows the parameters used. The length of the time window (interval) is set to 60 seconds. Thus the spread does not follow the short peak down at 14:04:45 but shows the deviation from the general trend by increased width.

The spread is used to abstract qualitative values of the curve. The qualitative value is changed only if both upper and lower margin of the spread are outside the previous qualitative region. This is a very conservative allocation strategy minimizing the changes in the qualitative value, but is mostly suitable for retrospective analysis.

For the purpose of intelligent alarming it might be desirable to plot the error bar on the rightmost end of the regression line instead of its center. In addition, alarms can also be triggered if only one margin of the spread crosses a certain limit e.g. if the upper margin of the spread enters the "extremely high"-region. Applying this procedure, bad data resulting in a wide spread cannot lead to delayed alarms, but might cause extraneous ones.

The advantage of the spread over other approaches lies in its dynamic adaptation to changing amounts of oscillations and missing data, which are very common in the clinical environment.

11.4.2 Grade Abstraction

While other authors like Shahar (Shahar & Musen, 1996) describe changes in the curve by two distinct qualitative values—gradient (e.g. increasing) and rate (e.g. fast)--we combine both in one value, the *grade*. It is the qualitative expression of the first deviation of the curve (e.g. fast increase, slow decrease) and can easily be derived from the slope of the regression lines calculated above. By drawing a spread for the slope too, its advantages (as described above) can be used for the abstraction of the grade too.

While current monitors mostly rely on the measured value of the parameters—their states—there is a strong demand for systems doing a more sophisticated analysis of the measured data. Defining alarms for qualitative values of the grade in addition to those for the state can help to avoid critical situations by drawing the physicians attention to problems before they cause a crisis. To arrive at a meaningful picture the grades measured over different periods of time together with the state must be considered for each parameter.

11.4.3 Bend Abstraction

When asked to comment on a curve many people describe it as a series of lines with bends of different sharpness in between. Motivated by this, we developed an method (Miksch & Seyfang, 1999) to break a series of data points into a sequel of bends with lines connecting them. Bends in a curve can be detected by looking at the second deviation of its graph. A minimum there indicates a bend to the right or down on the original curve, a maximum indicates a bend to the left or up (see figure 7).

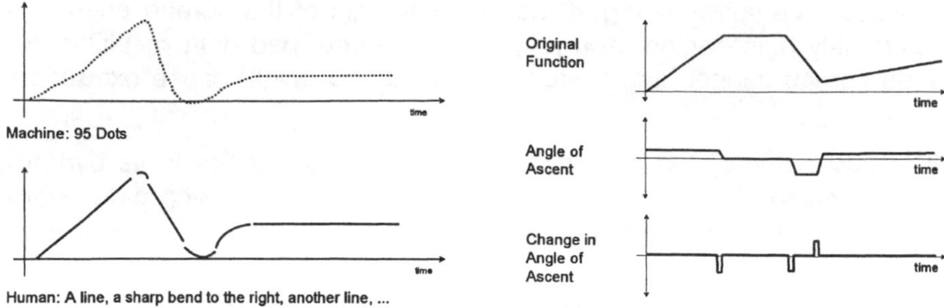

Figure 7. The bend abstraction. The basic idea in abstracting bends from a curve is, that humans describe as bends and lines what the devices supply as series of data points. Bends are defined as changes in the slope of the second deviation—in places, where the original curve makes a bend, its second deviation has an extremum.

To be more specific, first we calculate the angle of the slope of the original graph. Second, we calculate the slope of that curve. The resulting curve is called *indication function*. Each extremum or peek in the indication function represents one *bend*. From the sequel of the bends together with the original graph we derive *corners* and *lines*.

Each *bend* is described by the position of the corresponding extremum in the indication function, the height of the corresponding peak in the indication function, and the area of the peak.

The x-coordinate of the *corner* clearly equals the middle of the bend. The y-value could be the y-coordinate of the nearest point in the original curve, but to reduce influence of noise, it is necessary to take the average of some of its neighbors into account too in most cases. Integrating too many of them in the calculation will distort the result towards the inner side of the bend.

The *lines* between the bends can either be drawn just as connections of the corners of the curve, or they are calculated as a linear regression of the points of the original curve between two bends.

Which version of the above definitions is taken depends on the focus or preference of the users, which varies between different domains of application.

The data abstracted this way can be used in three different ways:

11.4.3.1 Direct Visualization

An example for the direct visualization of bends is shown in figure 8. Each bend in the original graph (at the top) is represented by a bar (on the bottom), who's height and area equals the height and area of the corresponding peak in the indication function (in the middle). This method is applicable to tasks, where the attention of the user must be drawn to relatively small irregularities in a periodic curve.

11.4.3.2 Symbolic Representation

The information about the bend can be expressed in list to make in accessible to symbolic reasoners like knowledge based systems or machine learning tools. This is important to bridge the gap between raw data delivered by monitors and knowledge bases using this knowledge in a high-level way.

The following Example describes a graph consisting of a line increasing by 20 degrees for 100 seconds followed by a narrow bend to the right and 30 seconds of decrease.

```
((line 100sec up 20°)
 (bow right narrow)
 (line 30sec down 30°))
```

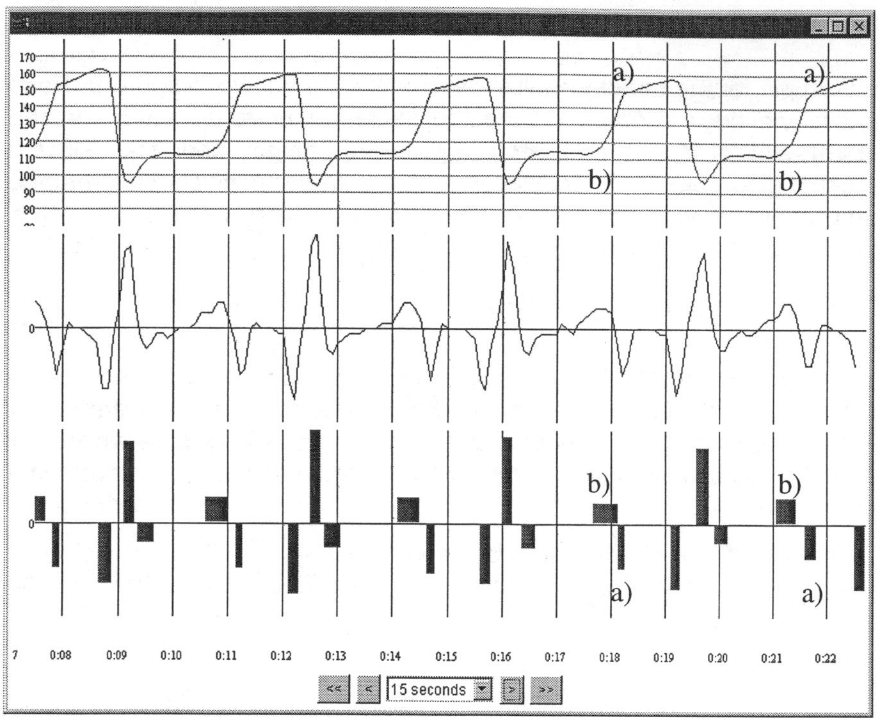

Figure 8. Visualization of bends. Starting at the top, we show the original graph, the indication function and the bars representing the significant bends. a) shows an example of an irregularity in the curve which a human could also detect if concentrating on every detail: the bend in the right-most oscillation is not as sharp as the corresponding one in the other oscillations. b) draws our attention to a feature not perceptible by looking at the raw data: the long-spread bow to the left of the second oscillation from the right is not as sharp as the others as indicated by inferior height of the bar. The corresponding part of the original curve does not seem different by itself. The significance of the features found in a) and b) depends on the domain knowledge about the data represented by the curve.

11.4.3.3 Interoscillation Reasoning

Many types of data recorded in the medical domain are periodic but varying. Deviations have natural, pathological, technical, or unexplainable origin. The field of signal processing provides a wide range of methods for both noise reduction and detection of deviations. However, they are designed for signals with technical origin, for which an exact mathematical model is available. Many signals recorded in medicine lack such an exact model. In some cases, there is a qualitative model, roughly describing the interdependencies of some parameters, but not supplying an exact formula for the calculation of the "real" values.

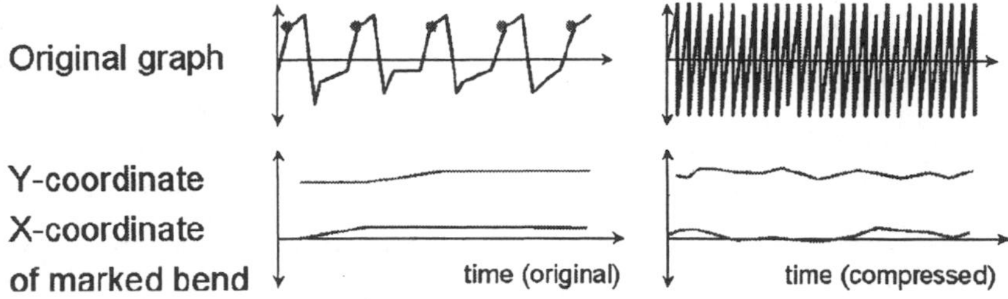

Figure 9. Visualizing the changes of the oscillation's shape. Plotting a bend's X-coordinate (its offset within the oscillation) or the Y-coordinate (the value of the original curve at this position) on a separate graph yields a very dense representation of the bend indicating all its changes and deviations clearly.

Another aspect is the format, in which the curve or function is described. Fast Fourier analysis, for example, describes periodic curves by a list of frequencies and their amplitudes. For a physician this is a very unusual way to look at an ECG.

As an alternative, we compare the position of each bend in an oscillation to its position in other oscillations. This yields information on the change of the oscillation's appearance over time which is rather intuitive, since it is in terms like "the second peak moved up by 10 % over the last minute". In many fields of application such formulations are compatible with the knowledge acquired by human experts when looking at curves (without the aid of computer systems).

On the one hand, plotting one dimension of a corner point in each instance of an oscillation as a separate curve yield a graph which gives a clear picture of the corner's development over time, even when the time axis is compressed (figure 9). On the other hand, this graph can be used as input to data abstraction to obtain qualitative information about the development of that detail of the oscillation.

As of this writing, we are examining the applicability of this approach to the fields of ECG and CTG.

11.4.4 Trend Curve Fitting

Often the aim of a treatment correlates with bringing the value of some parameter back to the normal region. In these cases the grade alone does not give full information. Instead we are interested in learning whether the value is improving i.e. approaching the normal region or not. An increase of a value which is too high has different semantics than an increase of a value which is too low.

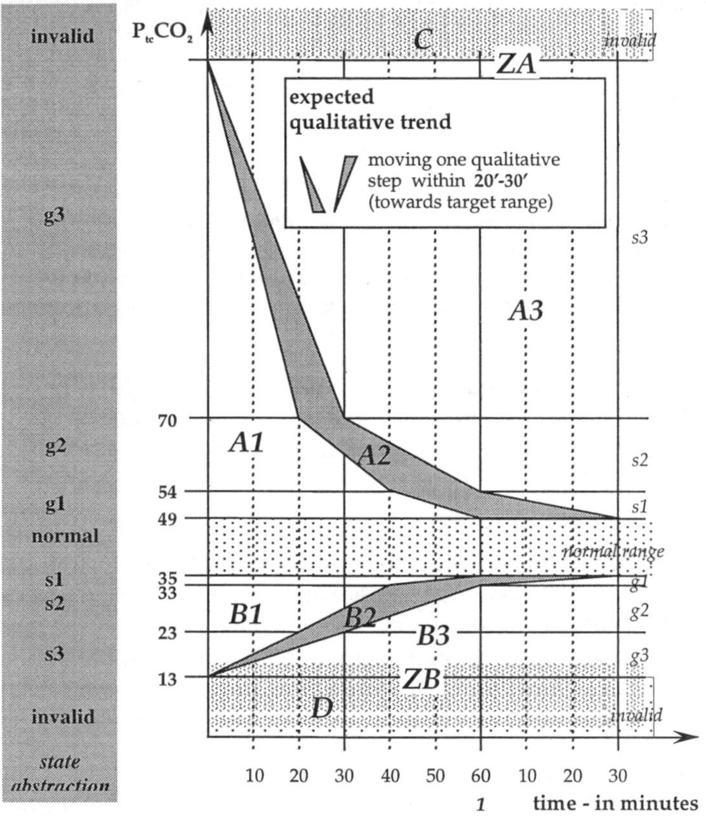

Figure 10. Expected improvement PtcCO2. Values which are too low should improves by one qualitative step within 10 to 20 minutes while values which are too high may take 20 to 30 minutes per step to improve.

In many cases there is also an estimation of how long it takes under normal conditions for the value to return to normal. So we can distinguish between normal improvement, too slow improvement and too fast improvement. Figure 10 shows the trends implemented in VIE-VENT. In this example, we demand that the value of $P_{tc}CO_2$ improves by one qualitative step within 20 to 30 minutes. The algorithm is explained in (Miksch et al., 1993). Table 2 summarizes the trends of a curve, depending on its state and rate of change.

values above the target range are	
A1	decreasing too fast
A2	decreasing normally
A3	decreasing too slow
ZA	staying constant
C	increasing dangerously

values below the target range are	
B1	increasing too fast
B2	increasing normally
B3	increasing too slow
ZB	staying constant
D	decreasing dangerously

Table 2. Schema of trend curve fitting in VIE-VENT.

11.4.5 Derived Status Information

In many cases the trend or state of a parameter does not itself give enough information. A rule base is needed to abstract more useful information from the basics.

The qualitative temporal abstraction of monitoring variables makes it easy to use simple rules to activate therapeutic actions. For example, rule *R8-therapeutic-actions* states, that we recommend an increase of both frequency and *PIP*, if the short-term trend of $P_{tc}CO_2$ is *A3*, *ZA*, or *C*, and its state is above normal, i.e. *s1*, *s2*, or *s3*, and the input is classified as correct.

```
(defrule R8-therapeutic-actions
activate-therapeutic-action-PtcCO2-ventilation"
   (phase (kind therapy_recommendation))
   (ventilation_phase (kind ippv))
   ?f1 <- (thp_recommendation ventilation)
   (qual_trend_category (parameter PtcCO2)
                        (kind_of_trend short)
                        (qual_trend A3|ZA|C))
   (qual_data_point_category (parameter PtcCO2)
                             (site tc)
                             (value s1, s2, s3))
   (causal-explanation-validation (parameter PtcCO2)
                                  (classification correct))
=>
   (retract ?f1)
   (assert (action (reason ventilation)
                   (BG PtcCO2)
                   (kind inc-f))
           (action (reason ventilation)
                   (BG PtcCO2)
                   (kind inc-pip))))
```

The essential preconditions for triggering therapeutic actions depend on the qualitative trend abstraction of the short-term trend (expressed as *qual_trend_category* in the rule *R8-therapeutic-actions*) and the qualitative state abstraction (expressed as *qual_data_point_category* in the rule *R8-therapeutic-actions*). If the qualitative state abstraction is *s1* or *s2* or *s3*, and the qualitative trend abstraction is *A3* or *ZA* or *C*, then therapeutic actions are recommended (increase ventilator settings). The second fact *ventilation_phase* in the left-hand side (LHS) of rule *R8-therapeutic-actions* refers to the mode of ventilation (i.e., IPPV) and indicates, that this rule belongs to the set of rules dealing with the phase of Intermittent Positive Pressure Ventilation). The last fact, *causal-explanation-validation*, supplies the necessary explanations of the data validation process, namely the classification of the particular validated parameter. The right-hand side (RHS) of rule *R8-therapeutic-actions* specifies the therapeutic actions. Each action-fact includes the kind of the recommended action and an explanation of the circumstances: the fact *(reason ventilation)* refers to "ventilation" process depending on the system model of ventilation), *(BG PtcCO2)* refers to the relevant parameter, namely the blood gas measurement, and *(kind ?x)* determines which particular action has to take place (e.g. *(kind inc-pip)* means, that an increase of the peak inspiratory pressure (*PIP*) is recommended).

11.5 Evaluation and Discussion

11.5.1 Empirical Evaluation

Within the VIE-VENT system (Miksch et al., 1993; 1996), we evaluated the effectiveness of the above data-validation methods presented in section 3 utilizing a particular evaluation scenario consisting of two steps (Horn et al., 1997): first, a visual inspection of the results of the data validation process, and, second, a formal evaluation of the validation results.

Our sample consists of 640786 seconds (approx. 177 hours) of data recordings from nine neonates. The age of the neonates was between four days and six weeks, the weight between 690 g and 3460 g.

In the first step, the data from the first six patients (approx. 115 hours) were used to tune the validation parameters, specifically to find suitable parameters for the stability check and the Højstrup method. Additional validation parameters, which could not be determined from the data recordings, were derived from the knowledge of expert neonatologists. We plotted the data curves and annotated the invalid data with rectangular markers below each curve, when our data-validation methods recognized errors. Two expert neonatologists examined the results. The parameters in our data-validation methods were tuned towards the overall goal of avoiding wrong therapeutic recommendations. As a consequence, the data-validation methods marked all measurements as invalid which depicted *unusable* signals. The remaining data (approx. 62 hours of recording) have been used to verify the correctness of the data-validation methods.

In the second step in our evaluation scenario we compared the data points found invalid by an expert neonatologist with the invalidation markers produced by VIE-VENT. Currently, no widely accepted "gold standard" exists to judge the correctness of the continuously assessed data of $P_{tc}O_2$, $P_{tc}CO_2$ and S_aO_2. Therefore, we relied on the judgement of the domain experts, experienced neonatologists.

For this evaluation study we took sequences of continuously assessed data which show some variation. We selected continuous sequences of 4320 seconds length which contain at least two invalidation markers from VIE-VENT.

From these sequences we randomly selected five sequences from different patients. The selected sequences were presented to the expert using high resolution plotting (without the invalidation markers of VIE-VENT). The expert marked those data points which he judged invalid. Table 3 gives the evaluation results from the comparison of the expert's and VIE-VENT's invalidation markers. VIE-VENT's perfect sensitivity is not surprising due to the tuning of the parameters towards recognition of all artifacts and unclear trends. The rather low specificity results from the overall goal to avoid wrong therapeutic recommendations. A further complication which lowers specificity is the fact, that the expert is able to see the future development of a parameter from the plot. In contrast, VIE-VENT operates in real-time. It has to wait for stability of a parameter until it is set back valid. This increases the number of false positives but is an effect caused by the constraints of real-time operation.

Parameter	*Sensitivity*	*Specificity*
S_aO_2	100%	88.9%
$P_{tc}O_2$	100%	83.2%
$P_{tc}CO_2$	100%	94.6%

Table 3. Evaluation of VIE-VENT's data validation procedures.

11.5.2 Discussion

The high-level abstraction methods presented in section 4 lead to the a series of opportunities both in visualisation and in interfacing knowledge-based systems.

11.5.2.1 Compact Visualization

Displaying only the important features of a graph in an abstract form in addition to the original graph allows for easy detection of trends and outliers which otherwise would be burried in the overwhelming impression of the data. Currently we are investigating into the application of various abstract data representations in the field of ECG-analysis and ventilation monitoring.

11.5.2.2 Bridge to Knowledge Representation

The abstracted information can be matched against conditions in a rule base. So the curves can be tagged according to a set of classifications stored in a knowledge base. This aspect is crucial for the integration of high-frequency data and symbolic systems such as symbolic machine learning, knowledge-based systems for intelligent alarming and a guideline execution system like the one developed in the Asgaard (Shahar, Miksch, & Johnson, 1998) project.

11.5.3 Overall Benefits

In the following we are summarizing the main benefits of our proposed methods:

11.5.3.1 Improving the Quality of Data

The data recordings assessed from various channels of devices are more erroneous than commonly expected. Applying our validation methods to the observed on-line and off-line data sets resulted in automatic elimination of most invalid measurements: false positive alarms were reduced and errors of data interpretation were minimized.

11.5.3.2 Communicating Various Kinds of Time-Stamped Data Lucidly

The physicians need an overview over a certain period of time and over various parameters which together give a more detailed, reliable, and comprehensible picture of the patient's condition. Our time-oriented data-abstraction methods transform a huge amount of numerical, time-stamped values into a convenient set of easy to understand qualitative descriptions of the patient's situation. This results in diminishing the information overload by visualizing the available information in a user specific and capable way: the physicians can recognize and predict a critical patient's condition more easily, which finally ensures a better treatment management.

11.5.3.3 Bridging to Higher-Level Reasoning

More sophisticated reasoning tasks need more advanced representations than numerical data or simple qualitative assessments. Our approach facilitates tagging various time-oriented data sets according to a set of qualitative and more intuitive classifications. These qualitative characteristics over time can be matched against conditions from a rule base, which results in more obvious and simple rule base. At the same time, this rule base enables more powerful reasoning components to be applied.

11.6 Future Research

Future work will focus on extending the methods' understanding of the underlying processes and on running elaborate evaluations.

11.6.1 Utilizing Qualitative Descriptions in Treatment Planning

Previous version of VIE-VENT used standard forward-chaining rules to formulate the knowledge about the data and its interdependencies. But application domains like artificial ventilation of neonates can only be described fully as a set of interweaving and interdependent treatment processes.

Several researches try to formalize that in knowledge-based systems. Still, for domains like ventilation in ICUs, most approaches do not seem powerful enough (Miksch, 1999). Instead, a framework for time-oriented modeling of treatment procedures (Shahar, Miksch, & Johnson, 1998) is needed to proper represent the domain knowledge, which can lead to even higher level abstraction of the data such as the assistance of the weaning process through recommendations for the settings of the respirator.

11.6.2 Repetitive Temporal Patterns

In dynamically changing environments, like ICUs, the basic temporal data-abstraction methods resulting in qualitative state, gradient, rate, or simple pattern description (compare (Shahar & Musen, 1996; Shahar 1997; Miksch et al., 1996)), are not sufficient.

High-level temporal data-abstraction methods are needed, which include a wide variability in the behavior of a parameter, variability in the time patterns a parameter shows, and specifications for relating different temporal patterns of different parameters. They have to be able to recognize and to describe recurring states, events, episodes, or actions (e.g. information about the frequency of temporal patterns in the past, like "three episodes of hyperoxemia during the last three hours occurred").

11.6.3 Further Evaluation

To achieve acceptance by practitioners it is crucial to run extensive evaluations both on recorded data and in real-time with all parts of the system. Currently, we are working on evaluation scenarios to examine the usefulness of our approach in the clinical setting of artificial ventilation of newborn infants.

11.6.4 Conclusion

We described methods to validate and to repair potentially unreliable time-oriented, high-frequency data and to abstract different kinds of qualitative descriptions over time from the validated but still partially untrustworthy data, in which some artifacts might remain unrecognized. Our methods presented were successful in overcoming the problems the medical staff is facing currently: first, to improve the quality of data to arrive at trustworthy data and, second, to ease the information overload caused by various channels of on-line and off-line data recordings. The methods support the medical staff to easily comprehend the various continuously and discontinuously assessed data utilizing different qualitative abstractions over time and combination thereof.

Our approach was evaluated on data from artificial ventilation of neonates and proved to reduce the number of wrong alarms while correcting most artifacts in the data.

Future research will focus on adding high-level treatment planning to the domain-knowledge base to implement an even deeper understanding of the processes lying behind the observed data. This will improve the performance especially in non-standard cases like life-threatening situations which cannot be described by a simple set of rules.

Acknowledgments

We thank Georg Duftschmid, Gerhilde Egghart, Klaus Hammermüller, and Robert Kosara for their contributions. This project is supported by "Fonds zur Förderung der wissenschaftlichen Forschung - FWF" (Austrian Science Foundation), P12797-INF. We greatly appreciate the support given to the Austrian Research Institute of Artificial Intelligence (OFAI) by the Austrian Federal Ministry of Science and Transport, Vienna.

References

Avent, R., and Charlton, J. 1990. A critical review of trend-detection methologies for biomedical monitoring systems. Critical Reviews in Biomedical Engineering 17(6):621-659.

Bellazzi, R.; Larizza, C.; Magni, P.; Montani, S.; and De Nicolao, G. 1999. Intelligent analysis of clinical time series by combining structural filtering and temporal abstractions. In Horn, W.; Shahar, Y.; Lindberg, G.; Andreassen, S.; and Wyatt, J., eds., Proceedings of the Joint European Conference on Artificial Intelligence in Medicine and Medical Decision Making, AIMDM'99, 271-280. Berlin: Springer.

Carlson, D.; Wallace, J.; East, T.; and Morris, A. 1993. Verification and validation algorithms for data used in critical care decision support systems. In Gardner, R., ed., Proceedings 19th Annual Symposium on Computer Applications in Medical Care (SCAMC'95). 188- 192.

Cios, K.; Pedrycz, W.; and Swiniarski, R. 1998. Data Mining Methods for Knowledge Discovery. Boston: Kluwer Academic Publishers.

Clancey, W. J. 1985. Heuristic classification. Artificial Intelligence 27:289-350.

Egghart, G. 1995. Validierung von In- und Outputdaten: Methoden und ihre Anwendungen in VIE-VENT. Master's thesis, Department of Medical Cybernetics and Artificial Intelligence, University of Vienna.

Fayyad, R., and Uthurusamy, R. 1996. Data mining and knowledge discovery in databases. Communications of the ACM 39:24-26.

Gardner, R.; Hawley, W.; East, T.; Oniki, T.; and Young, H.-F. 1992. Real time data acquisition: Experience with the medical information bus (MIB). In Clayton, P., ed., Proceedings of the Fifteenth Annual Symposium on Computer Applications in Medical Care, SCAMC-91. New York: McGraw-Hill.

Garfinkel, D.; Matsiras, P.; Mavrides, T.; McAdems, J.; and Aukburg, S. 1989. Patient monitoring in the operating room: Validation of instruments reading by artificial intelligence methods. In Kingsland, L., ed., Proceedings of the Thirteenth Annual Symposium on Computer Applications in Medical Care, SCAMC-89, 575-579. Washington, DC: IEEE Computer Society Press.

Haimowitz, I.; Le, P.; and Kohane, I. 1995. Clinical monitoring using regression-based trend templates. Artificial Intelligence in Medicine 7(6):473-496.

Højstrup, J. 1992. A statistical data screening procedure. Measurement Science & Technologie 4:153-157.

Horn, W.; Miksch, S.; Egghart, G.; Popow, C.; and Paky, F. 1997. Effective data validation of high-frequency data: Time-point-, time-interval-, and trend-based methods. Computer in Biology and Medicine, Special Issue: Time-Oriented Systems in Medicine 27(5):389-409.

Hunter, J., and McIntosh, N. 1999. Knowledge-based event detection in complex time series data. In Horn, W.; Shahar, Y.; Lindberg, G.; Andreassen, S.; and Wyatt, J., eds., Proceedings of the Joint European Conference on Artificial Intelligence in Medicine and Medical Decision Making, AIMDM'99, 271-280. Berlin: Springer.

Kay, S. 1993. Fundamentals of Statistical Signal Processing. Engelwood, New Jersey: Prentice Hall.

Keravnou, E. T. 1997. Temporal abstraction of medical data: Deriving periodicity. In Lavrac, N.; Keravnou, E.; and Zupan, B., eds., Intelligent Data Analysis in Medicine and Pharmacology. Boston: Kluwer Academic Publisher. 61-79.

Larizza, C.; Bellazzi, R.; and Riva, A. 1997. Temporal abstractions for diabetic patients management. In Proceedings of the Artificial Intelligence in Medicine, 6th Conference on Artificial Intelligence in Medicine Europe (AIME-97), 3 19-30. Berlin: Springer.

Lawless, S. 1994. Crying wolf: False alarms in a pediatric intensive care unit. Critical Care Medicine 22:981-985.

Miksch, S., and Seyfang, A. 1999. Finding intuitive abstractions of high-frequency data. In Miksch, S.; Andreassen, S.; Dojat, M.; Hunter, J.; Popow, C.; Rees, S.; and Thorgard, P., eds., Workshop "Computers in Anaesthesia and Intensive Care: Knowledge-Based Information Management", in conjunction with the Joint European Conference on Artificial Intelligence in Medicine and Medical Decision Making (AIMDM'99), 13-26.

Miksch, S.; Horn, W.; Popow, C.; and Paky, F. 1993. VIE-VENT: Knowledge-based monitoring and therapy planning of the artificial ventilation of newborn infants. In Andreassen, et al., S., ed., Artificial Intelligence in Medicine (Proceedings of the Fourth European Conference on Artificial Intelligence in Medicine Europe (AIME-93). Amsterdam: IOS Press.

Miksch, S.; Horn, W.; Popow, C.; and Paky, F. 1996. Utilizing temporal data abstraction for data validation and therapy planning for artificially ventilated newborn infants. Artificial Intelligence in Medicine 8(6):543-576.

Miksch, S.; Seyfang, A.; Horn, W.; and C., P. 1999. Abstracting steady qualitative descriptions over time from noisy, high-frequency data. In Horn, W.; Shahar, Y.; Lindberg, G.; Andreassen, S.; and Wyatt, J., eds., Proceedings of the Joint European Conference on Artificial Intelligence in Medicine and Medical Decision Making, AIMDM'99, 281-290. Berlin: Springer.

Miksch, S. 1999. Plan management in the medical domain. AI Communications, 4.

Quinlan, J. 1986. The effect of noise on concept learning. In Michalski, R.; Carbonell, J.; and Mitchell, T., eds., Machine Learning. An Artificial Intelligence Approach. Boston: Morgan Kauffmann. 149-166.

Shahar, Y., and Musen, M. A. 1996. Knowledge-based temporal abstraction in clinical domains. Artificial Intelligence in Medicine, Special Issue Temporal Reasoning in Medicine 8(3):267-98.

Shahar, Y.; Miksch, S.; and Johnson, P. 1998. The Asgaard Project: A task-specific framework for the application and critiquing of time-oriented clinical guidelines. Artificial Intelligence in Medicine 14:29-51.

Shahar, Y. 1997. A framework for knowledge-based temporal abstraction. Artificial Intelligence 90(1-2):267-98.

Sittig, D., and Factor, M. 1990. Physiologic trend detection and artificial rejection: a parallel implementation of multi-state kalman filtering algorithm. Computer Methods and Programs in Biomedicine 31:1-10.

Sittig, D., and Orr, J. 1992. Evaluation of a parallel implementation of the learning portion of the backward error propagation neural network: Experiments in artifact identification. In Clayton, P., ed., Proceedings of the Fifteenth Annual Symposium on Computer Applications in Medical Care, SCAMC-91, 290-294. New York: McGraw-Hill.

Sukuvaara, T.; Koski, E.; Maekivirta, A.; and Kari, A. 1992. A knowledge-based alarm system for monitoring cardiac operated patients - technical construction and evaluation. International Journal of Clinical Monitoring and Computing 10:117-126.

Uckun, S. 1994. Intelligent systems in patient monitoring and therapy management. International Journal of Clinical Monitoring and Computing 11:241-253.

van der Aa, J. 1990. Intelligent alarms in anesthesia. Master's thesis, Technische Universiteit Eindhoven, The Netherlands.

12 Data Mining the Matrix Associated Regions (MARs) for Gene Therapy

Gautam B. Singh[1] and Stephan Krawetz[2]
[1]Department of Computer Science and Engineering
Software and Information Technology Laboratory, Oakland University,
Rochester, MI 48309, U.S.A.
singh@oakland.edu
[2]Department of Obstetrics and Gynecology
Center for Molecular Medicine and Genetics
Wayne State University, School of Medicine
Detroit, MI 48201, U.S.A.
steve@compbio.med.wayne.edu

Unsupervised data mining holds considerable promise for knowledge discovery from biological databases that have continued their exponential growth over the last decade. In an application of unsupervised learning to gene therapy, our aim is to detect the elements of locus control that impart gene expression in a position-independent copy-number dependent manner. Incorporating these elements into gene therapeutics will move gene therapy from the bench to bedside. An example of such an element is the region known as the Matrix Association Region or MAR. Our limited knowledge of MARs has hampered formulating their detection using classical pattern recognition where the existence of lower level constituent elements is used to establish the presence of a higher level functional block. In contrast, MAR detection which utilizes the statistical estimation of "interestingness" of a sample has proven to be successful. This strategy has been implemented in the MAR-Finder software. Examples of its utility in identifying candidate MARs to guide the wet bench validation of MAR locations are presented. This strategy may be of general utility for the detection of other classes of regulatory signals when the data set describing a new type of functional element is limiting.

12.1 Understanding the Problem Domain

Every cell in an organism contains the same genetic information and expresses the same subset of genes for basic cellular function. In addition, there is a second set of genes that are uniquely expressed in each cell type. In this manner the functional role of that cell can be thought of as reflecting the partitioning of genes into compartments of those that can be expressed and those that cannot be expressed. The biological mechanism by which this is achieved is mediated by the presence of simple DNA sequence patterns that are predominantly found within the neighborhood of the gene locus (Kliensmith et al. 1995 and reviewed in Krawetz et al., 1999). These simple sequence patterns are embedded within the majority of nuclear non-coding DNA. This is in direct contrast to the 2% of the genome that corresponds to the protein coding regions.

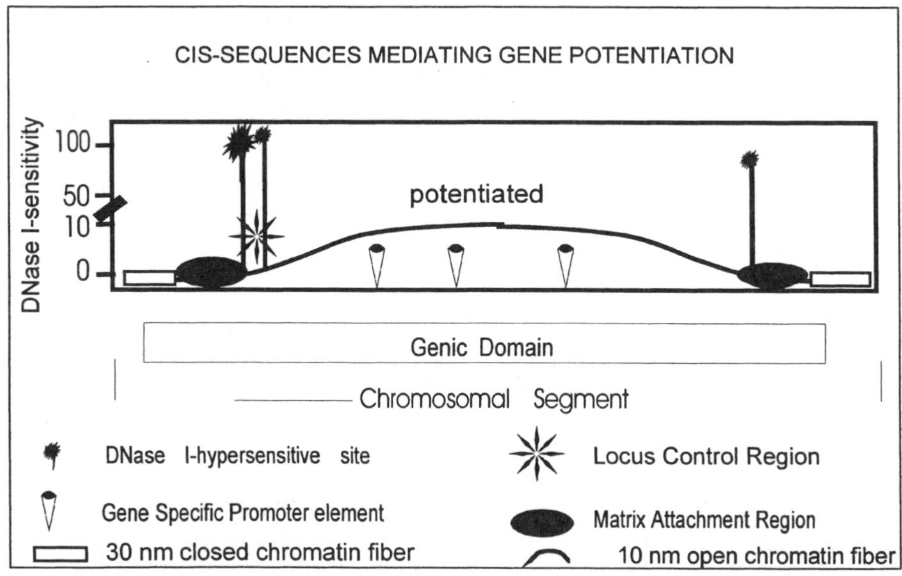

Figure 1. Cis-sequences mediating gene potentiation. As shown an open chromatin domain is contained within a 10nm chromatin fiber. This region is 10 times more sensitive to DNase I. The domain is bounded by regions of matrix attachment (filled ellipsoids) that appear at the transition of segment to the 30nm closed chromatin conformation (open boxes). Several DNase I hypersensitive sites (bursting stars) are contained within this domain. These sites are 100× more sensitive to DNase I. The gene specific promoter elements (triangles) are indicated. The Locus Control Region (LCR) is indicated as the open star coincident with hypersensitive sites and Matrix Attachment Regions.

Special sequences of regulatory importance such as introns, promoters, enhancers, Matrix Association Regions (MARs), and repetitive elements are found in these regions of non-coding DNA. Many of these regions contain patterns that represent functional control points for cell specific or *differential* gene expression (Kadonaga 1998;Roeder 1998), while others such as *repetitive* DNA sequence elements may serve as a biological clock (Hartwell et al. 1994) . These and numerous other examples indicate that the *patterns* embedded in the eukaryote DNA may play a vital role for its viability. Other examples of these patterns include the A+T or G+C rich regions, telomeric repeats of AGGGTT in human DNA, the rare occurrence or absence of dinucleotides, e.g.,TA and GC, and tetranucleotides, e.g., CTAG, and the GNN periodicity in the gene coding regions. Deviations from these patterns are usually deleterious to the viability of the organism. Thus, the DNA is not a homogeneous string of characters, but is comprised of a mosaic of sequence level motifs that come together in a synergistic manner to define the state of that organism.

The following four events of potentiation, initiation, elongation and termination are utilized as an ordered process for the successful transcription, i.e., the synthesis of RNA from a DNA template. First, potentiation, i.e. the change in the local chromatin conformation from a 30 nm fiber to an open structure that can be likened to the 10 nm fiber. As illustrated in Fig. 1, potentiation is the prerequisite for gene expression, as it serves to open that segment of the genome permitting access to the various transcription factors needed to transcribe the genes within this segment. Second, initiation, i.e., the binding of RNA polymerase to the gene marks the beginning of transcription. The third step elongation, the covalent addition of nucleotides to the growing polynucleotide chain then proceeds. Finally, the fourth, i.e., the termination of transcription is mediated by the recognition of the transcription termination sequence on the DNA template by the transcription machinery. This leads to the release of the DNA template and RNA product.

It is generally accepted that the structural properties of the nuclear DNA complex are responsible for maintaining the potentiated conformation of a gene-locus within a cell (Krawetz et al. 1999). As shown in Fig.1, the end-points of potentiated gene-loci are often attached to the nuclear matrix at points of contact known as Matrix Attachment Regions or MARs. The localization of loci to the nuclear matrix is thought to facilitate transcription by increasing the local concentration of transcription factors (reviewed in Cook 1999). In this manner by fixing a gene onto the nuclear matrix the problem of trans-factor interaction with the gene target is reduced from occurring in three-dimensional space to that occurring in two-dimensional space. This essentially increases the probability of an effective interaction for a productive transcription event by an order of magnitude.

Our understanding of the process of gene regulation is key to moving gene therapeutics from the bench to bedside. We have been collectively pursuing this objective for over 20-years and our efforts are beginning to bear fruit (Krawetz et al. 1999). This is evidenced by the surge in gene therapeutic protocols and the encouraging results that they have born. The least understood element in bringing gene therapeutics to the bench-side is that which controls the mechanism of potentiation. This holds the key to increasing the successful application of gene therapeutics as it renders the gene within each locus in a state that can be expressed. If we can harness this technology then we will possess the ability to seed our genome with therapeutics that will be appropriately maintained in an open conformation requisite for transcription. As discussed below, it is our hope that MARs will provide such as key.

12.2 Understanding the Data

The Matrix or Scaffold Attachment regions are relatively short (100-1000 bp long) sequences that anchor the chromatin loops to the nuclear matrix. MARs are often associated with the origins of replication (ORI). They usually possess a concentrated area of transcription factor binding sites (Boulikas 1993). Approximately 100,000 matrix attachment sites are believed to exist in the mammalian nucleus, where ~30,000-40,000 serve as ORIs (reviewed in Bode et al. 1996). MARs have been observed to flank the ends of genic domains encompassing various transcriptional units. It has also been shown that MARs bring together the transcriptionally active regions of chromatin such that transcription is initiated in the region of the chromosome that coincides with the surface of nuclear matrix (Bode et al. 1996;Nikolaev et al. 1996).

The success of the Human Genome Project (HGP) is dependent upon a continued effort to develop databases and tools that enable easy access and comparison of genome information. Several molecular biology databases have been created containing diverse information such as annotated biological sequences, 3D-structures, genetic and physical maps (Keen et al. 1992). As the HGP nears the completion of its first phase that is aimed at fully determining the approximately 3×10^9 characters of the human genome, the paradigm is shifting towards developing computational tools and algorithms that can assist in its analysis, interpretation and discovery of knowledge contained within these databases. At the time of this writing, the main genomic database,

GenBank, contains about 2.5 billion characters in DNA sequence data (excluding the annotations), in approximately 300 million DNA sequence records. The most common bioinformatics tasks that scientists routinely perform involves a search of this database with the hope of finding other reported sequences that bear resemblance to their query sequence. As the first phase, i.e., sequence acquisition of the Human Genome Project is nearing completion, it is expected that by year 2003 A.D., the next phase will focus on completing the transcript map and understanding the functional significance of the sequenced genes. It is anticipated that elements of locus control, like MARs, will be sought during this phase given their key role in genetic processes, and their localization to functional chromatin domains. Thus, a means to model these markers so that they could be placed on the genome sequence map would have significant ramifications from both a biological perspective as well as the development of new gene therapeutics.

MARs have been experimentally defined for several gene loci, including, the chicken lysozyme gene (Phi-Van et al. 1988), human interferon-β gene (Jade et al. 1995), human β-globin gene (Jarman et al. 1988), chicken α-globin gene (Farache et al. 1990), p53 (Deppert 1996) and the human protamine gene cluster (Kramer et al. 1996). Several motifs that characterize MARs have emerged although a MAR consensus sequence is not apparent. The motifs that are currently utilized are functionally categorized and represented as AND-OR patterns described below.

The following patterns have been known to be associated with the presence of Matrix Association Regions:

- *The Origin of Replication (ORI) Rule*: It has been established that replication is associated with the nuclear matrix, and the origins of replication share the ATTA, ATTTA and ATTTTA motifs.
- *Curved DNA*: Curved DNA has been identified at or near several matrix attachment sites and has been involved with DNA-protein interaction, such as recombination, replication and transcription (Boulikas 1993; Von Kries et al. 1990). Optimal curvature is expected for sequences with repeats of the motif, $AAAAn_7AAAn_7AAAA$ as well as the motif *TTTAAA*.
- *Kinked DNA*: Kinked DNA is typified by the presence of copies of the dinucleotide TG, CA or TA that are separated by 2-4 or 9-12 nucleotides. For example, kinked DNA is recognized by the motif TAn_3TGn_3CA, with TA, TG and CA occurring in any order.
- *Topoisomerase II sites:* It has been shown that Topoisomerase II binding and cleavage sites are also present near the sites of nuclear attachment. Vertebrate and Drosophila topoisomerase II consensus

sequence motifs can be used to identify regions of matrix attachment (Spitzner et al. 1988;Sander et al. 1985).

- *AT-Rich Sequences:* Typically many MARs contain stretches of regularly spaced AT-rich sequences in a periodic manner.
- *TG-Rich Sequences:* Some T-G rich spans are indicative of MARs. These regions are abundant in the 3'UTR of a number of genes, and may act as recombination signals (Boulikas 1993).

The base of patterns has been extended and now includes:

- *Consensus Motif:* The sequence TCTTTAATTTCTAATATATTTAGAA defined as the nuclear matrix STAB-1 binding motif, and
- *ATC Rule:* ATC rule (a stretch of 20 or more occurrences of H, i.e. A or T or C). The ATC rule was used in the analysis of Rice A1-Sh2 region by some researchers. Our own experience has shown that this rule is an effective indicator of regions with marked helix destabilization potential. This is associated with regions that are attached to the nuclear matrix.

The above rule base was derived from a compilation of 20 motifs. Their sequence interdependency is not known, but in most cases multiple motifs are utilized to create a functional MAR. Our current state of analysis makes it clear that at least three and possibly four independent types of MARs can be detected. These are MARs utilized as ORI's, (identified by the ORI rule), AT-rich MARs (identified by the AT-Rich rule and ATC rule) typified by lysozyme or β-interferon genes. MARs that are not AT-Rich as exemplified by those of the protamine locus and the MARs that are tissue specific.

12.3 Preparation of the Data

In such a general framework, a pattern description language is defined that has sufficient power to represent the variety of patterns likely to be discovered as our understanding about the DNA-protein interactions and the control of genetic machinery reaches a higher level of maturity. Also associated with each motif (and pattern) is the probability of its *random occurrence.* This value can be derived using the base composition of the sequence being analyzed (Staden 1988).

It is possible to employ a general set of DNA patterns using the AND-OR methodology. In such an AND-OR pattern specification methodology a disjunction (OR) of the conjunctions (AND) of the motifs detected in the sequence is used as the definition of the pattern being sought. The sequence level motifs serve as the lowest level *predicates* used to detect the presence of a higher level pattern. In general the following operations may be applied to the lower level motifs:

- Motif consensus sequence, m, represented as a regular expression of profile, or
- The logical OR of two motifs m_i and m_j, represented as $m_i \vee m_j$, or
- The augmented logical AND of two motifs m_i and m_j, represented as a $m_i \wedge_a^b m_j^2$ or
- The logical negation of a motif, m, represented as $\overline{m}$, specifying the absence of a given motif.

Motif Index	Motif Name	DNA Signature
m_1	ORI Signal	ATTA
m_2	ORI Signal	ATTTA
m_3	ORI Signal	ATTTTA
m_4	TG-Rich Signal	TGTTTTG
m_5	TG-Rich Signal	TGTTTTTTG
m_6	TG-Rich Signal	TTTTGGGG
m_7	Curved DNA Signal	AAAANNNNNNNAAAANNNNNNNAAAA
m_8	Curved DNA Signal	TTTTNNNNNNNTTTTNNNNNNNTTTT
m_9	Curved DNA Signal	TTTAAA
m_{10}	Kinked DNA Signal	TANNNTGNNNCA
m_{11}	Kinked DNA Signal	TANNNCANNNTG
m_{12}	Kinked DNA Signal	TGNNNTANNNCA
m_{13}	Kinked DNA Signal	TGNNNCANNNTA
m_{14}	Kinked DNA Signal	CANNNTANNNTG
m_{15}	Kinked DNA Signal	CANNNTGNNNTA
m_{16}	mtopo-II Signal	RNYNNCNNGYNGKTNYNY
m_{17}	dtopo-II Signal	GTNWAYATTNATNNR
m_{18}	AT-Rich Signal	WWWWWW

Table 1. Table of sequence level motifs: The set of motifs characterizing MARs constitute DNA-sequence signals or predicates upon which *rules* defining higher level patterns are constructed. Note that the IUPAC characters R,Y,W and K are defined as: R=A or G, Y=T or C,W = A or T and K=G or T.

The pattern specification methodology must account for the motif variability in its representation. Such a variability may be captured using the AND-OR rules. As an example, consider the rule to define the Origin of Replication of DNA. This can be based on an OR or the $\vee$ operator applied to the three motifs m_1 =ATTA, m_2 =ATTTA, and m_3=ATTTTA. The motif detectors bypass the AND layer in this case.

$$R_1 = m_1 \vee m_2 \vee m_3 \tag{1}$$

Similarly, the requirement for multiple motif occurrences can be specified using the AND or the $\wedge$ operator. An additional parameter is incorporated when using the AND rule to constrain the allowable gap between the two co-occurring motifs. For example, the AT-Richness rule can be formulated as the occurrence of two hexanucleotide strings, m_4=WWWWWW[3], that are separated by distance of 8-12 nt, using the augmented AND operator using $\wedge_{low}^{high}$ define the acceptable distance between the two motifs:

$$R_2 = m_4 \,\Lambda_8^{12}\, m_4 \tag{2}$$

Rule	Name	Definition	Probability
R_1	ORI Rule	$m_1 \vee m_2 \vee m_3$	$p_1 = \sum_{i=1}^{3} P_r(m_i)$
R_2	TG-Richness Rule	$m_4 \vee m_5 \vee m_6$	$p_2 = \sum_{i=4}^{6} P_r(m_i)$
R_3	Curved DNA Rule	$m_7 \vee m_8 \vee m_9$	$p_3 = \sum_{i=7}^{9} P_r(m_i)$
R_4	Kinked DNA Rule	$m_{10} \vee m_{11} \vee m_{12} \vee m_{13} \vee m_{14} \vee m_{15}$	$p_4 = \sum_{i=10}^{15} P_r(m_i)$
R_5	Topoisomerase Rule	$m_{16} \vee m_{17}$	$p_5 = \sum_{i=16}^{17} P_r(m_i)$
R_6	AT-Richness Rule	$m_{18} \wedge_8^{12} m_{18}$	$p_6 = P_r(m_{18}) \cdot (1-\exp(-5 \cdot P_r(m_{18})))$

Table 2. The set of biological rules defining patterns that were used for detecting structural MARs. The table also specifies the relationship between the DNA-motif probabilities, *P(m$_i$)*, and the rule probabilities, *p$_j$*. These higher level statistical association forms the basis for mining MARs from DNA sequences.

The significance of the occurrence of a pattern in a DNA sequence is inversely related to the probability that the pattern will occur purely by chance. The probabilities of random occurrences of the underlying predicates are mathematically combined to evaluate the probability of the random occurrence of a pattern specified by a given rule. As an illustrative example, the random occurrence probabilities for the given patterns described by the above two rules can be computed. This value for the set of acceptable patterns described by rule R_2 is based on the occurrence of *at least one motif* within an acceptable distance from the reference motif. These probabilities are computed as shown in Tables 1 and 2.

In similar manner, the random occurrence probability rules constructed on underlying predicates that are defined as *profiles* can be computed using generating functions (Staden 1988). As described, the rule probabilities are employed to estimate the statistical significance to the set of patterns that are detected in a given region of the DNA sequence. The database of higher level patterns used in detection of the Matrix Association Regions has been described (Singh et al. 1997;1998).

12.4 Data Mining for MAR Detection

Data mining is the method employed to search for interesting patterns in data. Such a search often takes place in large data sets where the likelihood of finding such patterns is greater than expected. As described (Klosgen 1992;Klosgen 1995), the data mining efforts aim at detecting *statistically significant* patterns, that are useful to the user since they are *not redundant*, *novel* in regards to user's previous knowledge, *simple* for the user to understand, and sufficiently *general* to the referred population.

When searching for patterns, one must strive for a balance between the *specificity* and *generality* of the patterns sought. Thus, a distinction is often drawn between the tasks of finding *patterns* and that of finding *models.* The distinction between these two terms is rather arbitrary. Generally, a model is a global representation of a structure that summarizes components underlying the data that explain how the data may have arisen. In contrast, a *pattern* is a local structure, perhaps relating to a handful of variables and a few cases. Such local patterns are often sought in the time-series data analysis (Keogh et al. 1997). One use of time series data analysis is for the analysis of stock market data to detect interesting patterns that are novel, useful, and simple enough for the investors to understand.

There are many different data mining algorithms (Crecone et al. 1993;Fayyad et al. 1996). They are classified according to whether they seek to build models or to find patterns. The methods aimed at building global models fall within the category of statistical exploratory analysis which, for example, led to the rejection of conventional wisdom that long term mortgage customers constitute a good portfolio. In a global sense, these customers constitute the group that were not able to find offers elsewhere, and may in fact be the not so good customers (Hand 1998). The second class of data mining methods seeks to find patterns by sifting through the data seeking co-occurrences of specific values of specific variables. It is this class of strategies that has led to the notion of data mining as seeking *nuggets* of information among the mass of data. The problem of detecting MARs from anonymous DNA sequence data falls within this category.

There is a difference between the pattern detection methods and the conventional diagnostic methods. One significant difference is that conventional diagnostic methods need a model to compare the data, while unsupervised pattern detection does not require such a model. Another difference is that the requirement in the pattern detection context is to search through very large collections of data and explore a large number of pattern shapes.

The search for MARs results from defining a group of patterns that are bonded together in order to form a biologically functional unit as per their similar function. After such a grouping, a search for the patterns in a given group can be performed to identify these regions in the query DNA sequence. If a large subset of members of a functionally related group of patterns is found in a specific region of the uncharacterized DNA sequence, one can begin to learn about its function. This process is called a *Functional Pattern Search* and is typified by the *MarFinder* system that performs a search for the group of patterns that are associated with Matrix Attachment Regions (MARS) (Singh et al. 1997).

It is quite intuitive to consider pattern-cluster density as a property defined along the *span* of a sequence. A *sliding window* algorithm can be applied for measuring this value, where the measurements are characterized by the two parameters, W and δ. The cluster-density is measured in a window of size W centered at location x along that sequence. Successive window measurements are carried out by sliding this window in the increments of δ nucleotides. If δ is small, linear interpolation can be used to join the individual window estimates that are gathered at $x, x+\delta, \ldots x+k\delta$. In this manner, a continuous distribution of the cluster-density is obtained as a function of x.

The task of estimating the density of pattern clusters in each window can be statistically defined as a functional inverse of the probability of rejecting the null hypothesis, that states that the frequency of the patterns observed in a given window is not significantly different from the expected frequencies from a random *W* nucleotide sequence of the same composition as the sequence being analyzed. The inverse function chosen as, $\rho = -\log(\alpha)$, where the parameter α is the probability of erroneously rejecting H_0. In other words, α represents the probability that the set of patterns observed in a window occurred purely by chance. The value of ρ is computed for both the forward and the reverse DNA strands since we do not know which strand or if both strands will be bound, the average of the two values is considered to be the density estimate at a given location.

In order to compute ρ, assume that we are searching for *k* distinct types of patterns within a given window of the sequence. In general, these patterns are defined as rules $R_1, R_2, \ldots, R_k$. The probability of random occurrence of the various *k* patterns is calculated using the AND-OR relationships between the individual motifs. Assume that these probabilities for *k* patterns are $p_1, p_2, \ldots, p_k$. Next, a random vector of pattern frequencies, *F*, is constructed. *F* is a *k-dimensional* vector with components, $F = \{x_1, x_2, \ldots, x_k\}$, where each component x_i is a random variable representing the frequency of the pattern R_i in the *W* base-pair window. The component random variables x_i are assumed to be *independently* distributed Poisson processes, each with the parameter $\lambda_i = p_i \cdot W$. Thus, the joint probability of observing a frequency vector $F_{obs} = \{f_1, f_2, \ldots, f_k\}$ purely by chance is given by:

$$P(F_{obs}) = \prod_{i=1}^{k} \frac{e^{-\lambda_i} \lambda^{f_i}}{f_i!} \quad where\ \lambda_i = p_i.W \tag{3}$$

The steps required for computation of α, the cumulative probability that pattern frequencies equal to or greater than the vector F_{obs} occurs purely by chance is given by Eq. 4 below. This corresponds to the one-sided integral of the multivariate Poisson distribution and represents the probability that the H_0 is erroneously rejected.

$$\alpha = P_r(x_1 \geq f_1, x_2 \geq f_2, \ldots, x_k \geq f_k)$$

$$= P_r(x_1 \geq f_1).P_r(x_2 \geq f_2) \ldots P_r(x_k \geq f_k)$$

$$= \sum_{x_1 = f_1}^{\infty} \frac{\exp^{-\lambda_1} \lambda_1^{x_1}}{x_1!} \cdot \sum_{x_2 = f_2}^{\infty} \frac{\exp^{-\lambda_2} \lambda_2^{x_2}}{x_2!}$$

$$\ldots\ldots \sum_{x_K = f_K}^{\infty} \frac{\exp^{-\lambda_K} \lambda_k^{x_K}}{x_k!} \qquad (4)$$

The p-value, α, in Eq.4 is utilized to compute the value of ρ or the *cluster-density* as specified in Eq. 5 below:

$$\rho = \ln\frac{1.0}{\alpha} = -\ln(\alpha) = \sum_{i=1}^{k}\lambda_i + \sum_{i=1}^{k}\ln f_i! - \sum_{i=1}^{k} f_i \ln\lambda_i$$

$$-\sum_{i=1}^{k}\ln(1+\frac{\lambda_i}{f_i+1}+\frac{\lambda_i^2}{(f_i+1)(f_i+2)}+....+\frac{\lambda^t_i}{(f_i+1)(f_i+2).....(f_i+t)}) \qquad (5)$$

The infinite summation term in Eq.5 quickly converges and thus can be adaptively calculated to the precision desired. For small values of λ_i, the series may be truncated such that the last term is smaller than an arbitrarily small constant, ε.

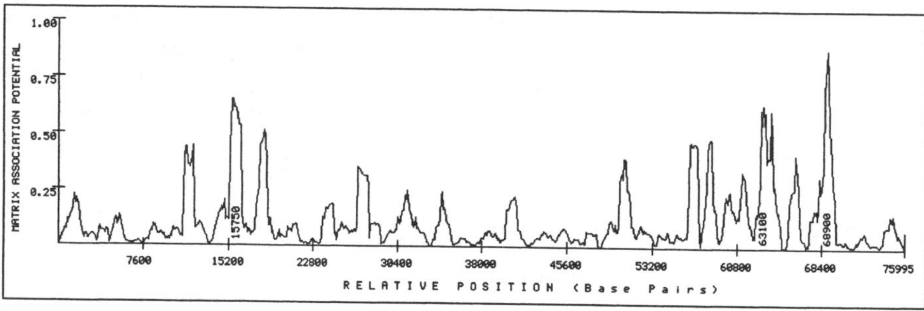

Figure 2. The analysis of human beta-globin gene cluster using the *MAR-Finder tool.* Default analysis parameters were used.

Fig.2 presents the output from the analysis of the human β-globin gene sequence. This statistical inference algorithm based on the association of patterns found within the close proximity of a DNA sequence region has been incorporated in the *MAR-Finder* tool. A java-enabled version of the tool described in (Singh et al. 1998) is also available for public access.

12.5 Evaluation of Discovered Knowledge

Several generalizations regarding the utility and interpretation of the data analysis by MAR-Finder have become apparent over the course its development and use as an analytical tool. As discussed above, one of the significant contributions from these analyses has been the classification of candidate MARs as a function of the distribution of MAR sequence motifs they possess (Kramer et al. 1996).

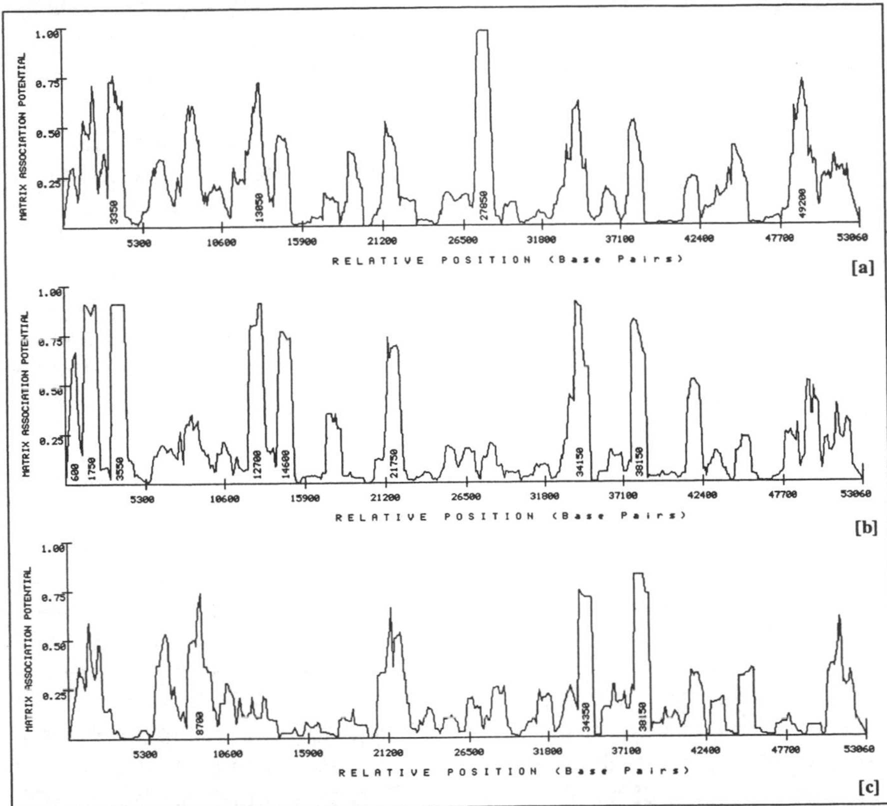

Figure 3. The results of analyzing the human protamine gene cluster using the MAR-Finder algorithm. Panel (a) shows the potential with all core rules selected, plus the optional ATC rule. Panel (b) shows the analysis results with all default core rules selected. Panel (c)provides the results for the default settings minus the ORI and AT-Richness rule.

This is best exemplified by AT rich MARs and ORI MARs. Both are examples of MARs with different biological function acting as either boundary elements or as origins of replication respectively. This has led to the strategy of initially scanning the query sequence with all available rules as a means to establish the potential class of MARs contained within the sequence selected for analysis. The distribution of identified elements and their local concentration can then be used to guide their initial classification and subsequent assessment of biological function. Experience has shown, that the initial classification scan is most efficiently carried out in three phases. First, sequences are examined with all the core (default setting) rules selected to establish the overall distribution of motifs. This is subsequently followed by scanning with the ORI and AT rich rules deselected in the presence and absence of the ATC rule. The relative contribution of each rule to the detection of that motif within the query sequence can then be assessed. Having, used the rule parameter selection to initially categorize the MAR, one then examines the distribution of probabilities using a low-threshold of detection. While this strategy may yield a high-false-positive rate, it ensures the detection of most MARs even when the individual MAR is at the limits of statistical detection (possess an expected value is at least e^{-8}). As shown in Fig.3 (multiple output showing the effect of the ORI, AT and ATC rules when examining the protamine locus), this strategy was effectively utilized to identify and classify the MARs of the PRM1 →PRM2 →TNP2 locus to the sperm-specific class (Kramer et al. 1998). It must be emphasized that the predictions of *MAR-Finder* can only provide a guide to biological verification (Kramer et al. 1997).

As shown in Fig. 4(a), a clustering of motifs with a low likelihood of occurrence by chance within any given region results in a single small region of very high MAR potential. As is the case with the T-Cell receptor gene locus, the one peak visible has an absolute potential value of 120. This roughly corresponds to a chance occurrence of the observed motifs at around 10^{-40}. During the normalization process, the other segments containing statistically significant candidate MARs are visually suppressed and upon initial inspection appear insignificant. This *MAR-Finder* tool can effectively compensate for this artifact by adjusting the saturation value of the display, i.e., the peak height to which all values are clipped and result the saturation (i.e. 100%) of data values. The data is then scaled to 100% of this value and visualization of the previously masked segments is then apparent. This correction was performed for the two ends of the T-Cell receptor gene and is shown in Figs. 4(b) and Fig. 4(c). In both of these cases, the potential values were clipped to 30, i.e. all values of MAR-Potential higher than 30 were saturated to this value. The remaining values were then normalized using this potential. The location of potential MARs has thus become apparent.

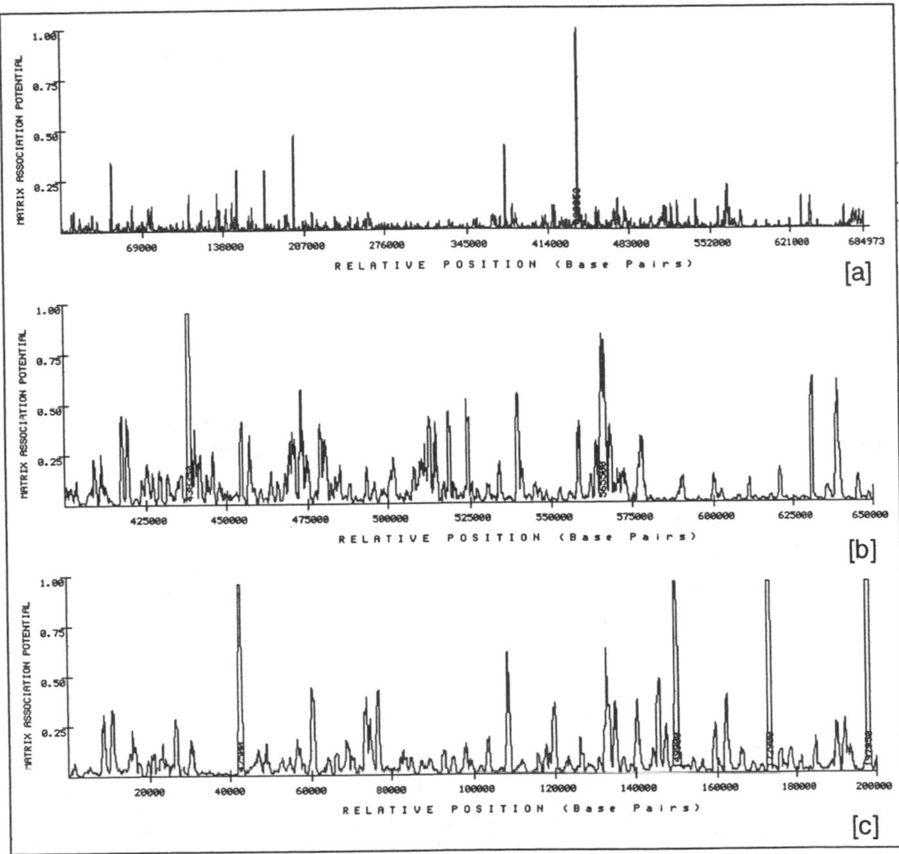

Figure 4. The results of analyzing the human T-cell receptor gene with MAR-Finder. In panel(a), the large peak (with the absolute potential value of 120) overshadows the lower, albeit significant, peaks. This peak is clipped to a value of 30 and the other peaks normalized accordingly. This enables us to visualize the locations of other candidate MARs in the two ends of this locus, as shown in panels (b) and (c).

MAR-Finder was originally conceived to examine sequences from cosmid sized (~ 40 kb) sequencing projects, the initial backbone of human genome project. The program default values of window length (1000), step size (100) and run length (3), i.e. number of concurrent steps were implemented accordingly. For cosmid sized or larger sequences, step size should be maintained at 100 bp, to minimize noise while permitting sufficient discrimination. In the case of shorter sequences ranging in size from 1,000 bp - 10,000 bp, a window size of 100 with a step of 10 usually yields optimum results. This is best illustrated below in the analysis of the β-interferon gene shown in Fig.5. The predicted locations of regions of matrix attachment correspond well with those experimentally determined and the predictions by SIDD (Stress Induced DNA Destabilization) program (Benham et al. 1997).

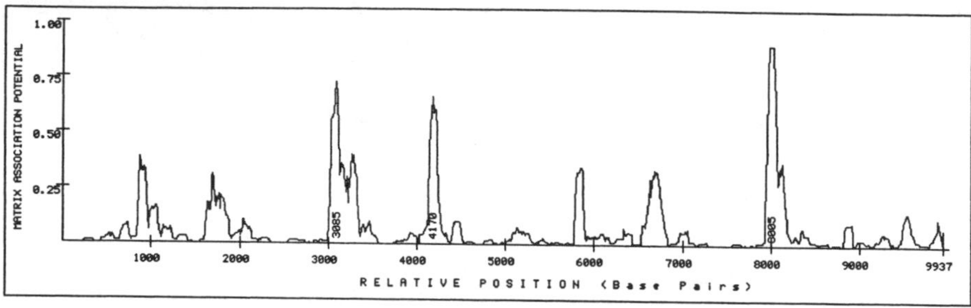

Figure 5. For shorter sequences, such as the Human-interferon gene shown above, the window size of 100 and step size of 10 is optimal.

The above examples of the application of *MAR-Finder* to these various classes of sequences has shown excellent correspondence when compared to the results obtained by wet-bench analysis (Kramer et al. 1996;1997;1998).

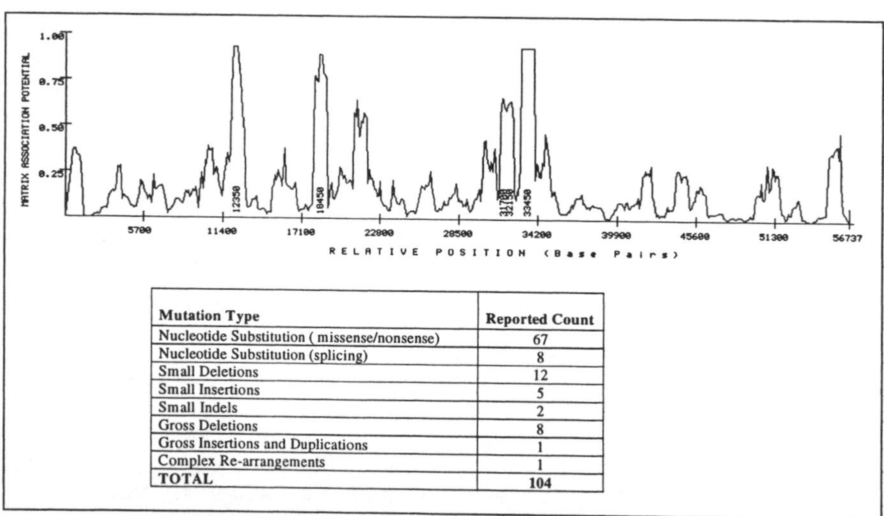

Mutation Type	Reported Count
Nucleotide Substitution (missense/nonsense)	67
Nucleotide Substitution (splicing)	8
Small Deletions	12
Small Insertions	5
Small Indels	2
Gross Deletions	8
Gross Insertions and Duplications	1
Complex Re-arrangements	1
TOTAL	104

Figure 6. The analysis of the Lesch-Nyhan syndrome HPRT gene shows that additional research is required to identify MARs such as those embedded in introns (positions 5534--6107). Interestingly, most peaks are coincident with known mutations in this human gene. Details are at: http://www.uwcm.ac.uk/uwcm/mg/search/119317.html.

However, there are cases where improvement is required. For example, consider that of the *hprt* gene, that when its function is impaired results in Lesch-Nyhan syndrome, a devastating self-multilating disease. In this case a MAR has been biologically defined to be contained within the first intron (positions 5534--6107) and has shown great promise when incorporated as an integral component of a gene therapeutic (Schnedider et al. 1998). However, as shown below in Fig. 6, when the hprt sequence was tested with *MAR-Finder*, this MAR region was not identified. This may reflect the fact that this MAR functions as an ARS (Autonomously Replicating Sequence) which is yet another type of MAR. Irrespective, other candidate MAR sequences have been identified by *MAR-Finder*. It is interesting to note that most of these candidates are coincident with known human mutations causing this disease. This would suggest that their biological assessment is warranted.

12.6 Using the Discovered Knowledge

There are two potentiative states, i.e., open or closed and two classes of potentiated open euchromatin, i.e., constitutive and tissue/cell-specific facultative. The constitutive class, e.g., those of the house-keeping genic domains, always maintain that segment of the genome in a transcriptionally favorable open chromatin conformation. In contrast, the tissue/cell-specific facultative class impose the open conformation onto a segment of the genome in a tissue/cell-specific manner. The two potentiative states, ready/open or off/closed, are correlated with the presence or absence of multiple factors interacting with element(s) that are far distal of their respective gene-specific promoters and enhancers at regions of locus control.

To date, three classes of elements that act as regions of locus control have been identified. This suggests that potentiation multiple and/or redundant means. The classes of elements are, MARs/SARs or the Matrix Attachment Regions/Scaffold Attachment Regions; SCSs or Specialized Chromatin Structures; and LCRs or Locus Control Regions (reviewed in Krawetz et al., 1999). These elements provide a dominant chromatin opening function that is an absolute requisite for transcription of this segment of the genome. In this manner phenotype is ultimately defined by gene potentiation.

It is estimated that mammalian somatic nucleus contains approximately 100,000 MARs of which 30,000 - 40,000 serve as origins of replication

(Bode et al. 1996). A substantial number appear to be localized towards the centromere (Strissel et al. 1996) and are only used for attachment in somatic cells. They are matrix independent in the male haploid gamete (Kramer et al. 1996). This begs the question: what is the function of the remaining MARs? One can begin to answer this question through the observation that MARs most often flank the ends of genic domains encompassing various genic units. It is reasonable to propose that the remaining 30,000 - 35,000 pairs of MARs in each cell, anchor the paired ends of the approximately 12,000 - 30,000 genic domains to the nuclear matrix. It is likely that this is not a simple coincidence that this is also the number of genes transcribed in each cell. If MARs act, or participate as regions of locus control, then it is likely that their reiteration throughout the genome provides a means to specifically tag genes for potentiation in that cell. If verified this may provide a means to facilitate and coordinate the expression of our genome. It will certainly help move gene therapy from the bench to bedside as it will ensure that the therapeutic adopts a cell-specific potentiated open chromatin conformation when integrated into the genome.

12.7 Conclusion

This chapter provides a summary of the various types of patterns that are present in DNA sequences that act as matrix attachment regions. We demonstrated that the task of detecting these patterns is possible due to the synergies between the availability of pattern database, a model for representing the patterns (such as profiles, or rules) and applying a search algorithm for their detection.

Acknowledgement

This work was supported in part by the NIH grant HD36512.

References

Benham C., Kohwi-Shigematsu T., and Bode J. 1997. Stress-induced duplex DNA destabilization in scafold/matrix attachment regions. *J. Mol. Biol.*, 274:181-196.

Bode J., Stenger-Iber M., Kay V., Schalke T. and Dietz-Pfeilstetter A. 1996. Scaffold/matrix attachment regions: Topological switches with multiple regulatory functions. *Crit. Rev. in Eukaryot. Gene Expr.*, 6(2&3):115-138.

Boulikas T. 1993. Nature of DNA sequences at the attachment regions of genes to the nuclear matrix. *J. cellular Biochemistry*, 52:14-22.

Cook P. 1999. The organization of replication and transcription. *Science*, 284:1790-1795.

Crecone N. and Tsuchiya M. 1993. Special issue on learning and discovery in databases. *IEEE Trans. Knowledge & Data Engg.*, 5(6), Dec.

Deppert W. 1996. Binding of MAR-DNA elements by mutant p53: Possible implications for oncogenic function. *J. Cellular Biochemistry*, 62:172-180.

Farache G., Razin S., Targa F., and Scherrer K. 1990. Organization of the 3'-boundary of the chicken alpha globin gene domain and characterization of a CR 1-specific protein binding site. *Nucleic Acid Res.*, 18:401-409.

Fayyad U., Piatetsky-Shapiro G., and Smyth P. 1996. From data mining to knowledge discovery: An overview. In U. Fayyad, G. Piatetsky-Shapiro, P. Smyth, and R. Uthuruswamy, editors, *Advances in Knowledge Discovery and Data Mining*, pages 1-34. AAAI Press, Menlo Park, CA.

Hand D. 1998. Data mining: Statistics and more? *The American Statistician*, 52(2):112-118.

Hartwell L. and Kasten M. 1994. Cell cycle control and cancer. *Science*, 266:1821-1828.

Jade J., Rios-Ramirez M., Mielke C., Stengert M., Kay V., and Klehr-Wirth D. 1995. Scaffold/Matrix attachment regions: structural properties creating transcriptionally active loci. *Intl. Rev. Cytology*, 162A:389-454.

Jarman A. and Higgs D. 1988. Nuclear scaffold attachment sites in the human globin gene complexes. *EMBO Journal*, 7(11):3337-3344.

Kadonaga J. 1998. Eukaryotic transcription: An interlaced network of transcription factors and chromatin-modifying machines. *Cell* 92:307-313.

Keen G., Redgrave G., Lawton J., Cinkowsky M., Mishra S., Ficket J., and Burks C. 1992. Access to molecular biology databases. *Mathematical Computer Modeling*, 16:93-101.

Keogh E. and Smyth P. 1997. A probabilistic approach to fast pattern matching in time series databases. In *Proc. Of the 3rd. Int'l Conf. On Knowledge Discovery and Data Mining*, pages 24-30. Menlo Park, CA: AAAI press.

Kliensmith L. and Kish V. 1995. *Principles of cell and molecular biology*. HarperCollins, 2nd. edition.

Klosgen W. 1992. Problems for knowledge discovery in databases and their treatment in the statistics interpreter EXPLORA. *Intl. Jou. For Intell. Sys.*, 7(7):649-673.

Klosgen W. 1995. Efficient discovery of interesting statements in databases. *J. Intell. Info. Sys.*, 4(1):53-69.

Kramer J. and Krawetz S. 1996. Nuclear matrix interactions within the sperm genome. *J. Biol. Chemistry*, 271(20):11619-11622.

Kramer J. and Krawetz S. 1997. PCR-Based assay to determine nuclear matrix association. Biotechniques, 22:826-828.

Kramer J., Admas M., Singh G., Doggett N., and Krawetz S. 1998. Extended analysis of the region encompassing the PRM1→PRM2→TNP2 domain: genomic organization, evolution and gene identification. *Jou. Of Exp.* Zoology, 282:245-253.

Krawetz S., Kramer J., and McCarry J. 1999. Reprogramming the male gamete genome: a window to successful gene therapy. *Gene*, 234:1-9.

Nikolaev L., Tsevegiyn T., Akopov S., L. Ashworth, and E. Sverdlov. 1996. Construction of a chromosome specific library of MARs and mapping of matrix attachment regions on human chromosome 19. *Nucleic Acid Res.*, 24(7):1330-1336.

Roeder R. 1998. The role of general initiation factors in transcription by RNA polymerase II. *Trends in Biochem. Sci.*, 21:327-335.

Phi-Van L. and Strätling W. 1988. The matrix attachment regions of the chicken lysozyme gene co-map with the boundaries of chromatin domain. *EMBO Journal*, 7:655-664.

Sander M. and Hsieh T. 1985. Drosophila topoisomerase II double stranded DNA cleavage: analysis of DNA sequence homology at the cleavage site. Nucleic Acid Res., 13:1057-1067.

Schnedider G., Morral N., Parks R., Wu Y., Koopmans S., Lansgton C., Graham F., Beaudet A., and Kochanek S. 1998. Gnemonic dna transfer with high capacity adenovirus vector results in improved in-vivo expression and decreased toxicity. *Nature Genetics*, 18:180-183.

Singh G., Kramer J., and Krawetz S. 1997. Mathematical model to predict regions of chromatin attachment to the nuclear matrix. *Nucleic Acid Res.*, 25:1419-1425.

Singh G., Stamper D., and Krawetz S. 1998. A web tool for detecting matrix association regions. *Trends in Genetcics*, 14(2):8. Java version available at http://www.futuresoft.org/MarFinder.

Spitzner J. and Muller M. 1988. A consensus sequence for cleavage by vertebrate DNA topoisomerase II. *Nucleic Acid Res.*, 16(12):5533-5556.

Staden R. 1988. Methods for calculating the probabilities of finding patterns in sequences. *Comput. Applic. Biosci.*, 5(2):89-96.

Strissel P., Espinosa R., III, Rowley J., and Swift H. 1996. Scaffold attachment regions in centromere-associated dna. *Chromosoma*, 105:122-133.

Von Kries J., Phi-Van L., Diekmann S., and Strätling W. 1990. A non-curved chicken lysozyme 5' matrix attachment site is 3' followed by a strongly curved DNA sequence. *Nucleic Acid Res.*, 18:3881-3885.

13 Discovery of Temporal Patterns in Sparse Course-of-Disease Data

Jorge C. G. Ramirez[1,2], Lynn L. Peterson[1], Diane J. Cook[1] and Dolores M. Peterson[2]

[1]Department of Computer Science & Engineering
University of Texas at Arlington, TX 76019-0015, U.S.A.
ramirez@cse.uta.edu
[2]HIV Clinical Research Group
Division of General Internal Medicine
University of Texas Southwestern Medical Center, TX 75235-9103, U.S.A.

Knowledge discovery in databases containing course-of-disease data for chronic illness is the thrust of the work detailed in this chapter. As seems to be typical of such databases, the data that is recorded is sparse and was collected with no concerted effort to maintain data quality. Despite this, we hypothesize that, given a database of clinical data for patients who had the same catastrophic or chronic illness, we can discover that subsets of these patients had a similar experience during the course of that disease. We use our experience in the development of the knowledge discovery system, Temporal Pattern Discovery System or TEMPADIS, to help understand the overall process of knowledge discovery in a medical database environment.

13.1 Understanding the Problem Domain

13.1.1 Determination of Objectives

The objective of the work is as stated above: Given a database that contains clinical data for patients diagnosed with the same catastrophic or chronic illness, we are interested in discovering patterns in the data which show that groups of patients had similar experiences during the course of the disease. This work is motivated by the knowledge that analysis of the course of such diseases can enhance provision of care, prognosis, monitoring, outcomes research, cost/benefit analysis, and quality assurance. Figure 1 diagrams the project plan, the steps used in the development of TEMPADIS.

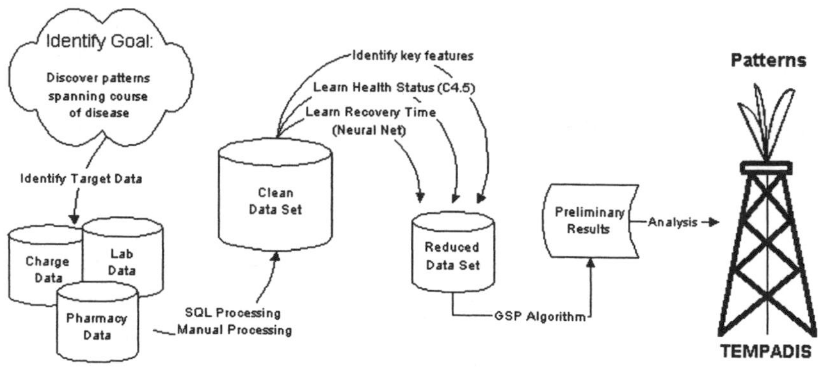

Figure 1. Overview of development of TEMPADIS

13.2 Understanding the Data

13.2.1 Description of the Data

Our domain is HIV disease. Our data collection is the Jonathan Jockush HIV Clinical Research Database, which was established in 1987 at the University of Texas Southwestern Medical Center at Dallas. The database contains data for over 8,500 patients of the Acquired Immune Deficiency Syndrome (AIDS) Clinic at Parkland Memorial Hospital, also in Dallas. The database consists of data collected from the hospital charge system, the pharmacy system, and the laboratory information system. In addition, some data is entered directly from patients' day sheets and charts.

The types of data available for our analysis include binary, numeric, symbolic and text data. The data fields that are recorded for each patient vary greatly between collection instances, and also vary between patients even for similar medical events.

Especially where laboratory, diagnosis, and therapy data are concerned, most of the data is temporal, i.e., there are multiple instances of the same data field with different dates and values for each instance. The significance of the temporal aspect, however, varies with the nature of the data. For example, for clinic or emergency room visits, or lab test results, the occurrence of an event and the order of occurrence relative to other events are important. For diagnoses or drug therapies, the duration of an event is just as important as the relative order of occurrence.

In summary, our task is to discover useful patterns in temporal, non-standard form, variable data-field, medical data.

13.2.2 Initial Exploration of the Data

The objective of our initial exploration of the data is to select a data set and to focus on a subset of variables. It is important to have enough data to contain significant patterns, and also to focus on as small a set of variables as will produce useful results in a reasonable amount of time.

We examine the database to characterize how long patients had been monitored and how many times they visited a medical facility. Of the over 8,500 patients in the database, there are many who had been monitored for only a short period of time. Several hundred had been seen for only a month or less. On the other hand there are several hundred that had been monitored for seven years or more. We need to find a group of patients on whom data had been collected for a significant length of time and often enough to have a significant detectable pattern. Approximately 1,100 of the patients had been monitored by the Parkland system for at least 4 years, with a minimum of 30 distinct dates when at least one type of event (i.e., charge, pharmacy, lab test result, etc.) was recorded. We randomly select groups of patients from these 1,100 patients for the results shown in this chapter. The number of patients used for any given task is discussed along with that task.

From the mass of available data, it is important to focus on a subset of the variables that are related to the knowledge to be discovered in the KDD process. To help focus, we sought a dozen key variables, and finally used twenty. This subset of the available data includes all encounters with patients, a subset of the laboratory results, and a subset of the pharmacy data. Later, in the data preparation phase of the KDD process, we add the final two variables that are measures of the patient's overall health status.

An encounter with a patient is represented by two variables. The first variable is the type of encounter (clinic visits, emergency room (ER) visits, and hospital stays). The second is the level of severity of the encounter. For example, it is not uncommon for patients to go to the ER, when they could have gone to the clinic had it been open. This type of visit would not be considered as severe as an ER trauma visit (e.g., gunshot wound). Conversely, patients sometimes go to the clinic when they really need to be hospitalized. Further, when hospitalized, the severity is different if the patient requires intensive care rather than placement on one of the regular wards. Therefore, each type of encounter has graded levels of severity.

An examination of the laboratory test data reveals that although there are literally thousands of different medical laboratory tests, some tests are recorded significantly more often than others throughout the database. When looking at the pharmacy data we find that 71 different drugs had been dispensed that were specific to HIV and/or HIV-related illnesses. Selection of subsets of these data is addressed in the discussion of data preparation.

13.2.3 Verification of the Quality of the Data

When examining the database from a data quality perspective, we find that the database contains duplicate laboratory data for several different time periods, i.e., that particular data was in fact loaded into the database twice during those time periods. We also discover that there are many errors in how the various prescriptions were recorded in the pharmacy's computer system. In an extreme example, one drug was coded 46 different ways throughout the pharmacy records.

Data for a single patient consists of entries for each day in which some medical event took place, e.g., visiting a medical facility, filling a prescription, obtaining lab results. By nature that data is sparse, i.e., thinly scattered or distributed, with respect to the attributes recorded and with respect to time. It is therefore apparent to us that the nature of the data (e.g., its sparseness, the obvious errors) is such that a major part of the effort involved in this knowledge discovery process has to come in the next phase, the preparation of the data.

13.3 Preparation of the Data

13.3.1 Data Cleaning

The purpose of the data cleaning step is to remove noise from the data or to develop a method for accounting for that noise, to look at strategies for coping with the sparseness of the data, and to handle any other known changes that need to be made. In our case, some identified problems can be cleaned up as a group by processing the database using straightforward SQL statements. This can be done to correct obvious errors like the same misspelling and/or miscoding of a drug in the pharmacy data that appears multiple times. Removal of duplicate records requires a manual search of the data. In one example, a charge for a single service was entered five times, and then corresponding records were entered to reverse the charge four times, with a net result of nine records for a single charge event.

Since the problems that can be cleaned up with SQL statements are easy, we can correct them for the entire database. However, handling the manual problems in the entire database would be too time-consuming. Therefore, we randomly selected a subset of 400 patients from our 1,100 described above in order to have a significant base of patients to work from without losing sight of the original goal of our project. A significant note to make at this point is that it required approximately 3 man-months to clean up those 400 patients' data. Our data cleaning was therefore limited to the correction obvious errors, and errors due to missing or incorrectly recorded data were not fixed.

13.3.2 Data Selection

The purpose of the data selection step is to find useful features to represent the data, depending heavily on the goal. This can involve using dimensionality reduction or transformation methods to reduce the effective number of variables under consideration or finding invariant representations of the data. Our goal is to use only a minimum number of key variables that well represented the clinical relevance of the data.

First, we reexamine the lab test results. We focus on variables that are most likely to be recorded on any given encounter and are important indicators of the health status of an HIV-infected patient. To make this determination we consulted the clinicians of the HIV Clinical Research Group.

The six variables selected are White Blood Cell (WBC), Hematocrit (HCT), Platelets (PLT), CD4 Absolute (CD4A), CD4 Percent (CD4P), and Lymphocytes (LMPH). These selections were made based on the fact that the first five of those variables are values that the clinicians look at first when examining a patient's lab results. The sixth, LMPH, is included because CD4P is calculated from WBC, LMPH and CD4A, so if CD4P is missing but the others were present, which is true especially in the early years of data collection, CD4P can be calculated.

Choosing a subset of the pharmacy data is a more challenging task. Since we want to find patterns that represent similar experiences during the course of disease, the most obvious solution is to group the drugs into categories according to the reason they were being prescribed. This yielded the following ten categories: Nucleoside Analogs, Protease Inhibitors, Prophylaxis Therapies, Intraveneous antibiotics, Anti-virals, Anti-pneumocystis pneumonia/toxoplasmosis, Anti-mycobacterials, Anti-wasting syndrome, Anti-fungals and Chemotherapies. The clinicians agree that this tracking of whether or not a patient is on a drug in a particular category on a given day is sufficient information for our purposes. The data selection process therefore yields 18 variables, or events, as shown in Table 1.

Figure 2 shows an example of a portion of a patient file after abstracting the basis for these 18 variables (i.e., in the figure, the drug data has not yet been translated to the ten drug category variables; drugs are still listed by individual drug code). Note that in this particular example the column in between Event Type and WBC, where Event Severity should be, is blank for each day, meaning that all of these samples are normal clinic visits or hospital days.

<u>Nature of the Event</u>
1. Event Type
2. Event Severity

<u>Blood Tests</u>
3. White Blood Cell (WBC)
4. Hematocrit (HCT)
5. Platelets (PLT)
6. CD4 Absolute (CD4A)
7. CD4 Percent (CD4P)
8. Lymphocytes (LMPH)

<u>Drug Categories</u>
9. Nucleoside Analogs
10. Protease Inhibitors
11. Prophylaxis Therapies
12. Intravenous antibiotics
13. Anti-virals
14. Anti-pneumocystis pneumonia/ anti-toxoplasmosis
15. Anti-mycobacterials
16. Anti-wasting syndrome
17. Anti-fungals
18. Chemotherapies

Table 1. The 18 Data Elements Extracted Directly From the Clean Data Set.

```
833 C  1.5 31.6  245  4.6    7 10  0
839 C  0.0  0.0    0  0.0    0  0  0
861 C  1.1 26.1  167  0.0    0 16  0
862    0.0  0.0    0  0.0    0  0  2 24: 30 38: 50
867 H  4.3 19.2  144  0.0    0 11  3  0:  3 22:  1 35:  2
868 H  2.2 26.2  144  0.0    0  5  3  0:  3 22:  1 35:  2
869    0.0  0.0    0  0.0    0  0  1 35: 60
874 C  1.3 32.4    0  0.0    0 17  0
889 C  1.1 30.4  154  0.0    0 36  0
890    0.0  0.0    0  0.0    0  0  3 22: 30 38: 50 39:480
923    0.0  0.0    0  0.0    0  0  1 39:480
933 H  3.6 20.4  182  0.0    0 11  3  0:  2 22:  1 39: 12
934 H  3.7 29.7  181  0.0    0  6  3  0:  3 22:  1 39: 16
935 H  1.6 27.9  186  0.0    0 11  3  0:  3 38:  2 39: 16
                 936 H  4.0 29.7  259  0.0    0  6  1  0:  3
937 H  2.7 24.1  246  0.0    0  9  1  0:  3
```

Figure 2. Portion of abstracted patient record. From left to right the columns are: Day, Charge Event Type (C = Clinic Visit, H = Hospital Room, Blank = drug dispensed only), WBC, HCT, PLT, CD4P, CD4A, LMPH, Number of Drugs Dispensed, Drug Code: Number Dispensed (repeated as necessary).

13.3.3 Constructing and Merging the Data

From a clinical point of view, there is still important information, which should be considered, that is not contained explicitly in these 18 variables. First, knowing that the “normal” value of lab results depends to some extent on the patient, we had previously developed a methodology for normalizing all the values for each patient so that comparisons could more appropriately be made with other patient's data (Ramirez et al. 1998). Each variable is treated separately for each patient. Each is normalized to a range of integers from –4 to +4. In this range, 0 is considered normal, and both -4 and +4 are indicative of severe illness (roughly equivalent to the number of standard deviations away from normal for that person). The methodology is based on statistical norms for the general population with adjustments made for the fact that immune-compromised patients tend to have lower than normal values. However, the methodology takes into account the fact that the normal value for any given patient may or may not be different, compared to the general population.

Second, the set of 18 variables does not explicitly contain a variable representing diagnosis. Diagnosis is the data element in the database that was collected in the least automated way. It was being manually entered directly from the patient day sheets each time the patient visited the clinic. However, the resources allocated to this task were not sufficient, and the recorded diagnosis data is rather incomplete. We therefore choose not to use the available diagnosis data for our discovery purposes, but instead develop another way to obtain equivalent information.

Based loosely on the way that the Centers for Disease Control classify the stages of HIV Disease, a new variable, health status, is added to the 18 previously selected variables to approximate the missing diagnosis data. This approach was recommended by the clinicians in the HIV Clinical Research Group. The five health status categories are shown in Table 2.

We use a machine learning technique called decision tree induction to learn rules for determining the health status value for any given patient on any given day. It is important to note that even though we use a machine learning technique to do this data reduction, this is not the data-mining step. In order to have a single variable that represents the general health status of the patient, we use decision tree induction to learn how to determine this value from a larger set of data.

Decision tree induction is commonly used for classification problems. Decision trees are built using varying rules about the information gained by splitting the remaining unclassified examples on each of the remaining unused attributes. In order to induce the tree for determining the correct health status value, we construct a set of data by randomly selecting four days from each of 100 patients and listing all drugs being taken on those days. Three clinicians rated the health status for each day, according to the categories listed in Table 2, based solely on the drug information. If there was a discrepancy among the clinicians' ratings, we went back to them and got a consensus.

1. Asymptomatic, not on any therapy
2. Asymptomatic, only on anti-HIV therapy
3. Immune system significantly damaged, on prophylactic therapy
4. Active opportunistic infection/illness
5. Severe/Life-threatening illness

Table 2. Health Status Categories.

We then use C4.5 (Quinlin 1993) to induce the decision tree. The inputs are the standard files required by C4.5. The names file contains the classes (which are the health status categories listed in Table 2), the attributes (the various drugs), and the attribute values (1 if currently on the drug and 0 otherwise). The data file contains the 400 samples with the attribute values and the class. We run C4.5 in iterative mode using the default parameters, except that we specify a 95% confidence level on the pruned tree. The resulting tree is converted to rules that are used to determine health status values. The health status field can now be inserted in each day of each patient's data as part of the data reduction preprocessing.

Now that we have a measure of health status, which gives us an idea of the current state of the patient, we need a measure that gives us a feel for how long the patient might remain in that state. The health status only tells what is currently wrong with the patient in a general way, but it gives no specific indication of how severe the current problem is. For example, health status could be 1, 2 or 3 and the patient could have the flu. A severity measure would provide a way to differentiate between that patient and another that has the same health status but no current illness. Further, a patient could have health status 5 and be near death or could be well on the way to recovery. Again, a severity measure would provide a means to differentiate between these two states. The combined information provided by the health status measure and a severity measure can provide a significant increase in the meaning not only of the current state of a patient, but also of a discovered pattern. The severity of the current event can be measured by determining how long it would take to recover from that event. However, again, this is not the type of information that appears in the database. Once again, we turn to a machine learning technique to inject information not already explicitly present in the database to enhance the discovery process.

Since neural nets have been used in a variety of ways in medical domains (Dombi et al. 1995; Frye et al. 1996; Izenberg et al. 1997; Mobley et al. 1995), including prediction of length of hospital stay, it is reasonable to assume we could use one to predict length of recovery time. The next task is to select the relevant inputs for determining some measure of recovery time. The inputs selected are shown in Table 3. An obvious first choice is our newly determined health status, which was developed to be a measure of the nature of the current illness.

No.	Input
1.	Days Since Previous Event
2.	Days Until Next Event
3-5.	Health Status (Previous, Current and Next Values)
6-8.	Event Type (Previous, Current and Next Values)
9-11.	Event Severity (Previous, Current and Next Values)
12-29.	Normalized Blood Test Values (Previous, Current and Next Values for each of WBC, etc.)

Table 3. Recovery Time Neural Net Inputs.

For additional inputs to the neural net, we include the current event type, since the output is a measure of how long it takes to recover from the current event. The current laboratory test results are also included. Further, in order to put the current event in context, we choose to include the same data related to the previous event and the next event, as well as the time since the previous event and the time until the next event.

For training cases, we randomly select six days from each of 50 patients. We then abstract the data needed for the neural net inputs. Again three clinicians rated the recovery time of the patients based solely on the information we would be providing to the neural net. We originally asked them to predict in number of days. When we saw a significant disparity in the predictions, we decided that we needed to decrease the granularity of the measure. Therefore, we use a scale of 0 to 5, where 0 to 4 represented estimated weeks to recovery, and 5 represented anything over 4 weeks. Again, where we found discrepancies, we went back to the clinicians for a consensus.

We use the NevProp3 neural net software (Goodman 1996), and its default 2/3-1/3 holdout, five sample cross validation. NevProp3 only allows for a single hidden layer. Within this context we experimented with various network structures. As shown in Table 4, the network with six hidden nodes performs the best, with an 85.3% correct prediction rate. The MeanSqErr is the mean of the squared differences between the predictions the model made and the target values designated by the clinicians, where 0 is best. R2 is commonly interpreted as the fraction of variance explained by the model, where 0 means that the model predicts the mean of the target values and 1 means that the model predicts the correct target value. This new knowledge, coupled with the health status, is then incorporated into the database for the purpose of giving more overall meaning to the data in the absence of an explicit diagnosis.

Hidden Nodes	MeanSqErr (Best=0)	R^2 (Best=1)	Predicted (Best=1)
4	0.216	0.886	0.713
5	0.181	0.905	0.813
6	0.140	0.926	0.853
7	0.174	0.909	0.810

Table 4. Results of Neural Net Training.

The result of the data preparation step is the reduced data set. This data set consists of 20 variables deemed to well represent the larger set of all data available. Figure 3 shows the results of the transformation of the data from Fig. 2. It is this set of data with 20 variables that is used in the data mining step.

833	C	3	0	-3	-1	0	-4	-4	-3	1	0	2	0	0	0	0	0	0	0
839	C	3	1	-9	-9	-9	-9	-9	-9	0	0	1	0	0	0	0	0	0	0
861	C	3	1	-4	-3	0	-9	-9	-1	0	0	2	0	0	0	0	0	0	0
867	H	4	4	0	-4	-1	-9	-9	-2	0	0	2	0	0	0	1	1	0	0
868		4	1	-2	-3	-1	-9	-9	-4	0	0	2	0	0	0	1	1	0	0
874	C	4	3	-4	-1	-9	-9	-9	0	0	0	2	0	0	0	1	1	0	0
889	C	4	2	-4	-2	-1	-9	-9	2	0	0	2	0	0	0	1	1	0	0
933	H	4	4	0	-4	0	-9	-9	-2	0	0	1	0	0	0	0	2	0	0
934	H	4	2	0	-2	0	-9	-9	-4	0	0	1	0	0	0	0	2	0	0
935	H	4	2	-3	-3	0	-9	-9	-2	0	0	1	0	0	0	0	2	0	0
936	H	4	2	0	-2	1	-9	-9	-4	0	0	1	0	0	0	0	2	0	0
937	H	4	2	-2	-4	0	-9	-9	-3	0	0	1	0	0	0	0	2	0	0

Figure 3. Portion of patient record after data preparation step. From left to right columns are: Day, Charge Event, Health Status, Recovery Time, six columns for normalized laboratory test results (-9 = not present) and ten columns for drug category data.

13.4 Data Mining

13.4.1 Selection of the Data Mining Method

The next task is selection of a method or methods to be used for searching for patterns in the data. This involves deciding which models may be appropriate and deciding which data mining method or methods match the goals of the KDD process. Model selection is usually based on what type of data is being mined, and mining method selection is based on what the end results needs to be, usually discovery or prediction.

We are trying to discover patterns in sequences of events across patients in a database. Patterns are represented in a form as shown in Fig. 4. This pattern contains six event-sets; each enclosed in curly braces. The first event-set is based on a clinic visit (EV C), the patients' health status is 3 on the scale of 1 to 5 described above (HS 3), and the recovery time measure is 0 on the scale of 0 to 5 described above (WTR 0). Further, only four of the six lab tests were run on this visit. These are (WBC 0), (PLT –1), (HCT 0) and (LMPH –3). The only one that would be of significant concern is the lymphocytes being considerably low at –3. The other two lab tests, CD4P and CD4A, can be seen in the third and sixth event-sets. Finally, the ten drug categories are represented by the binary values 0 or 1. In the first event-set, (onD 0000000000), means that none of the drug categories was currently being taken by the patients. However, in the third event-set, drugs from category 1, Nucleoside Analogs, and category 3, Prophylactic Therapies, are indicated as currently being taken.

```
< { (EV C ) (HS 3) (WTR 0) (WBC 0) (PLT -1) (HCT 0)
    (LMPH -3) (onD 0000000000) }
  { (EV E ) (HS 3) (WTR 2) (WBC 3) (PLT -1) (HCT 1)
    (LMPH 4) (onD 0000000000) }
  { (EV C ) (HS 3) (WTR 0) (WBC 1) (PLT 0) (HCT 0)
    (CD4P -3) (CD4A -1) (LMPH 0) (onD 1010000000) }
  { (EV C ) (HS 3) (WTR 1) (WBC -1) (PLT -1) (HCT 1)
    (LMPH 2) (onD 1010000000) }
  { (EV E ) (HS 3) (WTR 1) (WBC 2) (PLT -1) (HCT 1)
    (LMPH 4) (onD 0000000000) }
  { (EV C ) (HS 3) (WTR 1) (WBC 1) (PLT 0) (HCT 0)
    (CD4P -3) (CD4A -2) (LMPH 0) (onD 1010000000) } >
```

Figure 4. Typical pattern discovered by TEMPADIS.

In our review of the literature, we found that there are only a few data mining methods relevant for our goal (Agrawal and Srikant 1995; Mannila et al. 1995; Mannila and Toivonen 1996; Padmanabhan and Tuzhilin 1996; Srikant and Agrawal 1996). We chose Srikant and Agrawal's General Sequential Patterns (GSP) Algorithm (Agrawal and Srikant 1995; Srikant and Agrawal 1996) as the basis for the data mining method we would use.

The GSP Algorithm uses atomic events as the basis for building up sequences. In our domain an example of an atomic event, as seen in the example pattern above, would be (WBC 0), which is the occurrence of a White Blood Cell test result that is in the normal range for that patient. The database is searched for all atomic events that occur in the database, and then each atomic event is checked for support by the database. In our domain, support is the percentage of the patients in the database that had that event occur at least once. Only those events that meet the support threshold are "supported" by the database. We are using various support threshold levels from 5% (i.e., 1 of every 20 patients should support the pattern) to 33%. Those atomic events that survive are then combined as pairs, both as sequences and as concurrent occurrences. For example, if we have the atomic events (WBC 1) and (HCT 0) which are supported by the database, then the resulting combinations would be <{(WBC 1)(HCT 0)}>, which is a concurrent occurrence, and <{(WBC 1)} {(HCT 0}> and <{(HCT 0)} {(WBC 1)}>, which are sequences. All three are considered to be sequences of length two because they contain two atomic events. These sequences of length two are checked for support by the database. Only those with enough support contribute to what are called candidate sequences for the next iteration. Once the supported sequences are at least length two, the next generation of candidate sequences is created by joining together sequences that are supported at the previous length. For example, given supported sequences of length two:

```
<{(WBC 1) (HCT 0)}>
<{(HCT 0)} {(PLT -2)}>
<{(PLT -2) (CD4A -1)}>
```

Then we can generate two candidate sequences of length three:

```
<{(WBC 1) (HCT 0)} {(PLT -2)}>
<{(HCT 0)} {(PLT -2) (CD4A -1)}>
```

If both of those sequences are supported by the database, then we can generate the length four candidate sequence:

```
<{(WBC 1) (HCT 0)} {(PLT -2) (CD4A -1)}>
```

Note that the joined sequences must be exactly the same except for the first event of one and the last event of the other.

This continues until there are no candidate sequences that have support at the current level. We would say that the discovered pattern shown in Fig. 4 is of length 104, since it includes 104 atomic events, if you consider each drug type a separate event. This pattern would be discovered on the 104th iteration of the algorithm.

The GSP Algorithm also provides the windowing concept. The minimum and maximum gap (i.e., the allowable time between events for them to be considered to have happened consecutively) can be specified. In our domain, the minimum time between consecutive events would be 0 days, since we are interested in events that may happen on consecutive days (e.g., hospitalizations). Currently, we are using 90 to 120 days as the maximum gap. This range allows for a patient, who is going through a period of relatively good health, to only see the doctor every 2 to 4 months for follow-up visits. Otherwise, his or her sequence of event-sets would be partitioned (i.e., split into two parts at the point at which time between visits is greater than the maximum gap). This maximum gap, of course, allows for more frequent visits by those who are not so healthy. Further, the time window within which events can happen and still be considered to part of the same event-set can also be specified. In our domain, a window of 7 to 10 days is necessary to allow patients to come to have lab work done a week in advance of their next clinic appointment.

13.4.2 Building and Assessing the Model

The evaluation of the model and data mining method selections can result in modifications and refinements to the original selections. Further, upon seeing the exploratory results, hypotheses can be made about what are the realistic results of the particular KDD process. Our evaluation and the changes made as a result are explained in this section.

We ran our exploratory analysis on a modified version of the original GSP Algorithm model. Though the basic algorithm is the same, the details of implementation are different. The GSP algorithm was designed to work on sequences of events that either occurred or sequences of events that either occurred or did not, where the occurrence or lack thereof was significant to the patterns discovered. Also, none of the events had attributes. The differences in domains lead to several significant observations. In our domain, the occurrence of an event or lack thereof does not necessarily have any specific significance. The events themselves have attributes, especially when viewed from the event-set perspective. Finally, the shear numbers of events being dealt with computationally strains an algorithm that was designed to discover patterns at an individual event level. We concluded that our original modified-GSP implementation was insufficient (Ramirez et al. 1998). However, those experiments led us to propose our Event Set Sequence approach and a further modification to the GSP Algorithm. We call the system that implements this approach TEMPADIS, or the TEMporal PAttern DIscovery System.

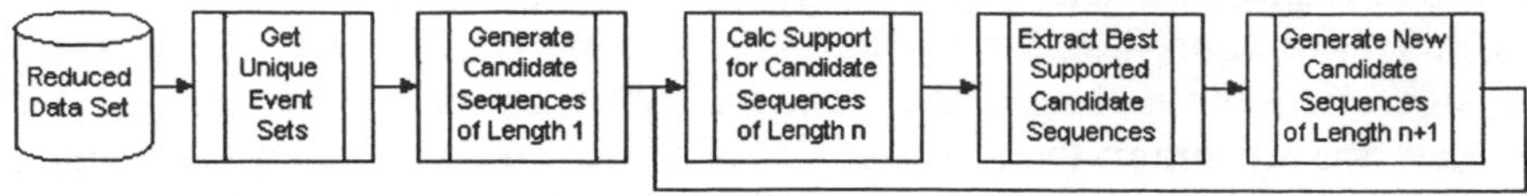

Figure 5. Algorithm for TEMPADIS.

Our concept of an event-set is based on the idea that the events in the database exist for one of three reasons: 1) some type of visit to a medical facility was made; 2) laboratory tests were performed; or 3) prescriptions were dispensed. Generally those events that happen on the same day or on days very close together are all related. For example, a patient who is having periodic check-ups may have lab tests done about a week prior to an appointment to ensure the test results will be available on the day they actually see the doctor. Further, they may not pick up a prescription until a day or two after seeing the doctor. Therefore, we have incorporated the time-windowing technique from the GSP Algorithm, that allows for those events to be considered as a single event-set. We use a set difference method that allows us to compare event-sets, looking at all 20 variables as a single unit. The algorithm for TEMPADIS is shown visually in Fig. 5 and listed below:

1. Read database
2. Get unique event-sets from database
3. curSeqs = GenerateNewSeqs from unique event-sets
4. while curSeqs

    4a. CalculateSupportInDatabase for curSeqs

    4b. supportedSeqs = ExtractBestSupportedSeqs from curSeqs

    4c. curSeqs = GenerateNewSeqs from supportedSeqs

   endwhile

Whereas GSP retrieved the unique atomic events, in step 2 we create a list of all of the unique event-sets in the database. In step 3, we put these unique individual event-sets into a sequence format of length one. Step 4 is to continue the algorithm as long as there are sequences to consider.

In step 4a, we determine the support for each sequence under consideration in the database. This is where our algorithm differs significantly from the original GSP. In GSP, the current sequence under consideration was supported by a specific instance in the database on an all or nothing basis, i.e., it supported it or it did not. Our algorithm is necessarily fuzzier than that.

There are many parameters that can affect what patterns are supported by the database. Above we mentioned the support threshold as being one. Within the CalculateSupportInDatabase function of step 4a there are several more. In this function, there is a critical sub-function called DegreeOfMatch. The method for determining the set difference can be varied and the weights of the individual elements of the set can be varied. For example, if a lab result is missing, in either the current sequence under consideration or in the particular database instance we are looking at for support, or both, then we give that a value of 50% support for that element of the event-set. The issue of missing drug data does not get addressed at all. If the drug is not present in the database, then there is no support for that element of the event-set, even if upon visual inspection of a patient's records we could reasonably assume they were on the drug at the time.

For the data that is present, we use a partial match system. For example, for WBC we might decrease the degree of match by 33% for each point difference on our scale of –4 to +4. In this example, if the current sequence under consideration has a value of -1, then the value in the particular database instance of -1 results in 100% match. The values of 0 or –2 result in a 67% match, and the values of 1 or –3 result in a 33% match. All other values (i.e., -4, 2, 3 and 4) result in a 0% match.

DegreeOfMatch then returns a value ranging from 0.0 to 1.0 for each event-set in the length of the sequence. TEMPADIS uses a weakest-link/average-link method for determining whether or not a sequence under consideration is supported by a given patient's data. For example, the weakest-link value might be set to 0.72, and the average-link value might be set to 0.80. This means that every event-set in the sequence must have at least 0.72 as its DegreeOfMatch, but the entire sequence must average at least 0.80 before it is considered to support the candidate sequence. The actual threshold values used were determined by empirical results, such that the results yielded a higher percentage of interesting patterns and still found patterns at all.

The last thing to consider in step 4a is the fact that each patient in the database might have multiple instances of support for a sequence currently under consideration. Because of this, and the fact that we want the best supported sequences to be found, each instance must have its support value calculated. Then only the highest value is saved for use in calculating the total support of the database for that sequence. These highest values are summed for all patients in the database that met the average-link threshold. If the sum is greater than the number of patients times the average-link value, then the sequence is considered to be supported by the database.

From the previous explanation, one might imagine that TEMPADIS is very computationally intensive, and it is. The algorithm is exponential in the length of the discovered patterns, and within that it is linear in the number of patterns of that length and linear in the number of patients. Therefore, as one of the many search control strategies that we have implemented, step 4b limits the number of sequences that can be carried over to the next iteration. We use a pruning method that considers a minimum number of sequences under which no pruning will be done, a maximum number over which pruning must be done, and a pruning factor, all of which can be varied.

Finally, step 4c generates the new set of sequences for consideration on the next iteration. We incorporate intelligent selection of the event-sets with which to attempt to lengthen the patterns. The intelligent selection is based on the event-sets that were present in the database immediately prior to and immediately after the best supported patterns within each individual patient. This list was saved during step 4a. Each sequence can spawn many new sequences during this step, including many duplicates. However, we use a hash tree to track the newly generated sequences and it discards duplicates as they are generated.

After all of the above steps of the knowledge discovery process are completed, we are finally ready to begin using TEMPADIS in the data-mining step. The data has been cleaned, preprocessed and reduced. We have incorporated knowledge learned from the database back into the database to give us more intelligent data from which to discover. We have developed a technique which reduces the computational complexity, and now we put our Event Set Sequence approach to the test.

We have stated that we use multiple methods of search control to reduce the computational complexity. When we begin the data mining, we implement search control strategies that will only look at patterns that are of interest. We initialize our search strategy during step 2, Get unique event-sets from database. If we are particularly interested in patterns with hospitalizations, then we only retrieve all unique event-sets that have a hospital stay as the visit type. If we are particular interested in patterns that have a specific trend in a specific variable then we screen for that trend during step 4c, GenerateNewSeqs.

13.5 Evaluation of the Discovered Knowledge

13.5.1 Assessment of the Results vs. the Objectives

At this point, we look at what was found and try to interpret it. This may again result in returning to a previous step to revise or fine-tune it. Once the algorithm has completed on a given set of parameters, the clinicians can examine the patterns for significance and meaning. The director of the HIV Clinical Research Group examined the example pattern, shown in Fig. 4, which was discovered by TEMPADIS. Her conclusion was:

> These [look] like fairly advanced patients in the era of poor or no anti-retroviral suppression of their viral loads. Therefore, they would be subject to any number of viral infections such as CMV "flares" which would likely make their lymphocyte counts go up. The cause of CMV flares is unknown but may be from any number of causes such as mild "colds", etc.

She observes that the patients have “poor or no anti-retroviral suppression of their viral loads.” This conclusion can be drawn from that fact that it was not until 1996 when Protease Inhibitors came into use for suppressing replication of the HIV, and it was only at that point when viral replication was successful repressed in large numbers of HIV patients. The pattern clearly shows no use of Protease Inhibitors (drug category 2) and shows only sporadic use of the other drug therapies. Her comments further reflect the relative flatness of all the variables except the white blood cells and the lymphocytes, which jump around significantly. Once a pattern is deemed to be significant or interesting, we can look at the specific patients that supported the pattern and do the various types of analysis mentioned above on this sub-population.

Simply discovering patterns in the database is not an issue, since TEMPADIS has discovered many patterns in our domain database. Discovering interesting patterns is the issue. In order to facilitate this type of discovery, we have begun implementation of a query module based on a set of questions the clinicians posed. These questions describe the types of patterns they would find interesting. Using those questions as a guide, we implement search control techniques to avoid discovering patterns that we well know should be in the database, but are not particularly interesting except for the fact that they validate the TEMPADIS's capability to discover valid patterns. However, these search control techniques still do not always bring about the desired results. It is true that even when we attempt to constrain the search, the results include many patterns that are not particularly interesting.

```
< { (EV C ) (HS 3) (WTR 0) (WBC -1) (PLT -1) (HCT 0)
    (CD4P -4) (CD4A -4) (LMPH 0) (onD 0010000000) }
  { (EV C ) (HS 3) (WTR 1) (WBC -2) (PLT 0) (HCT -1)
    (CD4P -4) (CD4A -4) (LMPH 0) (onD 1010000000) }
  { (EV C ) (HS 3) (WTR 1) (WBC 0) (PLT 0) (HCT 0)
    (CD4P 0) (CD4A 0) (LMPH 1) (onD 1010000000) }
  { (EV C ) (HS 3) (WTR 1) (WBC 0) (PLT 0) (HCT 0)
    (CD4P -2) (CD4A 0) (LMPH 1) (onD 1000000000) }
  { (EV C ) (HS 3) (WTR 1) (WBC -1) (PLT -1) (HCT 0)
    (LMPH 0) (onD 0000000)}
  { (EV C ) (HS 3) (WTR 1) (WBC -1) (PLT -1) (HCT 0)
    (CD4P 0) (CD4A 0) (LMPH 0) (onD 1000000000) } >
```

Figure 6. Discovered pattern with search control set for non-decreasing CD4A.

On the other hand, among the mass of discovered patterns are some that show that our original goal is met. TEMPADIS is able to discover useful concepts in our domain database. In Fig. 6, we see a pattern discovered when the search control was set for non-decreasing CD4A. This pattern is interesting for the fact that it is one of the few discovered that shows a group of patients that consistently maintained their drug therapy, and the result was the improvement in CD4A from –4 to 0 sustained over a period of time.

```
< { (EV C ) (HS 1) (WTR 1) (CD4A 0) (onD 0000000000) }
  { (EV C ) (HS 1) (WTR 0) (CD4A 0) (onD 0000000000) }
  { (EV C ) (HS 1) (WTR 0) (WBC 0) (PLT 2) (HCT 0)
    (CD4P -2) (CD4A 0) (LMPH 2) (onD 0000000000) }
  { (EV C ) (HS 1) (WTR 1) (CD4A 0) (onD 0000000000) }
  { (EV C ) (HS 1) (WTR 1) (CD4A 0) (onD 0000000000) }
  { (EV C ) (HS 1) (WTR 1) (WBC 0) (PLT 1) (HCT 0)
    (CD4P 0) (CD4A 0) (LMPH 0) (onD 0000000000) }
  { (EV C ) (HS 1) (WTR 2) (CD4A 0)
    (onD 0000000000) } >
```

Figure 7. Discovered pattern with search set to unchanged CD4A.

Figure 7 shows a pattern discovered while searching for unchanged CD4A. The intention of this query was to discover what other events were doing during a time period of stable CD4. Though the pattern seems unremarkable, it represents a group of patients that were not on any drug therapy and shows that the patients' condition seems to gradually be deteriorating due to a general trend of increased recovery time, despite the stable CD4.

13.5.2 Reviewing the Entire Knowledge Discovery Process

Having completed the KDD process for our database with our goal, we can evaluate the results. Fayyad, Piatetsky-Shapiro, and Smyth (Fayyad et al. 1996) provide some criteria for evaluating discovered patterns. They say that patterns should be understandable and novel, but that these concepts are subjective. They further state that the patterns should be "potentially useful", leading to some benefit to the user. They also note that the concept of interestingness (Silbershatz and Tuzhilin 1996) is an overall measure of the pattern value, combining factors such as validity, novelty, usefulness and simplicity, but can be explicitly defined, or manifested implicitly by the system itself.

It is clear from the presentation that the patterns in Figs. 4, 6 and 7 are understandable. In fact, they seem to represent specifically recognizable conditions. TEMPADIS is biased towards discovery of interesting patterns through the use of search control parameters that allow the user to specify what kinds of patterns would be interesting. As for the usefulness, that is the next step. Now that groups of patients can be identified by a pattern, those groups can be investigated for the purposes that the user originally had for specifying parameters that would yield patterns of that type.

Other measures that we considered for evaluation purposes include significance in terms of number of patients represented, and length of time covered by the patterns. With the parameters used for the pattern in Fig. 2, the pattern would have only had to represent one out of every sixteen patients in order to be discovered by TEMPADIS. However, this pattern actually represents one out of every 9.6 patients. Again with the parameters used for that particular run, this pattern likely spans a period of from 1 to 12 months. Examination of the 10 specific patients supporting the pattern shows that it actually varies from 5 to 10 months. Given that the majority of our patient data spans 48 to 60 months, patterns of this length are non-trivial.

Our experience with TEMPADIS reaffirms that this type of search problem easily becomes intractable. It is clear that this approach cannot be used to randomly sift through the database to discover whatever patterns might be out there. However, as stated earlier we are not interested in all the patterns that could be found. With careful use of search control,

TEMPADIS can be used to discover meaningful patterns in areas of specific research interest.

13.6 Using the Discovered Knowledge

13.6.1 Implementation and Monitoring Plans

Implementation depends on actions out of the control of this research group: acquisition of hardware, acquisition of database software, finding time for research nurses to supervise and insure quality of data entry, among others.

13.6.2 Overview of the Entire Project for Future Use and Improvements

Our overview of the project provides some lessons learned which can be passed on for future use by this group and others. We simply need to recognize the nature of medical data. It may have been stored for reasons (e.g., billing) that had nothing to do with the use in data mining to which it is currently being put. While it may serve its original function well, it certainly does not lend itself well to anything but simple analyses of a statistical nature. In contrast to medical imaging data or data collected with the *a priori* intent to do statistical analysis, this is typical of data sets from realistic domains collected for other purposes which are rarely "neat and tidy". Furthermore, this data was collected by a large number of people without concerted efforts to maintain consistency. A strong message that our experience sends, therefore, is that one should not minimize the need for data preparation, and the time and resources that this preparation will take.

One of the features of TEMPADIS that should be highlighted in this summary is the increased power that was gained using inexact discovery methods. Exact match will work for many domains, but should be questioned in the medical domain.

Our experience also shows the need to focus the search in the data mining step, to know what is being sought from the data and not simply to let data mining methods look in a database for patterns. Combinatorial explosion occurs easily with undirected search methods. This emphasizes the need to work closely with a domain expert who can focus the search based on the meaning of the data and the purpose of the search. As usual, the partnership between the computer scientist and the medical expert is key to a successful effort in medical knowledge discovery.

References

Agrawal R. and Srikant R. 1995. Mining sequential patterns. In: *Proc 11th Int Conf on Data Engineering*, 3-14

Dombi G.W., Nandi P., Saxe J.M., Ledgerwood A.M., and Lucas C.E. 1995. Prediction of rib fracture injury outcomes by an artificial neural network. *J of Trauma: Injury, Infection, and Critical Care*, 39(5):915-21

Fayyad U., Piatetsky-Shapiro G., Smyth P. 1996. From data mining to knowledge discovery in databases. *AI Magazine*, (Fall):37-53, AAAI, Menlo Park CA

Frye K.E., Izenberg S.D., Williams M.D., Luterman A. 1996. Simulated biologic intelligence used to predict length of stay and survival of burns. *J of Burn Care and Rehab*, 17(6):540-6

Goodman P.H. 1996. NevProp neural network software, version 3. University of Nevada, Reno (ftp://ftp.scs.unr.edu/pub/goodman/nevpropdir/index.htm)

Izenberg S.D., Williams M.D. and Luterman A. 1997. Prediction of trauma mortality using a neural network. *American Surgeon* 63(3):275-81

Mannila H., Toivonen H., Verkamo A.I. 1995. Discovering frequent episodes in sequences. In: *Proc 1st Int Conf on Knowledge Discovery in Databases*, AAAI Press, 210-15

Mannila H. and Toivonen H. 1996. Discovering generalized episodes using minimal occurrences. In: *Proc 2nd Int Conf on Knowledge Discovery in Databases*, AAAI Press, 146-51

Mobley B.A., Leasure R., Davidson L. 1995. Artificial neural network predictions of lengths of stay on a post-coronary care unit. *Heart and Lung* 24(3):251-6

Padmanabhan B., Tuzhilin A. Pattern discovery in temporal databases: a temporal logic approach. In: *Proc 2nd Int Conf on Knowledge Discovery in Databases*, AAAI Press, 351-4

Quinlan J.R. 1993. C4.5: programs for machine learning. Morgan Kaufmann

Ramirez J.C.G., Peterson L.L., and Peterson D.M. 1998. A sequence building approach to pattern discovery in medical data. In: Cook, DJ (Ed): *Proc 11th Int Florida Artificial Intelligence Research Symp Conf*, AAAI Press, 188-192

Silberschatz A. and Tuzhilin A. 1995. On Subjective Measures of Interestingness in Knowledge Discovery. In: *Proc 1st Intl Conf on Knowledge Discovery and Data Mining*, AAAI Press, 275-81

Srikant R. and Agrawal R. 1996. Mining sequential patterns: generalizations and performance improvements. In: *Proc 5th Int Conf on Extending Database Technology*, Springer-Verlag, 3-17

14 Data Mining-Based Modeling of Human Visual Perception

Luís Augusto Consularo[1], Roberto de Alencar Lotufo[2] and Luciano da Fontoura Costa[1]

[1]Cybernetic Vision Research Group IFSC-USP
São Carlos - SP, Brazil
{consul, luciano}@if.sc.usp.br
[2]DCA-FEE, UNICAMP
Campinas – SP, Brazil
lotufo@dca.fee.unicamp.br

In this article, data mining concepts and techniques are applied for evaluating the quality and impact of visual information. The main objectives are both to evaluate such images, and to derive mathematical-computational models of human perception of visual quality and impact for general applications in graphic design and image quality analysis. In addition, it is expected that such models and experiments can provide a basis for diagnosing some cognitive and neurological problems. The basic idea is that, once a model of such perceptions has been obtained by considering only normal subjects, it can be used as a comparison standard. While it is virtually impossible to consider a fully representative set of images, we have constrained the current approach, for simplicity's sake, to psychophysical experiments performed interactively through the internet, in which bitmap versions of some selected home pages in commercial sites are tachitoscopically presented, after which the subjects rate several quality-related parameters. At the same time, a series of measures of visual properties (features) are extracted from the considered home page bitmaps, including Fourier texture indicators, multiscale entropy and variance, fractal dimensions and color and gray level contrast. The genetic algorithm is applied to obtain interpolating surfaces which can be used as models for replicating the human visual perception of the image quality and impact. All the components of our investigation, from the internet-based psychophysical experiments to the mathematic-computational modeling, have been conducted in an integrated environment for data mining, called ΣYnergos. The obtained results have shown that human visual quality perception can be reasonably modeled even by using a limited set of relatively simple features.

14.1 Understanding the Problem Domain

The relevance of visual information and communication for human beings can not be over-stressed. By providing the broadest-band information channel from the external world into human perception, vision has achieved special importance to humans. According to D. Marr (Marr, 1982), vision is the process of identifying the objects present in a scene an their respective position. As such, vision has played an especially relevant role in shaping our behavior and interaction with the external world throughout the whole evolutionary process. That is not to say that vision is exclusive (all senses are important), but its predominant role can hardly be disputed. In the computer world, a particularly striking indication of the special importance of vision to humans has been provided by the evolution of the WWW. Although e-mail and ftp facilities had been available for a long time, it was only after the hardware and software advances had paved the way to fully visual an interactive environments that the Internet really took off. Indeed, the evolution of WWW environments has pointed out toward the use of more and more animations and 3D resources.

In spite of the importance of visual information, even the general related areas of graphic design, visual communication, movies, visual arts, marketing and visual literacy, seem to have relied on a predominantly subjective and incomplete understanding about the concepts and mechanisms underlying human visual perception. As observed by (Moriarty, 1995), even in marketing, where so much is at stake, little success has been achieved in understanding the meaning from visual messages. The main reasons identified by her are the difficulty of capturing visual meaning and the lack of well structured research addressing coding and categorization of visual concepts. Another indication of the complexity entailed by such an investigation is provided by Lieberman (Lieberman, 1995), who points out that even graphic designers have great difficulty in identifying the guidelines for a good and effective graphic design. In his investigations, Lieberman has verified that most of the transmission of expertise in this area is accomplished more effectively by visual examples of well-succeeded designs rather than by roles and texts. Indeed, such a scenario is hardly surprising, since human visual perception is highly complex, depending on an extremely large number of variables. For instance, the environment illumination, the size of the screen/monitor, and even the chair position and overall mood of a person can influence the way in which visual information is perceived. While the identification of the general tendencies underlying human appreciation of visual information is no doubt a very difficult endeavor, unlikely to be fully solved in the coming years, the recent advances in artificial intelligence, computer vision, psychophysics, visual neuroscience, as well as in software and hardware technologies, have provided exciting ways for improving our understanding of the way humans perceived visual information, even if in a relatively constrained fashion. Examples of recently obtained interesting results in visual communication-related areas include, but are by no means limited to: the study of visual semiotics an the production of meaning in advertising (Moriarty, 1995), the study of the influence of textures and contrast sensitivity on reading speed (Scharff et. al., 1999; Parker and Scharff, 1997), and the investigation of how text width and margins can affect the readability of GUIs (Youngman and Scharff, 1998).

The present article addresses the problem of obtaining mathematical models of the human judgement of a series of image quality parameters. Despite the broad range of implications of such investigations, here attention is directed toward the specific case of the evaluation of the graphic quality and impact of home pages. This is justified because such images are easily available from the Internet, and provide a reasonably varied sample of typical image contents.

The main motivation for obtaining such models include, but are not limited, to the following possibilities: (i) such models can yield insights about human perception; (ii) the obtained models can be used in order to automatically assess the quality of graphic design and image compression techniques, such as those broadly used for communications; and (iii) provide valuable information about the treatment and selection of visual properties, for instance while developing expert systems. Moreover, it is expected that once a model is obtained by considering only psychophysical data obtained from normal subjects, the visual perception model can be used as a standard for diagnosis of cognitive or neurological disorders.

The investigation and modeling of the whole process of human visual perception is particularly difficult and challenging because of the large number of involved variables. It is often convenient to classify such variables according to a complexity hierarchy. At the lower stages, we have the influence of basic visual properties, such as contrast, texture, color, and size. In the intermediate scale are included the overall shape of objects, their relative position, as well as the overall composition and balance of scenes. At the highest hierarchy, we include semiotics, contextual and cultural influences, such as the observers' mood, its background in pictorial art appreciation, and special cultural preferences and prejudices (see Moriarty, 1997). Interestingly, the neural hardware responsible for processing the elements along the above-identified hierarchy is distributed, roughly, from the back to the front of our cortex. Needless to say, our understanding of visual perception process considerably decreases when moving towards the higher hierarchies. Although elements in all hierarchies tend to act together in defining and influencing our visual perception, we have no alternative but concentrate on investigating such effects separately, often concentrating on the lower hierarchical elements. The success of such an approach is conditioned on our ability and the possibility of keeping stable as many as possible of the other elements during the psychological experiments. For instance, when investigating human visual perception, it is important to use always the same size of display, the same position of the head and eyes, the same room, and, if possible, the same time. Ideally, the only variables should be those we are interested in. However, despite all care and efforts, in practice it is often impossible to eliminate the influence completely of all secondary variables. As a matter of fact, much of the advances in human visual perception have been achieved through psychophysical investigations (see, for instance, Barlow, 1982; Goldstein, 1989; Levine and Sheffner, 1991), ranging form basic process controlling contrast perception to more sophisticated processes such as selective attention and active vision.

From the perspective of home page design and evaluation, it is important to start the investigation by considering what are the objectives to be fulfilled by the home pages. Although the main objective may vary from case to case (e.g. commercially oriented, communicating about scientific results, describing the activities of an institute, defending and ideological cause, warning people, and so on), the goal of home pages is often to transmit one or more messages to the broadest number of people, at least the broadest number of people in a specific community (see, for instance, Moriarty, 1997). The next important issue to be considered is the type of interaction characterizing WWW access and surfing. As observed by Rajani and Rosenberg (Rajani and Rosenberg, 1999), WWW interactions tends to be brief and oriented. Indeed, this hardly surprising, given the shared features between WWW and TV watching, which are both extremely dynamic environments. Indeed, as observed in (Rajani and Rosenberg, 1999) this could be due as consequence of such dynamic interactions. Given the extremely dynamic form of interaction, there is no time for analyzing more complex home pages. For such reasons, and also in order to constrain the range of neural process involved in the interpretation of the visual stimuli, our psychophysical experiments are conducted tachitoscopically.

The literature has shown some interesting statistical and psychological approaches relating visual complexity and aesthetic quality of landscapes. Some projects have been focused on mathematical and computational models (Orland, 1997), trying to find relationships between landscapes environmental features and respective image complexity. Among the proposed features we have: number of colors, number of edges, fractal dimension, standard deviation, entropy, Huffman encoding and run-length encoding (RLE). Riglis (Riglis, 1998) also highlights complexity measures such fractal dimension and compression measures, but including Klinger-Salingaros (Klinger and Salingaros, 1999) measures to visual complexity based on block symmetry of pixels of symbolic images. Bernaldez in (Bernaldez, 1987) performed a multivariate analysis of environmental features presented by landscape photographs where he concludes about independence among three feature dimensions: lightening, smoothness, and diversity. Synek in (Synek) on the other hand, synthesized landscape images at computer controlling their fractal dimensions and the presence of landscape elements, trying to relate preferences to the age of subjects and to explain evolutionary aspects of landscape images beauty evaluation.

The present article is organized in terms of the basic stages in developing the knowledge-based environment. It starts by describing how the image data was acquired from the www as well as how the psychophysical experiments were conceived. The method for data preparing is presented next, describing the approach to measure that images. The subsequent section, dealing on data mining, explains in detail the model construction. Following, a discussion about discovered knowledge is developed presenting the results and reviewing the entire project. Finally, the more promising results are highlighted and future improvements are proposed.

14.2 Understanding the Data

The experiment, performed from a web-site (http://iris.if.sc.usp.br), requests the subject to assign scores to visual quality parameters for each presented images (see Figure 1), which include a series of bitmaps extracted from actual WWW sites. The image size was normalized to 640x480 pixels. The first step in an experiment consists in filling a form with personal information (e.g. name and e-mail), that is followed by an explanation about the subsequent experiment. Next, the first image is presented on the screen, disappearing after four seconds, being replaced by an all-white image. This tachitoscopic effect is required in order the subject is little affected by the contextual information such as text, numbers or even iconic images, since they are not relevant to the undergoing investigation. Then, a form is presented asking the subject to assign scores to six visual qualities of the previously shown image. Special attention was focused on trying to normalize the experiment conditions, including distance from monitor, monitor dimensions, and the subjects profile.

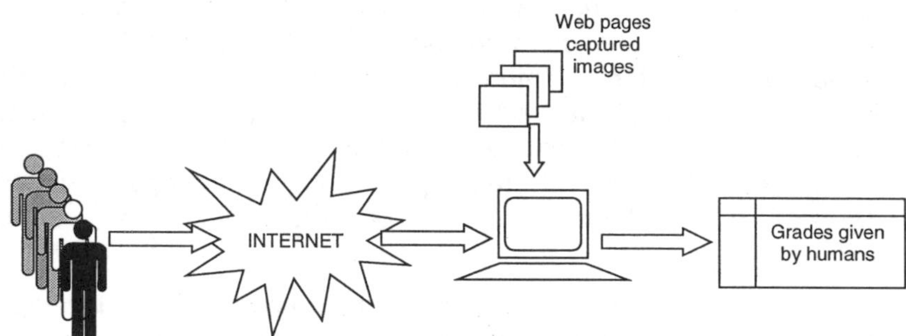

Figure 1. The subjects perform experiments on Internet.

14.3 Preparation of the Data

The measurements about the web page images were evaluated by using the image processing resources embedded into Σynergos, and stored into a table. N basic measures were extracted: gray-level distribution entropy and variance; Minkowski sausages (Coelho and Costa, 1996; Costa et. al., 1999); the Fourier spectrum and gray and color contrast. In fact, each of these features includes a set of measures. For instance, the entropy and variance extracted from a set of successively smoothed versions of the bitmap, implemented by using Gaussian low-pass filtering (Costa et. al. 1998). The Minkowski sausages correspond to a series of progressive dilations of the image, considering as structuring element spheres of increasing diameters. Radial and concentric histograms of the Fourier spectrum (Gonzales and Wintz, 1987) are used as indication of the orientation and spatial frequency distribution in the images. Global features were also obtained from the above ones, including the respective means and standard deviations, as well as time of life (of variance evolution along the spatial scale) and fractal dimensions (for Minkowski sausages). Each of these features is described in more detail below.

14.3.1.1.1 Entropy

The entropy of an image tells us about the information content. It is a concept inherited from information theory, having been used as measure of complexity, assuming the image formation as a stochastic process. It is defined as (Castleman, 1996):

$$H = S[I(a_k)] = -\sum_{k=0}^{K-1} P(a_k)\log(P(a_k)) \tag{1}$$

Where:
a_k is a gray level,
I is the image function,
$P(a_k)$ is the probability of find a gray level a_k on the image I.

Let H_σ be the entropy feature vector, where σ is the standard deviation of the Gaussian kernel function, and the smoothed image is $\hat{I}_\sigma$.

$$\hat{I}_\sigma = I * G_\sigma \tag{2}$$

Thus,

$$H_\sigma = S\{\hat{I}_\sigma(a_k)\}, \text{ for } \sigma = 0..N_H \tag{3}$$

where N_H is the number of scales.

The entropy averages (μ_H), and the standard deviations (σ_H), were also included into this feature vector.

14.3.1.1.2 Variance and Half-Life

The image variance is a simple statistical parameter obtainable from a bitmap which allows us to distinguish between images containing all ranges of gray levels from those presenting just a few ones. It is useful for detecting photographic images (high variance) and drawings (such as schematics and diagrams) in home pages. The variance can be calculated as:

$$V = \sigma^2\{I(x,y)\} = E[I^2(x,y)] - E^2[I(x,y)] \qquad (4)$$

where:
x, *y* are pixel position coordinates,
I is the image function
E(*I*) is the expected value of image *I*.

The multi-scale variance (Bruno et. al., 1998) was also considered in the present work. By multi-scale, it is understood that the variance is calculated for a series of successively smoothed versions of the original bitmap, implemented by using Gaussian smoothing with increasing standard deviations (spatial scales). When the evolution of the variance is considered in terms of the successive spatial scales, the half-life of the evolution can also be considered as an additional feature. The half-life is based on the exponential decay time, being defined as:

$$\sigma_{half-life} = \sigma\{(V_{\sigma=0})/2\} \qquad (5)$$

While a short half-life will indicate several small structures in the image, longer half-lives will reveal the presence of large structures or lack of texture in the bitmap. For the same smoothed image from (6):

$$V_\sigma = Var\{\hat{I}(x,y)\} \quad \text{for } \sigma = 0..N_V \qquad (6)$$

where N_V is the number of scales evaluated for variance.

Statistical global parameters such as the average of variance (μ_V) and the respective standard deviations (σ_V) were also considered as features.

14.3.1.1.3 Spectral Description (Radial and Concentric)

Spectral descriptors express the distributions of orientations and spatial frequencies in the image, being typically used to characterize texture (Gonzales and Wintz, 1987). While low frequencies mean more uniform areas (as far as the gray-level distribution is concerned), on the other hand, high frequencies typically characterize edges or some kind of noise. In order to obtain these descriptors, it is necessary to evaluate the image Fourier transform. So, given an image $f_I(x, y)$ and its Fourier transform, $\Im\{I(x, y)\} = F_I(u, v)$, it is possible to extract from the respective power spectrum $|F_I(u, v)|$ two projections: radial and concentric, illustrated in Figure 22 and Figure 3, respectively.

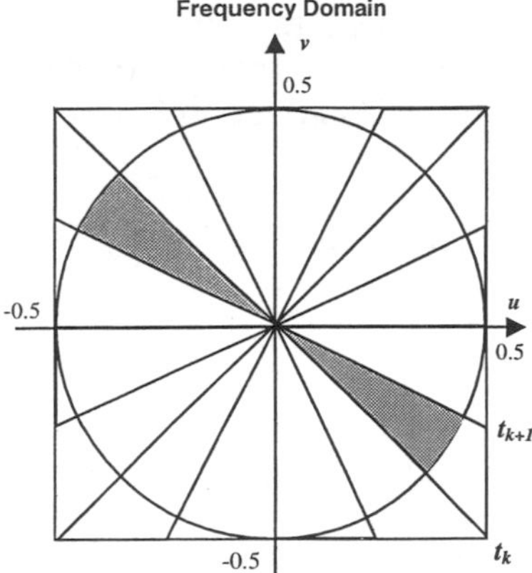

Figure 2. Representation of the radial descriptor regions on frequency domain.

The radial projection is obtained by adding the spectrum space along radial sectors, as illustrated in Figure 2.

$$S_{rad}[k] = \sum_{\arctan(v/u)=t_k}^{\arctan(v/u)=t_{k+1}} F_I(u,v), \text{ for } \sqrt{u^2+v^2} < 0.5 \tag{7}$$

Where $k = [0..N_{sectors}-1]$ and $N_{sectors}$ depend on angle step adopted.

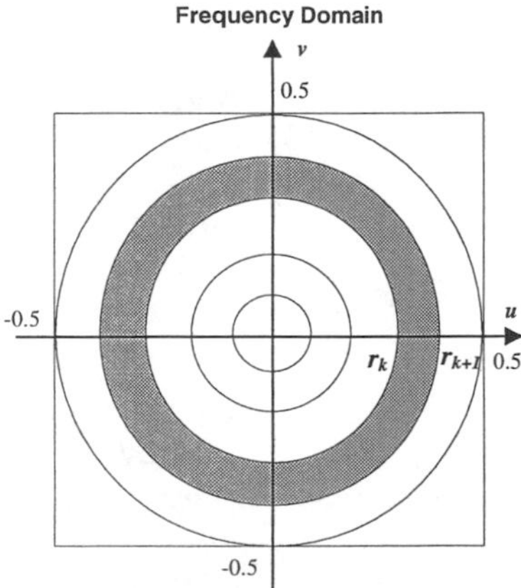

Figure 3. Representation of the concentric descriptor regions on frequency domain.

The concentric spectral descriptors, on the other hand, integrate the frequency domain according to concentric circles, generating a feature vector $S_{conc}[k]$. This process is illustrated in Figure .

$$S_{conc}[k] = \sum_{\sqrt{u^2+v^2}=r_k}^{\sqrt{u^2+v^2}=r_{k+1}} F_I(u,v), \text{ for } \sqrt{u^2+v^2} < 0.5 \tag{8}$$

where $k = [0..N_{stripes}-1]$.

14.3.1.1.4 *Minkowski Sausages and Fractal Dimension*

Fractal dimension is a measure frequently used for characterizing textures because of its ability to express self-similarity and spatial coverage. A nice introduction to fractals and fractal dimension can be found in (Warfel, 1998). The Minkowski-Bouligand method to evaluate fractal dimension represents, among the several methods, a good tradeoff between computational overhead and accuracy. Its implementation can be performed by successive dilations by a circular or spherical structurant element of two-dimensional or three-dimensional objects (Coelho and Costa, 1996; Costa et. al., 1998; 1999). These dilations can be performed by using mathematical morphology approaches or by Fourier Transform properties. However, the Fourier transform in three dimensions is computationally prohibitive, forcing us to think about more effective morphological strategies. Let $I_{2D}(x,y)=k$, where $0 \leq k < 256$ be a two-dimensional image. It can be treated in terms of the following 3D extension:

$$I_{3D}(x,y,z) = \begin{cases} 0, \text{if } I_{2D}(x,y) \neq k \\ 1, \text{if } I_{2D}(x,y) = k \end{cases} \text{ and}$$

$$S_r(x,y,z) = \begin{cases} 1, \text{if } \sqrt{x^2+y^2+z^2} < r \\ 0, \text{otherwise} \end{cases} \tag{9}$$

where
k means the gray level intensity, and r the radius of sphere as structurant element

Now, it is possible to dilate a spherical element along the image surface, counting the number of covered voxels. Hence, denoting I_r as the volume of the dilated image for a sphere with radius r, and $\oplus$ as the dilation operator, the process can be expressed as (10).

$$I_r = I_{3D} \oplus S_r \tag{10}$$

In order to speed up this process, instead of counting the covered voxels, empty spheres have been adopted as structuring elements, in such a way the dilated object becomes hollow. Now, the covered volume can be more effectively determined by identifying the upper and lower limits of the dilated region along the *z*-axis, starting from the top and bottom of the image, respectively. Therefore, denoting *Ones(I) = (position of the upper limit) – (position of the lower limit)* as the number of ones in the dilated surface, the feature vector containing this counting for dilations with spheres of radius *r*, *M[r]*, can be written as (11).

$$M[r] = Ones(I_r) \tag{11}$$

Global statistics (average and standard deviation) of this vector as well as the fractal dimension was also considered as features. The fractal dimension can be calculated by linearly interpolating the Log-Log representation of *M[r]* in terms of *r*, and taking as the fractal dimension the value 3 – (slope of the interpolated line).

14.3.1.1.5 Gray-Level and Color Contrast

The gray level contrast is here estimated by differences between cross-neighborhoods of a pixel. Thus, given the source image $I(x,y)$, a new image of average differences $D_{gray}(x, y)$ is formed as:

$$D_{gray}(x, y) = \frac{(4I(x, y) - (I(x+1, y) + I(x, y+1) + I(x-1, y) + I(x, y-1)))}{4} \tag{12}$$

The histogram $H_{gray}(a_k)$ of $D_{gray}(x, y)$ provides the contrast feature vector. Statistics (average and standard deviation) are also evaluated and included into the feature vector.

The color feature vector is evaluated similarly, but the source image for differences consists of scalar products of vectors in the RGB space. The RGB space is defined in terms of three components: $I_R(x, y)$ for red, $I_G(x, y)$ for green, and $I_B(x, y)$ for the blue channel, i.e.:

$$\vec{v}_{(x,y)} = \left(I_R(x,y) \quad I_G(x,y) \quad I_B(x,y)\right) \tag{13}$$

The average scalar product between the cross-neighborhood values is calculated as:

$$D_{RGB} = \frac{(\vec{v}_{(x,y)} \cdot \vec{v}_{(x+1,y)} + \vec{v}_{(x,y)} \cdot \vec{v}_{(x,y+1)} + \vec{v}_{(x,y)} \cdot \vec{v}_{(x-1,y)} + \vec{v}_{(x,y)} \cdot \vec{v}_{(x,y-1)})}{4} \quad (14)$$

High values for such scalar product indicates uniform color regions, lower values corresponding to non-uniform regions. The histogram of D_{RGB} provides the feature vector expressing color contrast.

14.4 Data Mining

14.4.1 The Σynergos

The Σynergos system was proposed in 1998 (Bruno et. al, 1998) as a laboratory for experiments in visual processing and perception, including data mining, validation of concepts and techniques, and determination of optimal parameters and configurations of visual processing techniques. The basic idea underlying Σynergos is the integrated and complementary application of many paradigms in computer science, mathematics, vision research, artificial intelligence, distributed systems, databases and Internet, to name but a few. It is expected that the overall result of combining such concepts and techniques will be greater than the sum of the parts when used separately (synergetics). Of course, what is at stake here are investigations of specific problems, not the full fledged integration of all such concepts. For instance, the Σynergos system has already been implemented in a distributed system and successfully applied to a series of situations, including: modeling the human judgement of pictorial complexity (Bruno et. al., 1999), validating the classification of neural cells in terms of their respective complexity (Bruno et. al., 1998), and also as a means of deriving calibration curves to be used for obtaining proper parameter configurations when applying curvature-based contour segmentation (Consularo et. al., 1999). All these applications have been characterized by the use of optimization techniques, such as the genetic algorithm, as a means of searching for sub-optimal configurations. The specific configuration and methods that are being considered in the Σynergos systems in order to address the current issue is described in the following section.

14.4.2 The Approach

The perception about some sensation involves a plethora of issues, and to model it is a painful task. This current work aims to model constrained but unknown situations: the visual impact of web pages design. As related below, the experimental framework provides subjective evaluations about a selected set of web pages and a feature vector holding measures about captured images from web pages. The idea here is extract a model to predict a commonsense about visual impact. This could be extended for any images category, but the focus on web pages will allow us to confront experts feelings given by prolific literature, including those about press design (Dondis, 1973).

Modeling perception demands a reference in order to validate the approach. Here we adopt as reference the psychological response provided by humans, treating the perception modeling as a reversal-engineering problem (see Figure 44). Therefore, the typical human subject is treated as a black box receiving as visual stimuli the home-pages bitmaps. The output is given by the grades assigned by the subjects with respect to some specific visual quality (e.g. complexity, color harmony, and artistic quality). The sought model involves extracting a set of meaningful features from the stimuli, which are processed in some convenient way in order to produce an answer that, hopefully, is in agreement with what would be typically given by a human subject.

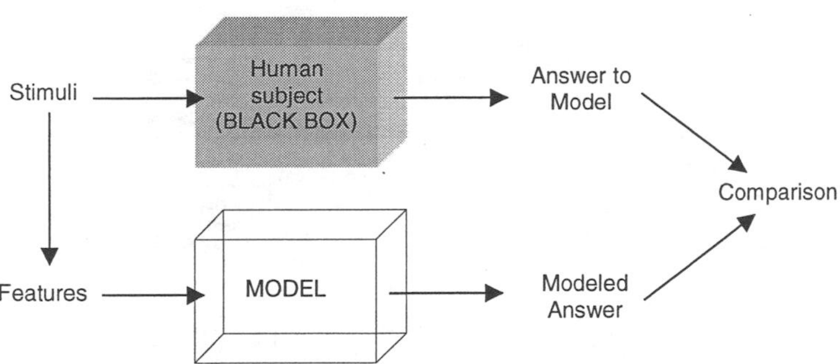

Figure 4. The modeling approach.

The visual quality parameters considered in this work are expected to reflect the quality and impact of web pages as perceived by people while assessing them. The basic idea is to identify a set of features, as well as a mathematical model, upon which a reasonable estimation of the respective perceptual response could be obtained. The considered quality parameters are: pleasantness, color balance, originality, artistic quality, the motivation to further explore the home page, and the estimated time each subject though necessary to stay in the home-page.

The psychophysical experiment and the adopted features are described in the following sections, respectively.

The mathematical model should act on the selected features in order to provide a reply that is statistically in agreement with the human perception. This approach entails two important issues: (i) select a reasonable way to combine the features, yielding the overall rate; and (ii) tune this model by considering the results obtained by the psychophysical experiment. These two issues are discussed in more detail in the following.

14.4.3 Generalization

The adopted modeling approach consists simply in interpolating a set of selected features for each quality parameter being considered. So, given a set of images, the model operation can be summarized as searching for interpolating coefficients which when applied to new images can optimize the agreement between its response and the respective human assessment (see Figure 55). This process will be henceforth called generalization.

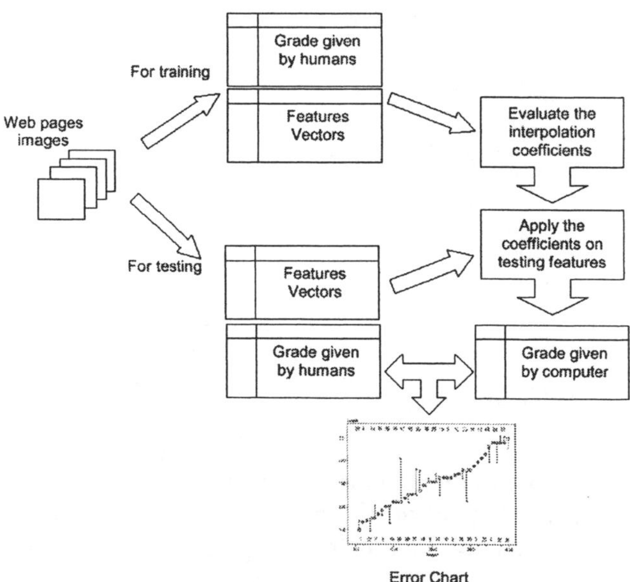

Figure 5. Applying the model.

This generalization can be performed according to the following alternative ways: (1) artificial neural networks; (2) grammatically structured information, (3) models based on parametric equations, or still by (4) interpolation, the alternative adopted in the present approach. A great diversity of interpolation methods can be found in the scientific literature (Powell, 1981). Ideally, the method used in the present work should:

- be able to deal with an arbitrary number of dimensions;
- be able to interpolate irregularly spaced points;
- not imply intensive computations.

Guided by the above conditions, a flexible interpolation method was sought, the chosen method being known by diverse names such as thin plate splines, surface splines, biharmonic interpolation, or radial basis function, just to cite a few of them (Duchon, 1977; Sandwell, 1987; Powell, 1994). The thin plate splines (TPS) is usually applied to surface interpolation because of its ability to minimize the bending energy of a surface. Another of its important features is the smoothing imposed by the biharmonic equation solution, mainly for high dimensional spaces. Powell developed a nice theory about two dimensions applications of TPS, which Sandwell applied to solve biharmonic equation (Powell, 1994; Sandwell, 1987). That article served as reference for MathWorks in the implementation of a routine for irregular grid points interpolation (griddata()) (Mathworks, 1992). Duchon showed the multidimensional possibilities of TPS, guided by some constraints (Duchon, 1977). Buhmann showed the feasibility of Radial Functions as a quasi-interpolant basis for scattered data (Buhmann et. al., 1995). Hegland developed methods implementing TPS interpolation for Data Mining applications using finite elements, but with a limitation: this is an interactive algorithm possibly violating the third requirement above (Hegland et. al., 1998). Mees developed a suitable approach assuming as radial basis function the distance itself (Mees et. al., 1992). This latter approach was adopted in the current work, being described in the following.

The data considered in the interpolation are those obtained in the psychophysics experiment. Each image I_k yield a vector formed by the perception scores (u_k) and a feature vector (v_k), as described above. The perception score was averaged and both u_k and v_k were normalized to the [-1, 1] range. A fixed amount of images was used as reference (v_i), and another set of images was considered for testing (ξ_j). The important question now is to select a suitable set of visual features to be used in the interpolation. More specifically:

- How many features are needed to interpolate the averaged perceptual scores in order to minimize the error when compared to another set of arbitrary images?
- What are these features?

Therefore, to answer these questions, the set of reference images was divided into two groups, one for training (*i*), and other for tests (*j*). So, naming v_i the feature vector for image *i*, defined in a multidimensional space (*d* dimensions), and being u_i a function resulting from v_i which could be thought as a thin surface $f(v_i)$ interpolating these points. This surface can be applied to the test images *j*, whose feature vector is represented by ξ_j, in order to obtain the artificial scores values η_j. Now what remains is to evaluate all combinations of features, interpolating them, while searching for the minimum error. However, this is not so simple. As observed in Section 5, there are at least $d = 152$ possible features to combine, yielding the following number of cases:

$$\sum_{j=2}^{d} \binom{d}{j} = 2^d - d \tag{15}$$

where
d is the number of features (or dimension of interpolation space) and *j* indexes the number of combinations.

Since this is often a prohibitive quantity, some optimization algorithm has to be considered. Here we adopted the genetic algorithm, to be described in Section 4.4.

The basic idea in the adopted interpolation method is to find a weight vector *w* (representing the mathematical model) which operates on ξ_j resulting in η_j. This could, at the simplest instance, be treated as a linear system, but this solution would only express a much simpler linear relationship than that proposed by Weber and Fechner (Gordon, 1989).

Bookstein (Bookstein, 1989), solving the partial difference equation known as the biharmonic equation (Powell, 1994), found a variational problem whose solution is given by splines polynomials such as:

$$f(\vec{v}) = \sum_{i=1}^{N} c_i \phi(\|\vec{v} - \vec{v}_i\|) \tag{16}$$

where
c_i =coefficients strength of the smoothness of Radial Basis Function $\phi(\|r\|)$.
N = the amount of control points, i.e., the available measurement points.

The choice of the function $\phi(\|r\|)$ can be done with some freedom, but the function $\phi(\|r\|) = r^2\log(r)$ (Powell, 1994) is the ideal if the goal is to minimize the bending energy on a thin plate. Here, r is the norm of space in question. Euclidean distance (17) is adopted henceforth. We also consider Mees' approach, which allows more freedom by adding a linear polynomial to $f(v)$ (Mees et. al., 1992). This increment allows a skew strength around orthogonal axis given in terms of a and an offset parameter b in one direction. So $f(v)$ now looks like (18).

$$r = \|\vec{u} - \vec{v}\| = \sqrt{\sum_{k=1}^{d} (u_k - v_k)^2} \tag{17}$$

$$f(\vec{v}) = \sum_{i=1}^{N} c_i \phi(\|\vec{v} - \vec{v}_i\|) + \vec{a} \cdot \vec{v} + b \tag{18}$$

The coefficients can be found by imposing the boundary condition (Mees et. al., 1992):

$$\sum_{i=1}^{N} c_i = 0 \qquad \textit{and} \qquad \vec{c} \cdot \vec{v} = 0 \tag{19}$$

Expressed in matrix notation, this equation becomes:

$$\begin{bmatrix} u_1 \\ u_2 \\ \vdots \\ u_N \\ \hline 0 \\ 0 \\ \vdots \\ 0 \\ 0 \end{bmatrix} = \left[\begin{array}{cccc|cccc:c} 0 & \phi(\|\vec{v}_1 - \vec{v}_2\|) & \cdots & \phi(\|\vec{v}_1 - \vec{v}_N\|) & v_{11} & v_{12} & \cdots & v_{1d} & 1 \\ \phi(\|\vec{v}_1 - \vec{v}_2\|) & 0 & \cdots & \phi(\|\vec{v}_2 - \vec{v}_N\|) & v_{21} & v_{22} & \cdots & v_{2d} & 1 \\ \vdots & \vdots & \ddots & \vdots & \vdots & \vdots & & \vdots & \vdots \\ \phi(\|\vec{v}_1 - \vec{v}_N\|) & \phi(\|\vec{v}_2 - \vec{v}_N\|) & \cdots & 0 & v_{N1} & v_{N2} & & v_{Nd} & 1 \\ \hline v_{11} & v_{21} & \cdots & v_{N1} & 0 & 0 & \cdots & 0 & 0 \\ v_{12} & v_{22} & \cdots & v_{N2} & 0 & 0 & \cdots & 0 & 0 \\ \vdots & \vdots & & \vdots & \vdots & \vdots & \ddots & 0 & 0 \\ v_{1d} & v_{2d} & \cdots & v_{Nd} & 0 & 0 & \cdots & 0 & 0 \\ \hdashline 1 & 1 & \cdots & 1 & 0 & 0 & \cdots & 0 & 0 \end{array}\right] \begin{bmatrix} c_1 \\ c_2 \\ \vdots \\ c_N \\ \hline a_1 \\ a_2 \\ \vdots \\ a_d \\ \hdashline b \end{bmatrix} \tag{20}$$

Where

$\phi(\|\vec{v}_i - \vec{v}_k\|) = \|\vec{v}_i - \vec{v}_k\|^2 \log(\|\vec{v}_i - \vec{v}_k\|)$,

$\vec{u}$ is the vector containing the scores assigned to each image.

N is the total of trained images, and

d is the number of dimensions or features.

For simplicity's sake, the linear system (20) can be written as

$$\begin{bmatrix} \vec{c} \\ \vec{a} \\ b \end{bmatrix} = \begin{bmatrix} \phi & V & 1 \\ V^T & 0 & 0 \\ 1 & 0 & 0 \end{bmatrix}^{-1} \begin{bmatrix} \vec{u} \\ 0 \\ 0 \end{bmatrix} \quad \text{or } \vec{w} = G^{-1}\vec{u} \tag{21}$$

This expression will allow us to apply the *w* vector in order to obtain the interpolation for new data sets, providing an estimation of the perceived quality. The distances between the given and desired points have now to be evaluated (22).

$$\begin{bmatrix} \eta_1 \\ \eta_2 \\ \vdots \\ \eta_M \end{bmatrix} = \left[\begin{array}{cccc|cccc:c} \phi(\|\vec{\xi}_1 - \vec{v}_1\|) & \phi(\|\vec{\xi}_1 - \vec{v}_2\|) & \cdots & \phi(\|\vec{\xi}_1 - \vec{v}_N\|) & \xi_{11} & \xi_{12} & \cdots & \xi_{1d} & 1 \\ \phi(\|\vec{\xi}_2 - \vec{v}_1\|) & \phi(\|\vec{\xi}_2 - \vec{v}_2\|) & \cdots & \phi(\|\vec{\xi}_2 - \vec{v}_N\|) & \xi_{21} & \xi_{22} & \cdots & \xi_{2d} & 1 \\ \vdots & \vdots & & \vdots & \vdots & \vdots & & \vdots & \vdots \\ \phi(\|\vec{\xi}_M - \vec{v}_1\|) & \phi(\|\vec{\xi}_M - \vec{v}_2\|) & \cdots & \phi(\|\vec{\xi}_M - \vec{v}_N\|) & \xi_{M1} & \xi_{M2} & & \xi_{Md} & 1 \end{array}\right] \left[\begin{array}{c} c_1 \\ c_2 \\ \vdots \\ c_N \\ \hline a_1 \\ a_2 \\ \vdots \\ a_d \\ \hdashline b \end{array}\right] \tag{22}$$

The next step is to search the best *d* which minimizes the difference between the evaluated perception and the perceived sensation scores, in order not only to answer the question (1), but also to indicate the best features to be used, hence answering also the question (2).

14.4.4 The Search

As mentioned before the search space for this problem is great and an effective searching strategy has to be applied. Several strategies exist in literature, all them implying specific advantages and shortcomings. Methods like "brute force" (Gen and Cheng, 1997), evolutionary algorithms (Bäck, 1996), simulated annealing (Kirkpatrick et. al., 1983), or uphill/downhill searches (Gen and Cheng, 1997), or hybrid strategies as tabu search (Glover, 1997), have been proposed in the literature. The problem implied by the adopted modeling approach is characterized by the following characteristics: (1) an unknown search space; (2) the solution may not be unique or not exist; (3) a clear goal is available (i.e. to minimize the error while estimating the scores). These characteristics make the Genetic Algorithm (GA), proposed by Holland as a search strategy that mimics the Darwinian evolution process (Holland, 1962), a good choice. Since Holland's original insight, every sort of approaches and applications has made of the GA a very popular stochastic search algorithm. The GA considered in this work, which corresponds to one of its simplest variants, is described in (Goldberg, 1989; Gen and Cheng, 1997). However, the choice of some parameters and specifications deserves some additional comments. The population is formed by individuals or chromosomes, where each one, in the current case, represents a feature vector. This feature vector or chromosome means a combination of features (genes) that must be tested and evaluated. Let $f_i = \{b_1 b_2 \cdots b_d\}$ be a binary vector whose elements (genes) can assume two values: $b_k = 0$ means the feature is not being considered, and $b_k = 1$ means that the feature is being considered. Again, d is the maximum number of features tested simultaneously.

The initial population can be initialized at random or by considering previous knowledge about the solution space. Since the final number of features has been verified to be close to 15, the initial population is defined by combinations of 10 randomly selected features. As already observed the goal here is to minimize the distance between the human and modeled perceptions regarding each quality parameter. This evaluation is achieved after the interpolation, as described in previous session, and compared in terms of the Euclidean distance between the original perception vector $p = [\rho_1 \quad \cdots \quad \rho_M]^T$ and the evaluated perception $q = [\eta_1 \quad \cdots \quad \eta_M]^T$. The goal function can thus be expressed as:

$$\varphi(f_i) = \sqrt{\sum_{i=1}^{M} (\eta_i - \rho_i)^2} \tag{23}$$

After evaluation, the individuals are sorted in ascending order by φ and the first half is selected for recombination, which is done in terms of two types of evolutionary operators: the crossover and the mutation. The adopted crossover was the multi-point crossover (Goldberg, 1989), aiming a faster convergence. The mutation is a simple change of gene status, i.e., if 0 assumes 1 and if 1 assumes 0. Each operation follows a probability rate, one for crossovers and other for mutations. The assessment continues until a suitable value for the goal function is reached or the variance of goal function value at population is small enough or zero.

14.5 Evaluation of the Discovered Knowledge

The modeling process was carried out for all perceived sensation parameters. Before training, it was necessary to test the Radial Basis Function (RBF) to be used in the interpolation. Since Mees (Mees et. al., 1992) warns about bad choices for the interpolating function, which could generate more errors than others – see Equation (20), special attention was focused on considering several functions, obtained by varying the exponent for the radial basis function, in the GA and also implementing a surface viewer. The consistency of the linear system implied by the interpolation (Equation (20)), was checked during the GA, being unconsidered in case of inconsistency.

In order to assess the performance of the GA approach, brute force selection of the features, i.e. trying all possible options for two and three features on a 154 total amount of features was applied. Only the "pleasantness" quality parameter was considered in this investigation. Histograms of the Euclidean distance (ED) between interpolated answer and the experiment answer, i.e. the estimation error, were calculated for the following cases: (i) $\phi(||r||) = r$; (ii) $\phi(||r||) = r^2\log(r)$; (iii) $\phi(||r||) = r^3$ and (iv) $\phi(||r||) = r^{½}$.

The thus obtained distributions were compared, and the resulting histograms are shown in Table 1 and Table 2. It is clear from the results for $\phi(||r||) = r$ and $\phi(||r||) = r^{½}$ that there is a range (2.5 < Euclidean distance < 4.5) allowing smaller errors for both space dimensions (2 and 3 dimensions). However, for $\phi(||r||) = r^2\log(r)$ and $\phi(||r||) = r^3$, greater Euclidean distance values become more common as warned in (Mees et. al., 1992). For r^3, the higher errors are probably caused by the smoothness implied by this larger exponent.

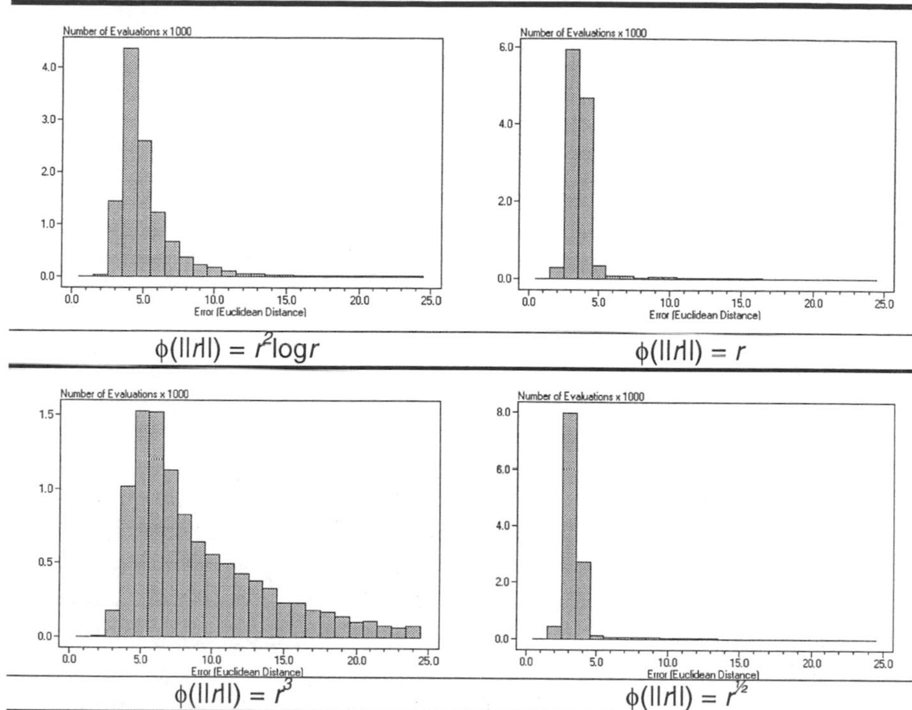

Table 1. Error histograms for originality using the brute force method for combinations of two features.

In addition to the error histograms, the brute force investigation has also provided insight about the selected features and minimum errors in the case of two and three features, which are shown in Table 3 and Table 4, respectively. It is clear from these table that the color contrast for the interval $229.5 \leq d < 242.25$ has always been chosen as one of the features.

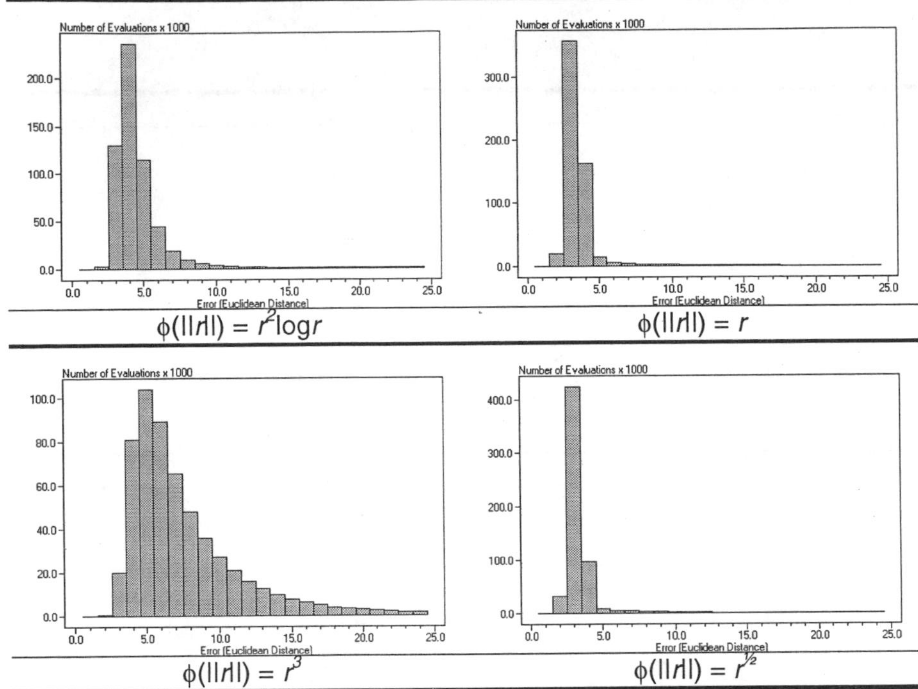

Table 2. Error histograms for originality using the brute force method for combinations of three features.

As explained in the previous sections, the adopted modeling approach aims to minimize the number of used features. Even when not considering the number of features in the goal function, few (between 14 and 18) features have been selected. It has also been verified that the obtained number of feature does not vary too much along repeated evolutions considering randomized initial conditions. The evolution, including 225 generations, was performed over a random population, but constraining the number of initial combined features for each individual. The random initializations implied slow evolution, but converged to the similar number of features and goal function values. Several numbers of initial combinations were tried, but a value about 10 allowed faster executions. Table 5 shows the estimations obtained by the best solution, with respect to each sensation. The image sequence in the horizontal axis is obtained by sorting the bitmaps in terms of their averaged assigned scores (from the psychophysical experiment). These scores are represented by squares, in such a way that filled squares represent the images used for training and the squares+dots correspond to the reference and estimated values, respectively. The number sequence at the top and bottom of each graph represent the code of the considered images.

The genetic algorithm, using the binary representation of features by 152 genes for each chromosome, was applied over a population containing 200 individuals. Independent evolutions were performed for each sensation parameter. The mutation rate was 0.01 and the crossover rate 0.7. The multi-point crossover broke the chromosome in eight points. Instead, of using the convergence as a stopping condition, the process was always concluded after 225 generations, in order to standardize among the several-modeled sensations.

The evolution results have shown good performance for some perceived qualities, being reasonable for the others. Similar performances were also obtained by the brute force method. Qualities such as originality and artistic quality have proven to be more amenable to the adopted modeling approach, producing more agreement with the psychophysical experiment. This success was characterized in terms of the number of selected features and the best obtained error (goal function), i.e., small error reveals a good agreement between the original and estimated scores for the diverse qualities. Although Table 5 does not identify the features, the selected features are presented for the brute force method, in Table 3 and Table 4. For instance, the color contrast range [229.5, 242.25] and spectral descriptor ranges are frequently chosen by the technique.

FBR $\phi(\|r\|)$	Selected Features		Mininum Error
$r^2 \log r$	RGB Contrast Histogram ($229.5 \leq d < 242.25$)	Concentric Spectrum Histogram ($0.79 \leq s < 0.94$)	1.1562
R	RGB Contrast Histogram ($229.5 \leq d < 242.25$)	Concentric Spectrum Histogram ($1.88 \leq s < 2.04$)	1.1467
r^3	RGB Contrast Histogram ($229.5 \leq d < 242.25$)	Radial Spectrum Histogram ($0.1 \leq s < 0.125$)	1.3405
$r^{1/2}$	RGB Contrast Histogram ($229.5 \leq d < 242.25$)	Concentric Spectrum Histogram ($2.83 \leq s < 2.98$)	1.0750

Table 3. The selected features and minimum errors for the several considered radial basis interpolating functions (considering two features).

FBR $\phi(\|r\|)$	Selected Features			Mininum Error
$r^2 \log r$	RGB Contrast Histogram ($178.5 \leq d < 191.25$)	RGB Contrast Histogram ($216.75 \leq d < 229.5$)	Radial Spectrum Histogram (in rad) ($2.36 \leq s < 2.51$)	0.9815
R	RGB Contrast Histogram ($229.5 \leq d < 242.25$)	Concentric Spectrum Histogram (Variance)	Radial Spectrum Histogram (in rad) ($0.47 \leq s < 0.62$)	0.8895
r^3	RGB Contrast Histogram ($229.5 \leq d < 242.25$)	RGB Contrast Histogram (Variance)	Radial Spectrum Histogram (Variance)	1.0374
$r^{1/2}$	RGB Contrast Histogram ($229.5 \leq d < 242.25$)	Radial Spectrum Histogram ($0.47 \leq d < 0.63$)	Concentric Spectrum Histogram (Variance)	0.9250

Table 4. The selected features and minimum errors for the several considered radial basis interpolating functions (considering three features).

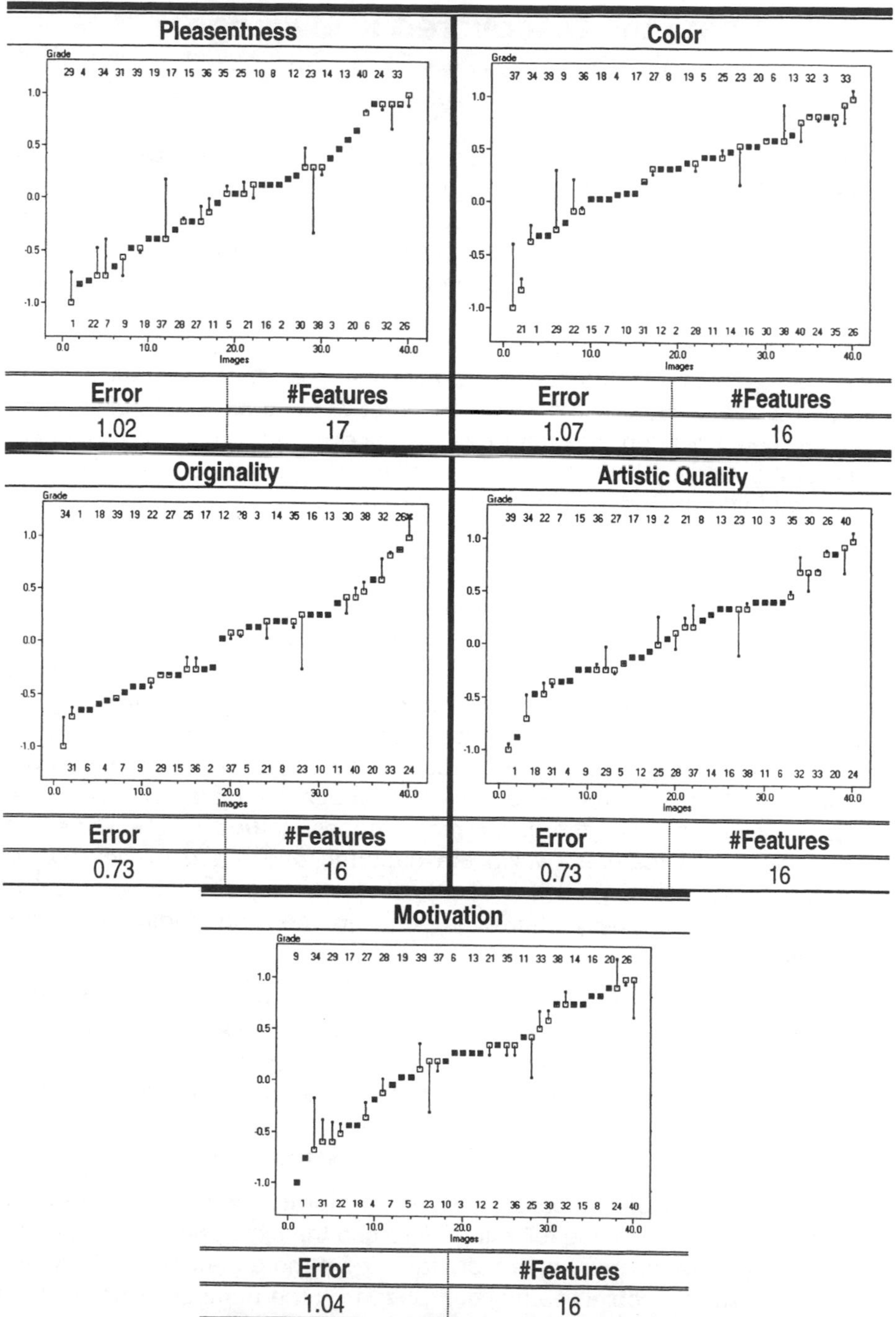

	Error	#Features
Pleasentness	1.02	17
Color	1.07	16
Originality	0.73	16
Artistic Quality	0.73	16
Motivation	1.04	16

Table 5. Errors for training pleasentness, color, originality, artistic quality, and motivation.

14.6 Using the Discovered Knowledge

Texture, contrast, visual information, and other image properties can be measured by using a great diversity of features. However, to infer their relationship with human visual perception demands some care. The visual perception modeling is a complex problem that has to be addressed in several fronts (such as neuroscience, psychology, computer vision, information theory, among others), the current approach representing an attempt to integrate several of these possibilities. One of the problems with such modeling approaches is that the important features are not known a priori. Here, we considered a set of features which, given their nature, could play an important role in modeling the perception. Indeed, one of the results allowed by the modeling approach is to infer, given the selected features, which of them are more relevant.

One of the most important results of the present work has been the verification that reasonably good models of visual quality perception by humans can be obtained by the considered approach. This is particularly surprising because such perceptions are very likely affected by subjective factors, such as personal preferences and cultural biases. On the other hand, the considered qualities certainly rely, as it was substantiated by our experiments, upon some basic visual attributes, shared my most people, such as complexity and balance. This result is particularly relevant for our initial objective of using the adopted approach for diagnosis. In other words, deviations from the basic, more broadly shared mechanisms and combinations of features, which are captured and made explicit by the model, can possibly yield indications of some cognitive or neurological deficits. This possibility, however, has to be confirmed by further investigations.

It is expected that more accurate and complex models of such visual perceptions can be obtained by considering hierarchical structures, possibly involving non-linear interactions, which could be constructed by applying the genetic algorithm constructively along the many hierarchical levels. Such models will also need to incorporate mechanisms capable of coping with the context and shapes in the presented images.

Regarding some of the possible specific improvements to the reported approach, we suggest the following: (*i*) to use the exponent k as part of the genes in the evolutionary approach, favoring a more general modeling; (*ii*) use an alternative objective function based on the number of hits instead of the overall Euclidean distance, which could enhance the generalizing ability of the obtained models; and (*iii*) consider models explicitly relating the diverse visual qualities, which could allow the inference of more comprehensive and compact rules.

Acknowledgements

Luciano da F. Costa is grateful to FAPESP (Procs 94/3536-6 and 94/4691-5) and CNPq (Proc 301422/92-3) for financial support. Luis A. Consularo is grateful to CNPq (Proc 143725/96-3) for financial support.

References

Bäck, T. 1996. Evolutionary Algorithms in Theory and Practice. Oxford University Press.

Barlow, H. 1982. The Senses. Cambridge University Press.

Bernaldez, F.G. 1987. Children's Landscape Preferences: From Rejection to Attraction. Journal of Environmental Psychology. 7:169-76.

Bookstein, F.L. 1989. Principal Warps: Thin-Plate Splines and the Decomposition of Deformations. IEEE Trans. on Pattern Analysis and Machine Intelligence, (11)6:567-85

Bruno, O.M., Cesar Jr., R.M., Consularo, L.A. and Costa, L.F. 1998. Automatic Feature Selection for Biological Shape Classification in Σynergos. in: Proceedings of SIBGRAPI'98, IEEE Comp. Soc., 363-370.

Bruno, O.M., Cesar Jr., R.M., Consularo, L. A. and Costa, L.F. 1999. Σynergos – Synergetic Vision Research, Real-Time Systems. (submitted)

Buhmann, M.D., Dyn, N. and Levin, D. 1995. On Quasi-Interpolation by Radial Basis Functions with Scattered Centres. Constructive Approximation. 11:239-254.

Castleman, K. 1996. Digital Image Processing, Prentice-Hall.

Coelho, R.C. and Costa, L.F. 1996. On the Application of the Bouligand-Minkowski Fractal Dimension for Shape Characterization, Applied Signal Processing, 3:163-176.

Consularo, L.A., Cesar Jr., R.M. and Costa, L.F. 1999. Σynergos and its Application to Contour Segmentation. in: Proc. of III Workshop on Cybernetic Vision, IFSC-USP, 77-83.

Costa, L.F., Cesar Jr., R.M., Coelho, R.C. and Tanaka, J.S. 1998. Analysis and Synthesis of Morphologically Realistic Neural Networks, in: Poznanski, R. (Ed) Modeling in the Neurosciences: From Ionic Channels to Neural Networks, Harwood Academic Publishers.

Costa, L.F., Manoel, E.T.M. and Tanaka, J.S. 1999. A New Model for Neural Curvature Detection and its Investigation in Terms of Neuromorphometric Measures, in: Proc. of III Workshop on Cybernetic Vision, IFSC-USP, 18-24.

Dondis, D.A. 1973. A Primer of Visual Literacy, MIT Press.

Duchon, J. 1977. Splines Minimizing Rotation-invariant Semi-norms in Sobolev spaces. in: Lectures Notes in Mathematics. 571:85-100.

Gen, M. and Cheng, R. 1997. Genetic Algorithms and Engineering Design, John Wiley and Sons.

Glover, F. and Laguna, M. 1997 Tabu Search. Kluwer.

Goldberg, D. 1989. Genetic Algorithms in Search, Optimization, and Machine Learning, Addison-Wesley.

Goldstein, B. 1989. Sensation and Perception. Wadsworth Pub. Co.

Gonzales, R.C. and Wintz, P. 1987. Digital Image Processing, Addison-Wesley.

Gordon, I.E. 1989. Theories of Visual Perception, John Wiley and Sons.

Hegland, M., Roberts, S. and Altas, I. 1998 Finite Element Thin Plate Splines for Data Mining Applications. Mathematical Methods for Curves and Surfaces II, 245-252.

Holland, J. 1962. Outline for a logical theory of adaptive systems. J. of Assoc. Comput. Mach., 3:297-314.

Kirkpatrick, S.; Gelatt, C.D. and Vecchi, M.P. 1983. Optimization by simulated annealing. Science, 220:671-680

Klinger, A. and Salingaros, N.A. 1999. A Pattern Measure. Univ. Texas at San Antonio. (http://www.math.utsa.edu/sphere/ salingar/PatternMeasure. html)

Levine, M.W. and Sheffner, J.M. 1991. Fundamentals of Sensation and Perception. Brooks/Cole ITP.

Lieberman, H. 1995. The Visual Language of Experts in Graphic Design. In: Proc. of 11th Int. Symp. on Visual Languages. IEEE Comp. Soc. Press. (http://www.computer.org/ conferen/vl95/ talks/T1.html)

Marr, D. 1982. Vision: A Computational Investigation into the Human Representation and Processing of Visual Information. W.H. Freeman and Co.

Mathworks Inc. 1992. Matlab Reference Guide, The Mathworks Inc.

Mees, A.I., Jackson, M.F. and Chua, L.O. 1992. Device Modeling by Radial Basis Functions. IEEE Trans. on Circuits and Systems-I: Fundamental Theory and Applications. (39)1:19-27.

Moriarty, S. 1995. Visual semiotics and the production of meaning in advertising. (Visual Communication Division of AEJMC http://spot.colorado.edu/ ~moriarts/vissemiotics.html)

Moriarty, S. 1997. A Conceptual Map of Visual Communciation. Journal of Visual Literacy, (17)2:9-24. (http://spot.colorado.edu/~moriarts/ conceptmap.html).

Orland, B., Weidemann, E., Larsen, L. and Radja, P. 1997. Exploring the Relationship between Visual Complexity and Perceived Beauty. Image Systems Lab. (http://www.imlab.uiuc.edu/complex/index.html)

Parker, B.A. and Scharff, L.F.V. 1997. Influences of contrast sensitivity on text readability in the context of a graphical user interface. 1997. (http://hubel.sfasu.edu/research/agecontrast.html).

Powell, M. J. D. 1981 Approximation Theory and Methods. Cambridge University Press.

Powell, M.J.D. 1994 The uniform convergence of thin plate spline interpolation in two dimensions, Numerische Mathematik, 68:107-128.

Rajani, R. and Rosenberg, D. 1999. Usable?.. Or Not?.. Factors affecting the usability of web sites. Computer-Mediated Communication Magazine, 6:1. (http://www.december.com/cmc/mag/current/ toc.html)

Riglis, E. 1998 Modeling Complexity in Visual Images, PhD Report, Image Systems Engineering Laboratory, Heriot-Watt University, Edinburgh, UK.

Sandwell, D.T. 1987. Biharmonic spline interpolation of GEOS-3 and SEASAT altimeter data, Geophysical Research Letters, 2:139-142.

Scharff, L. V., Ahumada, A. J., and Hill, A.L. 1999. Discriminability Mea-sures for Predicting Readability. in: Rogowitz, B. and Pappas, T. Eds., Human Vision and Electronic Imaging, IV, SPIE Proc., 270-277.

Synek, E. Evolutionary aesthetics: Visual Complexity and the Development of Human Landscapes Preferences. (Ludwig-Boltzmann Institute for Urban Ethology, Vienna, Austria. http://evolution.humb.univie.ac.at/institutes/urbanethology/student/html/erich/synekpro.html)

Warfel, M. 1998. Fractals. (http://www.cee.cornell.edu/~mdw/fractal.html).

Youngman, M. and Scharff, L.F.V. 1998. Text width and margin width influences on readability of GUIs. in: Proc. of the 12th Nat. Conf. on Undergraduate Res., 2:786-789.

15 Discovery of Clinical Knowledge in Databases Extracted from Hospital Information Systems

Shusaku Tsumoto

Department of Medical Informatics
Shimane Medical University, School of Medicine
Izumo 693-8501, Japan
tsumoto@computer.org

Abstract. Since early 1980's, the rapid growth of hospital information systems stores the large amount of laboratory examinations as databases. Thus, it is highly expected that knowledge discovery and data mining(KDD) methods will find interesting patterns from databases as reuse of stored data and be important for medical research and practice because human beings cannot deal with such a huge amount of data. However, there are still few empirical approaches which discuss the whole data mining process from the viewpoint of medical data.In this chapter, KDD process from a hospital information system is presented by using two medical datasets. This empirical study show that preprocessing and data projection are the most time-consuming processes, in which very few data mining researches have not dicussed yet and that application of rule induction methods is much easier than preprocessing.

15.1 Introduction

Medical practice and research has been changed by rapid growth of life science, including biochemistry and immunology(Levinson, 1996). The mechanism of a disease can be explained as a biochemical process or cell disorder and the diagnostic accuracy of medical experts is increasing due to the development of laboratory examinations. However, it is also true that data analysis is very indispensable to generating a hypothesis. For instance, discovery of HIV infection and Hepatitis type C were inspired by analysis of clinical courses unexpected by experts on immunology and hepatology, respectively (Fauci et al, 1997). Although the life science has been rapidly advanced, mechanisms of many diseases are still unknown: especially, neurological diseases were very difficult to analyze because their prevalence is very low (Adams and Victor, 1993). Even the mechanism of diseases with high prevalence, such as cancer, is partially known to medical experts. In this sense, medical research always need a good hypothesis, which is one of the most important motivations to data mining and knowledge discovery for medical people.

Also, another aspects interest medical researchers in data mining. Since early 1980's, the rapid growth of hospital information systems (HIS) stores the large amount of laboratory examinations as databases (Van Bemmel, and Musen, 1997). For example, in a university hospital, where more than 1000 patients visit from Monday to Friday, a database system stores more than 1 GB numerical data of laboratory examinations for each year. Furthermore, storage of medical image and other types of data are discussed in medical informatics as research topics on electronic patient records and all the medical data will be stored in hospital information systems within the 21th century. Thus, it is highly expected that data mining methods will find interesting patterns from databases as reuse of stored data and be important for medical research and practice because human beings cannot deal with such a huge amount of data.

In this chapter, knowledge discovery and data mining (KDD) process (Fayyad, et. al, 1996) for two medical datasets extracted from a hospital information system is presented. This empirical study show that preprocessing and data proejction are the most time-consuming processes, in which very few data mining researches have not dicussed yet and that application of rule induction methods is much easier than preprocessing.

This chapter is organized as follows. Section 2 makes a brief explanation of data selection. Section 3 and 4 presents data cleaning and data reduction as preprocessing processes. Section 5 shows application of rule induction method. Section 6 gives interpretation of induced rules by domain experts. Section 7 discusses the whole KDD process from the viewpoint of computational time. Finally, Section 8 concludes this chapter.

15.2 Data Selection

In this chaper, we use the following two datasetsfor data mining, which are extracted from two different hospital information systems. One is bacterial test data, which consists of 101,343 records, 254 attributes. This data includes past and present history, physical and laboratory examinations, diagnosis, therapy, a type of infectious disease, detected bacteria, and sensitivities for antibiotics. The other one is a dataset on the side effect of steroid, which consists of 31,119 records, 287 basic attributes. This data includes past and present history, physical and laboratory examinations, diagnosis, therapy, and the type of side effects. The characteristic of the second dataset is that it is a temporal database: although it includes 287 basic attributes, 213 attributes of which have more than 100 temporal records. These datasets are obtained through the first to third steps of KDD process: data selection, data cleaning and data reduction.

In the first step of KDD process, these databases are extracted from two different hospital information systems. Since each hospital information systems(HIS) is developed by a different company, each data structure is very different. On one hand, the HIS in a municipal hospital for bacterial test databases, is based on a simple relational database, the tranformation of data into a table is a very simple task as a SQL query process. Query is given as a single condition described as "select records if any bacterial tests has been examined." On the other hand, the HIS in a university hospital for side-effect of the steroid is based on a b-tree type database, the selection process is more complicated. Since the builtin process of transformation is very slow, we decided to write a program for translation by ourselves. In this case, selection is described as a conditon: "select records if a steroid therapy is given for more than one month.

Table 1 gives results for data selection: the second column shows the total size of HISs when data were selected (December, 1998). The third column presents the size of data selected from HIS. Finally, the fourth column gives the computational time required for data selection. Since each HIS is implemented on different computers, it may be difficult to compare each computational time, but those values suggests that time is not dependent on the selected data, but on the total HIS size.

Datasets	HIS size	Target Data	Time Required
Bacterlal Test	1,275,242(52GB)	361,932(14GB)	2.3 Days
Side-Effect	2,631,549(100GB)	135,749(6GB)	7.3 Days

Table 1. Data Selection Results.

15.3 Data Cleaning as Preprocessing

After data selection, data cleaning is required since the data obtained from the first step are not clean, including data records not suitable for data analysis. Even though these records are selected by matching the query condition, they do not include enough amount of information. In the case of bacterial tests, some patients have information about bacterial tests, but they made very few laboratory examinations. On the other hand, in the case of side effects, some patients have a record on steroid therapy, but they made two or three examinations for each year since the status of allergic diseases was stable and the patients do not suffer from any side-effects. These data may be removed if the queries in the first step are refined. However, it should be pointed out that the refinement of queries is not so a easy task because we have many types of insuitable data, which is difficult to predict and will occur not only due to the factors of patients but also due to the factors of medical doctors. For example, some patients may not come to the outpatient clinic when they recover from allergic disorders. Some doctors may tell the patients not to come to the clinic so often. In some cases, some patients are found to suffer from very a severe disease and they should be admitted to a university hospital. In other cases, patients may move from a university hospital to a municipal hospital. Many factors not included in a database, mainly social factors, will be a cause for degrading the cleaness of data.

Thus, it is much easier to clean the data not by using complex queries but by using simple statistics. Since each domain has attributes indispensabe to evaluating the status of patients, the number of attributes used to describe each record is a good index for removing not-clean records. So, we define the two-fold cleaning steps as shown in Figure 1: first we select the records which have no missing values in the pre-defined indispensable attributes. Then, we calculate how many attributes in the remaining attributes are used to describe the records in the first step. If the number of attributes used for a case is not sufficient, then this case will removed. For those steps, the indispensable attributes and the threshold for the second selection are given a priori by domain experts.

In the case of bacterial tests, 254 attributes are very important. Furthermore, 27 attributes are indispensable to describe each case. Thus, in the data cleaning step, first select the records which have missing values in the 27 attributes. Then, calculate how many attributes have missing values in remaining 227 attributes. If 75% of them are missing , then remove these records. In the case of steroid side-effects, the same strategy is applied. 74 non-temporal attributes are indispensable and 217 temporal attributes are used for second selection.

Procedure Data Cleaning

Given Parameters: a list of all indispensable attributes:

a threshold for second selection: δ

begin

Select a record;

if all the indispensable attributes are recorded, **then**

begin

Calculate the ratio of attributes used in remaining attributes:r ;

If ($r \geq \delta$) **then** Store the record;

end

end. {Procedure Data Cleaning};

Figure 1. An Algorithm for Data Cleaning.

Datasets	Data	Cleaned Data	Time Required
Bacterlal Test	361,932(14GB)	101,343(3GB)	5.2 Days
Side-Effect	135,749(6GB)	31,119(1,5GB)	2.5 Days

Table 2. Data Cleaning Results.

Table 2 summerizes results for data cleaning. The second column shows the number of records selected in the data selection. The third column shows the size of data after the data cleaning process is applied. The fourth column gives the computational time required for the whole steps.

15.4 Data Reduction and Projection as Preprocessing

15.4.1 Data Projection for Bacterial Test Database

From the viewpoint of table processing, data cleaning can be viewed as cleaning steps in the direction of records, that is, in the direction of *row*. On the other hand, data reduction can be viewed as cleaning steps in the direction of attributes, that is, in the direction of *column*. Although the data cleaning process is a time-consuming process, it takes much more time to reduct and project data in clinical databases due to the characteristics of biological science, including medicine. The tradition of classification in biology tends to have a large scale of classification systems. For example, let us consider the classfication of bacteria. If we look at the classification tree of bacteria, more than millions of bacteria are classified neatly in one classification tree. However, the number of bacteria on which we want to focus in medicine is very few, compared with this total classification. But, even the number of bacteria used in bacterial tests are too many, compared with the total number of classes used in data mining techniques. In the case of bacterial test database, 1194 kinds of bacteria and other bioorganism are used as a target class. If conventional classification or statistical methods are applied to this data, most of induced rules or patterns may be useless because these methods tend to extract knowledge for differentiation between 1194 classes. These tendencies are unexpected for medical experts who want to have more generalized results.

Thus, generalization of such over-classified attributes is required to discover rules which are easy for medical experts to interpret. For bacterial test databases, a simple concept hierarchy shown in Figure 2 was used for generalization of values. All the bioorganism are classified into 1124 bacteria and 70 non-bacteria bioorganism. Then, 1124 bacteria are classified into aerobic (973) and anaerobic (151). From the levels below, which is not shown in this figure, conventional bacterial classification sytem is used for construction of tree, into which totally five levels of hierarchy is implemented.

For each data mining task, we set up which hierarchical level is suitable for data analysis. For example, if we want to extraact knowledge about differentiation between aerobic and anaerobic bacteria, we have to tranform the values in the attribute into these two values. If we want to focus on the diffentiation between stereptococcus and other aerobic bacteria, we have to tranform the values into several generalized values on the level of the suitable classficaiton. If simple classificaiton knowledge is required, binarization of attributes is recommended because binarization can easily capture the positive and negative aspects for differential diagnosis for a target class.

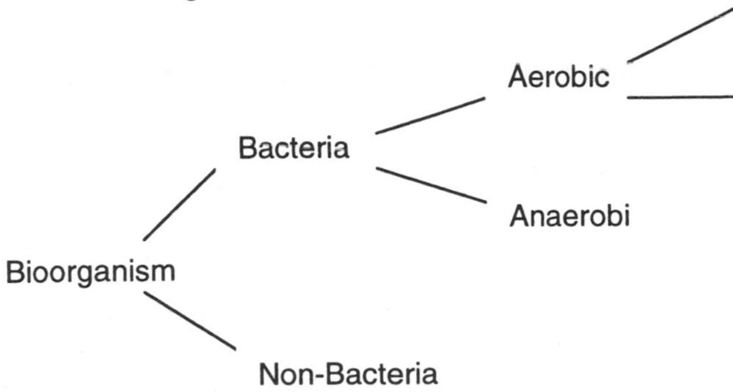

Figure 2. A Concept Hierarchy for Bacteria.

Although data projection for this dataset is parallel with data mining process, we show how much time is needed for each data projection in Table 3.

Projection Level	Total Values	Generalized Values	Time Computation	Time Construction
2. (Bacteria)	1194	2	24 hours	1.0 Days
3.	1194	5	25 hours	1.4 Days
4	1194	52	26 hours	3.0 Days
5	1194	175	27 hours	7.0 Days
6	1194	1194	0	-

Table 3. Generalization of Bacteria.

The first column denotes the level of concept hierarchy used for generalization. The second one shows the number of total values for compairson. Ther third column gives the number of total values for generalization.The fourth column gives computational time for generalization. Finally, the fifth column gives time for construction of a hierarchical tree by interaction between data analyzers and domain experts. Especially, since a construction of hierarchical tree can be viewed as a knowledge acquisition process, as discussed in (Buchanan and Shortliffe, 1984), it cannot be automated.

In addition to this hierarchical tree, the following hiearchical tre is also needed for generalization of this dataset: a classification tree for chronic diseases which each patient suffers from. This process also takes 7 days to complete the tree structure with domain experts.

15.4.2 Data Reduction for Steroid Side-Effect Database

15.4.2.1 Characteristics of Medical Temporal Databases

Since incorporating temporal aspects into databases is still an ongoing research issue in database area (Abiteboul, et. al., 1995), temporal data are stored as a table in hospital information systems (H.I.S.) with time stamps. Table 4 shows a typical example of medical data, which was retrieved from H.I.S. The first column denotes the ID number of each patient, and the second one denotes the date when the datasets in this row is examined. Each row with the same ID number describes the results of laboratory examinations, which were taken on the date in the second column. For example, the second row shows the data of the patient ID 1 on 04/19/1986. This simple database show the following characteristics of medical temporal database:

(1)The Number of Attributes are Too Many. Even though the dataset of a patient focuses on the transition of each examination (attribute), it would be difficult to see its trend when the patient is followed for a long time. If one wants to see the long-term interaction between attributes, it would be almost impossible. In order to solve this problems, most of H.I.S. systems provide several graphical interfaces to capture temporal trends (Van Bemmel and Musen, 1997) However, the interactions among more than three attributes are difficult to be studied even if visualization interfaces are used.

(2) Irregularity of Temporal Intervals. Temporal intervals are irregular. Although most of the patients will come to the hospital every two weeks or one month, physicians may not make laboratory tests at each time. When a patient has a acute fit or suffers from acute diseases, such as pneumonia, laboratory examinations will be made every one to three days. On the other hand, when his/her status is stable, these test may not be made for a long time. Patient ID 1 is a typical example. Between 04/30 and 05/08/1986, he suffered from a pneumonia and was admitted to a hospital. Then, during the therapeutic procedure, laboratory tests were made every a few days. On the other hand, when he was stable, such tests were ordered every one or two year.

ID	Date	GOT	GPT	LDH	γ-GTP	TP	Edema
1	19860419	24	12	152	63	7.5	-
1	19860430	25	12	162	76	7.9	+
1	19860502	22	8	144	68	7.0	+
1	19860506						
1	19860508	22	13	156	66	7.6	-
1	19880826	23	17	142	89	7.7	-
1	19890109	32					-
1	19910304	20	15	369	139	6.9	-
2	19810511	20	15	369	139	6.9	-
2	19810713	22	14	177	49	7.9	-
2	19880826	23	17	142	89	7.7	-
2	18980109	32					-

Table 4. An Example of Temporal Database.

(3)Missing Values. In addition to irregularity of temporal intervals, datasets have many missing values. Even though medical experts will make laboratory examinations, they may not take the same tests in each instant. Patient ID 1 in Table 4 is a typical example. On 05/06/1986, medical physician selected a specific test to confirm his diagnosis. So, he will not choose other tests. On 01/09/1989, he focused only on GOT, not other tests. In this way, missing values will be observed very often in clinical situations.

15.4.2.2 Data Reduction Using Moving Average Method

The way to how to deal with medical temporal databases is discussed in (Tsumoto, 1999). Tsumoto introduces extended moving average method, which automatically set up the scale of the temporal interval. For example, if the scale factor is set to be 2, then the temporal interval for moving average is calculated from 2, 4, 8, 16, and so on. Each temporal interval is called *window*.In general, let s and y_i denote a scale factor and a value for laboratory test. Then moving average for y is defined as:

$$\overline{y} = \frac{\sum_{i=1}^{s^n} y_i}{s^n},$$

where n denotes an integer which is set up for temporal interval. Thus, s^n gives the size of window.

One of the disadvantages of moving average method is that it cannot deal with categorical attributes. To solve this problem, we will classify categorical attributes into three types, whose information should be given by users. The first type is *constant*, which will not change during the follow-up period. The second type is *ranking*, which is used to rank the status of a patient. The third type is *variable*, which will change temporally, but ranking is not useful. For the first type, extended moving average method will not be applied. For the second one, integer will be assigned to each rank and extended moving average method for continuous attributes is applied. On the other hand, for the third one, the temporal behavior of attributes is transformed into statistics as follows.

First, the occurence of each category (value) is counted for each window. For example, in Table 4, *edema* is a binary attribute and variable. In the first window, an attribute edema takes {-,+,+,-}.(Missing values are ignored for counting. So, the occurence of - and + are 2 and 2, respectively.Then, each conditional probability will be calculated.In the above example, probabilities are equal to p(-lw1)=2/4 and p(+lw1)=2/4.

By using this method, data of the first patient in Table 4 is summerized into Table 5 when the window size is set up to 2^8(=256) days. The last row, the period of which is denoted by infinity(∞) means the average of total data, that is, the average of the maximum window

ID	Period	GOT	GPT	LDH	γ-GTP	TP	Edema (+)	Edema (-)
1	1	23.25	11.25	153.5	68.25	7.5	0.5	0.5
1	2	23	17	142	89	7.7	0.0	1.0
1	3	32					0.0	1.0
1	4						0.0	1.0
1	5	20	15	369	139	6.9	1.0	0.0
1	∞	24	12.83	187.5	83.5	7.43	0.43	0.57

Table 5. Final Table with Moving Average for 2^8(=256) Days.

For further discussion on data reduction of temporal data, the readers may refer to (Tsumoto, 1999).

15.4.2.3 Results of Data Reduction for Steroid Side Effects

Steroid side-effects is known as long-term side-effects, usually observed when a patient takes steroid for more than several years. Thus, to capture long-term effects, the window size is set to 2^7(=128) and 2^8(=256). It is true that a significant amount of temporal information is lost by using data reduction, but we should remember that the first objective of data mining is to find simple useful and unexpected patterns from data. As discussed in 4.2.1, medical temporal data suffer from many types of irregularities. Table 6 shows the computational time required for data summerization.

Window Size	Computational Time
2^7(=128)	12.0 hours
2^8(=256)	8.0 hours
∞	7.0 hours

Table 6. Computational Time for Data Summerization.

It is notable that this table shows the trade-off relationship between the window-size and computational time: if the window-size is smaller, the computational time grows much larger.

15.4.3 Total Time Required for Data Reduction

In summary, Table 7 gives the total time required for data reduction and projection for each data set, including knowledge acquisition process. The second column gives the type of preprocessing. The third column shows total time required for each process. Finally, the fourth column shows the time required for acquisition of knowledge from domain experts.

Dataset	Preprocessing	Total Time	Time for Acquisition
Bacterial Test	Projection	15.25 Days	7.0 Days
	Summarization	2.3 Days	0

Table 7. Total Time Required for Data Reduction.

This table suggests the generalization of values in attributes should be a time-consuming process, especially when domain knowledge is given.

15.5 Rule Induction as Data Mining

After the third step, rule induction based on rough set model (Pawlak, 1991) was applied to two medical datasets. Tsumoto (1998, 2000) extends rough-set-based rule induction methods into probabilistic domain. In this section, we make a briefly explanation about definition of probabilistic rules and an algorithm based on this definition. Although many interesting theoretical results about rule induction are easily proved by rough set framework, we concentrate on the minimal requirements for this chapter. For further discussion, the readers may refer to (Polkowski and Skowron, 1998).

15.5.1 Definition of Rules Based on Rough Sets

15.5.1.1 Rough Set Notations

In the following sections, we use the following notations introduced by (Skowron and Grzymala-Busse, 1993), which are based on rough set theory (Pawlak, 1991). These notations are illustrated by a small database shown in Table 8, collecting the patients who complained of headache.

No.	Age	Location	nature	Prodrome	nausea	M1	Class
1	50-59	Occular	persistent	No	no	yes	m.c.h.
2	40-49	Whole	persistent	No	no	yes	m.c.h.
3	40-49	Lateral	throbbing	No	yes	no	Migraine
4	40-49	Whole	throbbing	Yes	yes	no	Migraine
5	40-49	Whole	radiating	No	no	yes	m.c.h.
6	50-49	Whole	persistent	No	yes	yes	Psycho

DEFINITIONS: M1: tenderness of M1, m.c.h.: muscle contraction headache, migraine:classic migraine, psycho: psychogenic headache.

Table 8. An Example of Database.

Let U denote a nonempty, finite set called the universe and A denote a nonempty, finite set of attributes, i.e., $a: U \rightarrow V_a$ for $a \in A$, where V_a is called the domain of a, respectively. Then, a decision table is defined as an information system, $\mathbf{A}=(U, A \cup \{d\})$. For example, Table 1 is an information system with $U=\{1,2,3,4,5,6\}$ and $A=\{age, location, nature, prodrome, nausea, M1\}$ and $d=class$. For $location \in A$, $V_{location}$ is defined as $\{occular, lateral, whole\}$.

The atomic formulae over $B \subseteq A \cup \{d\}$ and V are expressions of the form $[a=v]$, called descriptors over B, where $a \in B$ and $v \in V_a$. The set $F(B,V)$ of formulas over B is the least set containing all atomic formulas over B and closed with respect to disjunction, conjunction and negation. For example, $[location=occular]$ is a descriptor of B. For each $f \in F(B,V)$, f_A denote the meaning of $f \in A$, i.e., the set of all objects in U with property f, defined inductively as follows.

1. If f is of the form $[a=v]$, then, $f_A=\{s \in U \mid a(s)=v\}$
2. $(f \wedge g)_A= f_A \cap g_A$; $(f \vee g)_A= f_A \cup g_A$; $\neg f_A= U- f_A$

For example, $f=[location=whole]$ and $f_A=\{2,4,5,6\}$. As an example of a conjuctive formula, $g=[location=whole] \wedge [nausea=no]$ is a descriptor of U and g_A is equal to $g_{location,nausea}=\{2,5\}$.

15.5.1.2 Definition of Accuracy and Coverage

By the use of the framework above, classification accuracy and coverage, or true positive rate is defined as follows.

Definition. Let *R* and *D* denote a formula in *F(B,V)* and a set of objects which belong to a decision *d*. Classification accuracy and coverage(true positive rate) for R →d are defined as:

$$\alpha_R(D) = \frac{|R_A \cap D|}{|R_A|} (= P(D|R)),\ \kappa_R(D) = \frac{|R_A \cap D|}{|D|} (= P(R|D)),$$

where *|S|*, $\alpha_R(D)$, $\kappa_R(D)$ *and P(S)* denote the cardinality of a set *S*, a classification accuracy of *R* as to classification of *D* and coverage (a true positive rate of *R* to *D*), and probability of *S*, respectively.

In the above example, when *R* and *D* are set to *[nau=1]* and *[class=migraine]*, $\alpha_R(D)$=2/3=0.67 and $\kappa_R(D)$=2/2=1.0.
It is notable that $\alpha_R(D)$ measures the degree of the sufficiency of a proposition, *R* →*D*, and that $\kappa_R(D)$ measures the degree of its necessity. For example, if $\alpha_R(D)$ is equal to 1.0, then R →D is true. On the other hand, if $\kappa_R(D)$ is equal to 1.0, then *D* → *R* is true. Thus, if both measures are 1.0, then R ↔D.

15.5.1.3 Probabilistic Rules

By the use of accuracy and coverage, a probabilistic rule is defined as:

$$R \xrightarrow{\alpha,\kappa} d \quad s.t. \ R = \wedge_j [a_j = v_k],\ \alpha_R(D) \geq \delta_\alpha \ and \ \kappa_R(D) \geq \delta_\kappa,$$

This rule is a kind of probabilistic proposition with two statistical measures, which is an extension of Ziarko's variable precision model(VPRS)(1993).

It is also notable that both a positive rule and a negative rule are defined as special cases of this rule, as shown in the next subsections.

15.5.2 Algorithms for Rule Induction

An algorithm for rule induction is shown in Figure 3, which is a modification of the algorithm introduced in PRIMEROSE-REX(Tsumoto, 1998).

This algorithm will work as follows. (1)First, it selects a descriptor $[a_i=v_j]$ from the list of attribute-value pairs, denoted by L_1. (2) An index i is set to 1. (3) Until L_i becomes empty, the algorithm repeats the following procedures: (a) A formula $[a_i=v_j]$ is removed from L_i. (b) The algorithm checks whether the coverage $\kappa_R(D)$ is larger than the threshold. If the coverage is larger, the algorithm further checks whether the accuracy $\alpha_R(D)$ is larger than the threshold or not. If so, then this formula is included a list of the conditional part of probabilistic rules. Otherwise, it will be included into *M*, which is used for making conjunction of attributes in the future. (4) When L_i is empty and *M is not empty*, the next list L_{i+1} is generated from descriptors in the list *M*. If *M* is empty, the algorithm quits.

For example, when we take class as a decision attribute, attribute-value pairs the coverage of which is larger than 0.5 are: [age=40-49](0.67), [loc=whole] (0.67), [nature=persistent] (0.67), [nausea=no] (1.0), and [M1=yes] (1.0). The values of accuracy for them are 0.5, 0.67, 1.0, and 0.75, respectively. Therefore, if the thresholds for coverage and accuracy are set to 0.5 and 0.75, [nausea=no] and [M1=yes] are selected as the conditions of probabilistic rules and [age=40-49], [nature=persistent] and [loc=whole] are stored in a list *M*. In the next step, the conjunction of these three pairs is used. However, three conjunctions do not satisfy the condition of accuracy and coverage, so they will be discarded. Finally, two rules are obtained: [nausea=no]→m.c.h., and [M1=yes] →m.c.h.

15.5.3 Application of Rule Induction Methods

The algorithm introduced in the last section was implemented on the Sun Spaarc station and was applied to the above two medical databases, the information of which is summarized in Table 9. For rule induction, the thresholds for accuracy and coverage are set to 0.5 and 0.5, respectively.

```
procedure Induction of Probabilistic Rules;
  var i: integer;  M, Li: List;
  begin
    L1:= (a list of all attribute-value pairs);  i:=1; M:={};
    for i:=1 to n do   /* n: Total number of attributes in a database */
     begin
      while (Li ≠{}) do
       begin
```

```
          Select one pair R=∧ [a_i=v_j] from L_i ;
          L_i := L_i - {R} ;
          if (κ_R(D) ≥ δ_α) then do
             if (α_R(D) ≥ δ_α) then do
                      S_ir := S_ir ∪ {R};  /* Include R in a list of Rules */
             else M := M ∪ {R};
        end
      if (M={}) quit.
      else
        L_{i+1}:= (A list of the whole combination of the conjunction
                formulae in M);
      end
  end {Induction of Probabilistic Rules};
```

Figure 3. Induction of Probabilistic Rules.

Data	Size	Attributes	Induced Rules	Computational Time
Bacterial Test	101,343 (3GB)	254	24,335	60 hours (2.5 Days)
Side-Effects	31,119 (1.5GB)	287	14,715	18 hours (0.75 Days)

Table 9. Summary of Data Mining.

For bacterial test databases, six attributes for which domain experts want to find simple pattern are assigned to decision attributes. For side-effect databases, one attribute (side-effect) is assigned to a decision attribute. Table 9 summarizes the results of data mining. The second and third columns give information about data. The fourth column shows the number of rules induced by rule induction methods. Finally, the fifth column presents the computational time required. It is notable that the computational time is rather small, compared with computational time.

15.6 Interpretation of Induced Rules

After the data mining step, we obtain many rules to be interpreted by medical experts. Even if the amount of information is very small compared with the original databases, it still takes about one week to evaluate all the induced rules.

15.6.1 Induced Rules of Bacterial Tests

Of 24,335 rules, only 114 rules are unexpected or interesting to medical experts. From these discovered results, nine rules are shown below.

1. β-lactamase(+) → Bacteria_Detection (+)

   (Accuracy: 0.667, Coverage: 0.541)

2. β-lactamase(3+) → Bacteria_Detection (+)

   (Accuracy: 0.702, Coverage: 0.553)

These two results are interesting from the viewpoints of history of bacterial infection. Since penicillin has been introduced as antibiotics, many bacteria have acquired to generate enzymes that decompose penicillin, called β-lactamase. The above two results show that such penicillin-resistant bacteria can be more easily found than penicillin-sensitive ones.

3. Pneumonia→ Bacteria_Detection (-)

   (Accuracy: 0.826, Coverage: 0.12)

4. Fever (BT>39) → Bacteria_Detection(-)

(Accuracy: 0.790, Coverage: 0.11)

5. Malignant Tumor → Bacteria_Detection (-)

(Accuracy: 0.77, Coverage: 0.13)

These three results are unexpected by medical experts. As for the third rule, it is well known that bacterial infection is the main cause for pneumonia. However even if pneumonia comes from the bacterial infection, it would be difficult to detect bacteria. Concerning the fourth rule, high fever suggests that the degree of infection is high. However, it would be difficult to detect bacteria even if the degree is high. Finally, in the case when a patient suffers from malignant tumor, he/she may suffer from a severe infection due to immunological insufficiency. However, it may be difficult to detect bacteria for this case.

6. Fusobacterium → PCG(Sensitive) (Accuracy: 0.92, Coverage: 0.26)

7. MRSA → VCM(Sensitive) (Accuracy: 0.89, Coverage: 0.12)

8. Tonsilitis → Aug(S) (Accuracy: 0.84, Coverage: 0.10)

These three results show the unexpected relationships between bacteria and antibiotics. As for the first two cases, the values of accuracy are unexpected. It is well known that although most of Fusobacterium and MRSA are sensitive to PCG and VCM, respectively, these results show that some substantial part of these bacteria have already been resistant to those antibiotics.

9. Neurology → MRSA (Accuracy: 0.6, Coverage: 0.4)

The final rule shows the relationship between the ward and the bacteria. Unexpectedly, there is a strong relationship between the neurological ward and MRSA infection, which may cause a very serious infection.

Those unexpected/interesting rules are feedbacked to the municipal hospital which donates a dataset to us and the staff in the hospital is evaluating them.

15.6.2 Induced Results of Steroid Side-Effects

Of 14,715 rules, only 106 rules are unexpected or interesting to medical experts. From these discovered results, four rules are shown below

For simplicity, these rules are given in the summarized form, though they are originally represented as the conjunction of temporal attributes.

1. [Steroid>3.0years] & [Headache(+)>0.5] →Glaucoma

(Accuracy : 0.97, Coverage: 0.85)

2. [Headache(+)>0.5] →Glaucoma

(Accuracy: 0.61, Coverage: 1.0)

These two results show that headache is an important sign for glaucoma due to steroid side-effect.

3. [Steroid>2.5years] & [Blurred Vision(+)>0.75] → Cataract

(Accuracy: 0.85, Coverage: 0.78)

4. [Steroid>5years] & [SEX=Female] → Osteoporosis

(Accuracy: 0.77, Coverage: 0.9)

These two results show that if a patient takes steroid for more than two years, the side effects may be frequently observed.

Those unexpected/interesting rules are also feedbacked to the university hospital, which donates a dataset to us, and the staff in the hospital is evaluating them.

15.7 Discussion

After the data interpretation phase, about one percent of induced rules are found to be interesting or unexpected to medical experts. In this section, the total KDD process is reviewed with respect to computational time.

15.7.1 Summary of Time Required for KDD Process

Table 10 shows the total time required for KDD process. Each column shows two data sets for each process. Each row includes computational time required for each process. Totally, it takes about one month and three weeks to complete the whole KDD process for bacterial test database and side-effect database, respectively. It is notable that more than 60% of the process is devoted to the three preprocessing processes: data selection, cleaning and reduction. Especially, as for the bacterial test dataset, 22.75 days (79.5%) are used for three processes. It is because domain knowledge should be acquired for generalization of data, as discussed in Section 3. On the other hand, only 4 to 8 percent of total time is spent for data mining process. In the case of bacterial test database, only 2.5 days (8%) is used for rule induction. Therefore, these empirical results suggest that the main KDD processes should be preprocessing rather than discovery of patterns from data.

KDD Process	Bacterial Test	Side-Effect
Data Selection	2.3	7.3
Data Cleaning	5.2	2.5
Data Reduction	15.25	2.3
Data Mining	2.5	0.75
Data Interpretation	7.0	7.0
Total Time	32.25	19.85

Table 10. Total Time Required for KDD Process.

Another important point is that data interpretation is also time-consuming process, compared with data mining process because it needs interpretation by domain experts. In summary, if we want to make KDD process faster, then we should consider the automation of processes which needs interaction between computers and domain experts. Especially if domain knowledge is easily incorporated into the program, the computational time for the third step may be significantly improved. Therefore, more intensive research on automation of data preprocessing is required for future research.

15.7.2 Summary of Data Interpretation

Table 11 presents the number of induced rules and rules which are interesting to medical experts. Surprisingly, only small portion of induced rules are related with discovered knowledge. This results also suggest that data interpretation is still a difficult process even if all the rules have a very simple representation. One of the reasons why data interpretation is difficult is that too many rules are generated because we use several hundred attributes for rule induction. However, if we reduce the number of attributes, we may delete the possibility to find unexpected rules.

One way to solve this problem is to define the measures for interestingness or unexpectedness of rules (Hilderman and Hamilton, 1999). However, since these measures strongly depends on the applied domain and they are used for selection of attributes, it may be not so different from the selection of attributes by human experts. So, the other way to solve this problem is to ask domain experts to give more information about attributes, such as the rank of importance. If the attributes are selected according to this rank, strong rules with lower rank attributes may be unexpected or interesting to medical experts. It would be a future work to incorporate such decision process of medical experts for the selection of attributes into KDD process.

	Induced Rules	Interesting Rules
Bacterial-Test	24,335	114 (0.47%)
Side-Effect	14,715	106 (0.72%)

Table 11. Summary of Induced Rules and Interpretation.

15.8 Conclusions

In this chapter, we present KDD process for two medical databases extracted from two hospital information systems. This empirical study shows that data selection, cleaning and reduction occupied about 80% and 61% of total time required for bacterial test and steroid side-effect data, respectively and that these three steps are the most time-consuming processes, in which very few data mining researches have not discussed yet. On the other hand, application of rule induction methods is much easier than preprocessing, which occupied only 8 and 4% of time for bacterial test and steroid side-effect data, respectively. About one hundred rules for each data are found to be interesting for medical experts, though they are a small part of induced rules. Therefore, it would be two important future directions discovered from this empirical research. One is the more intensive study on the automation of preprocessing. The other one is the studies on the automation of data interpretation.

References

Adams, R.D. and Victor, M. 1993. *Principles of Neurology, 5th edition*, McGraw-Hill, New York.

Abiteboul, S., Hull, R., and Vianu, V. 1995. *Foundations of Databases*, Addison-Wesley, New York.

Buchanan, B.G., and Shortliffe, E.H. *Rule-Based Expert Systems*, Addison-Wesley, New York, 1984.

Fauci, A.S., Braunwald, E., Isselbacher, K.J. and Martin, J.B. (eds.) 1997. *Harrison's Principles of Internal Medicine (14th Ed)*, McGraw Hill, New York.

Fayyad, U., Piatetsky-Shapiro, G. and Smyth, P. 1996. The KDD Process for Extracting Useful Knowledge from Volumes of data. *CACM*, 39: 27-34.

Levinson, W.E. and Jawetz, E. 1996. *Medical Microbiology & Immunology : Examination and Board Review (4th Ed)*, Appleton & Lange.

Hilderman, R.J. and Hamilton, H.J. Heuristic Measures of Interestingness. In: *Proc. 3rd European Conference on Principles of Knowledge Discovery and Data Mining* (PKDD), LNAI 1704, Springer Verlag, 232-241.

Holt, J.G. (Ed.) *Bergey's Manual of Systematic Bacteriology (Vol 1)* Lippincott, Williams & Wilkins.

Pawlak, Z. 1991. *Rough Sets*, Kluwer Academic Publishers.

Polkowski, L. and Skowron, A. 1998. *Rough Sets in Knowledge Discovery* Vol.1 and 2, Physica-Verlag.

Skowron, A. and Grzymala-Busse, J. 1994.From rough set theory to evidence theory. In: Yager, R., Fedrizzi, M. and Kacprzyk, J.(eds.) *Advances in the Dempster-Shafer Theory of Evidence*, John Wiley & Sons, New York, 193-236.

Tsumoto, S. 1998. Automated extraction of medical expert system rules from clinical databases based on rough set theory, *Information Sciences*, 112, 67-84.

Tsumoto, S. 1999. Rule Discovery in Large Time-Series Medical Databases. In: *Proc. 3rd European Conference on Principles of Knowledge Discovery and Data Mining* (PKDD), LNAI 1704, Springer Verlag, 23-31.

Tsumoto, S. 2000. Automated Discovery of Positive and Negative Knowledge in Clinical Databases based on Rough Set Model., *IEEE EMB Magazine* (in press).

Van Bemmel,J. and Musen, M. A.1997. *Handbook of Medical Informatics*, Springer-Verlag, New York.

Ziarko, W. 1993. Variable Precision Rough Set Model. *Journal of Computer and System Sciences* 46:39-59.

16 Knowledge Discovery in Time Series Using Expert Knowledge

Fernando Alonso[1], Juan P. Caraça-Valente[1], Ignacio López-Chavarrías[1] and Cesar Montes[2]

[1]Departement of Languages & Systems
[2]Department of Artificial Intelligence, Facultad de Informática
Universidad Politécnica de Madrid, Campus de Montegancedo
Boadilla del Monte, Spain

In this chapter, we describe the process of discovering underlying knowledge in a set of isokinetic tests, using the expertise of a physician specialised in isokinetic techniques in several phases of discovery. An isokinetic machine is basically a physical support on which patients exercise one of their joints, in this case the knee, according to different ranges of movement and at a constant speed. The data on muscle strength supplied by the machine are processed by an expert system that has built-in knowledge elicited from an expert in isokinetics. It cleans and pre-processes the data and conducts an intelligent analysis of the parameters and morphology of the isokinetic curves. Data mining methods based on the discovery of sequential patterns in time series and the fast Fourier transform by means of which to find similarities and differences among exercises were applied to the processed information to characterise injuries and discover reference patterns specific to populations. The results obtained were applied in two environments: one for the blind and another for elite athletes.

16.1 Introduction

Historically, medicine has been a crucial domain for computer science applications. Many well-known models and methods have been designed to solve medical problems. The sheer volume of the data for collection, the need for better procedures and techniques to assist physicians in their work and, generally, the need for subtle or routine processes to be automated are some of the reasons behind this state of affairs.

Data Mining is not an exception. A better comprehension of medical data is a must for improving medical effectiveness. Moreover, there is a shortage of good models for certain injuries that could reduce the rate of wrong decisions being made in a host of fields.

In this chapter, we describe some of the results of R&D in the field of physiotherapy and, more specifically, in muscle function assessment based on isokinetic data. Physicians collect these data using a mechanical instrument called an isokinetics machine. This machine can be described as a piece of apparatus on which patients perform strength exercises, which has the peculiarity of limiting the range of movement and the intensity of the effort at a constant speed (which explains the term isokinetic). Data concerning the strength employed by the patient throughout the exercise is recorded and stored by the machine so that the physician can analyse and visualise the results using specialised computer software.

The information supplied by an isokinetics machine has a lot of potential uses: muscular diagnosis and rehabilitation, injury prevention, training evaluation and planning, etc. However, the software built into these systems and the isokinetic-based diagnosis techniques themselves still have some significant handicaps that have detracted from the success of this field:

- The software provides only a graphical representation of the massive data flow supplied by these systems. The physician is left to analyse this with no further help. This is not a simple task, as it depends almost exclusively on the personal experience of the therapist.
- Obviously, as the output is a graphical representation of strength data, blind physicians are unable to use these methods to their full potential.
- Novice therapists have enormous difficulties in interpreting and understanding these graphs, as no further interpretation is provided.
- Lastly, but certainly most important of all, data are not analysed to improve the procedure as a whole. Decisions are guided by the therapist's instinct, as there are no injury models that can be used as a reference. Moreover, the few simple models that do exist have merely been stated by experts and are not founded on rigorous data analysis. Hence, the massive data flow supplied by these systems have not been fully exploited.

The I4[1] line of projects is aimed at conducting a more comprehensive analysis of the data output. This involves intelligent understanding and interpretation of the strength curves obtained through the isokinetic exercises on which the assessments are based.

Due to the generality of the goal and the above-mentioned problems, the solution should combine both practitioner expertise and the knowledge that could be discovered within the data. This led us to opt for a knowledge discovery (KD) process based on Brachman and Anand's approach (Brachman and Anand, 1996) from the interactive point of view and on (Fayyad et al., 1996) with regard to procedure, albeit adapted to the peculiarities of our particular problem. In the following sections, we describe the problem and the problem-solving process in more detail.

16.2 Understanding the Problem Domain

The assessment of muscle function has been a primary goal of medical and sports scientists for decades. The main objectives were to evaluate the effects of training and the effectiveness of rehabilitation programs (Gleeson and Mercer, 1996) (Kannus, 1994).

The release of isokinetic systems meant that a group of muscles could be safely exercised to full potential throughout the entire range of movement. Used for diagnostic purposes, these systems can calculate the strength generated by the muscle during exercises of this sort at each point along the arc of movement. This is tantamount to a complete dynamic assessment of muscle strength, which can be represented graphically.

The methods for assessing muscle strength using isokinetic techniques are well established in the field of injury rehabilitation and medical monitoring, especially of top-competition athletes, as they provide an objective measurement of one of the basic physical conditions that is extremely important in a wide range of sports.

However, as mentioned in the introduction, the performance of the software built into these systems (e.g., LIDO) still does not make the grade

---

[1] I4 stands for Intelligent Interpretation of Isokinetic Information and has been developed in conjunction with the Spanish National Centre for Sports Research and Sciences (hereinafter referred to as CNICD) and the School of Physiotherapy of the Spanish National Organisation for the Blind (hereinafter referred to as EFONCE).

as far as isokinetic test interpretation is concerned. This means that the massive data flow supplied by these systems cannot be fully exploited. And, of course, physicians with impaired vision cannot use these systems at all.

The I4 project materialised to solve this problem and identify the underlying knowledge in this massive data flow. Three objectives were defined for this purpose:

a) *Equip the isokinetic system with a knowledge-based system (KBS) that would perform an intelligent analysis of the strength curves output by the isokinetic test on which the assessments are based.* This would be a valuable aid for the examining physician in detecting a possible injury. Additionally, the system was equipped with a user interface and aids and appliances for the blind, by means of which to analyse graphical and numerical strength data. This provides for the results to be interpreted by blind physicians in particular.

b) *Characterise injuries.* Taking into account the huge amount of isokinetic tests produced and stored in a database, we aimed to class this information concerning patient characteristics. The objective was to output some sort of pattern that would characterise the injuries. This was to be used to typify the injuries occurring and thus be able, if possible, to make a correct diagnosis of the injury. Data mining techniques based on the discovery of sequential patterns in time series were applied for this purpose.

c) *Create reference models.* The third objective involved discovering standard patterns that characterised specific population types taken from the isokinetic data already prepared and stored in the database. For example, the process of evaluating a particular athlete against a standard curve, specific to his or her sport, is a very effective means of assessing the athlete capacity and potential for the sport they intend to go in for.

16.2.1 Overview of the System

Figure 1 shows the architecture of the I4 system from the viewpoint of its functionalities. The isokinetics machine includes the LIDO Multi-Joint II system, which supplies the data of the isokinetic tests run on patients. Patients will be in a seated position and the movement is made within a 0 to 90°C flexion/extension arc of their right or left leg (see Figure 2). The LIDO system records the angle and the strength employed by the patient. As shown in Figure 1, after the isokinetic tests have been completed by the LIDO system, the first operation performed by I4 is to decode, transform and format the data files output by LIDO into a more standard format and to correct any inaccurate or incomplete particulars. This is the only I4 module that depends on the LIDO isokinetics system, which means that this would be the only module that would require changes if I4 were to be adapted to another isokinetics system.

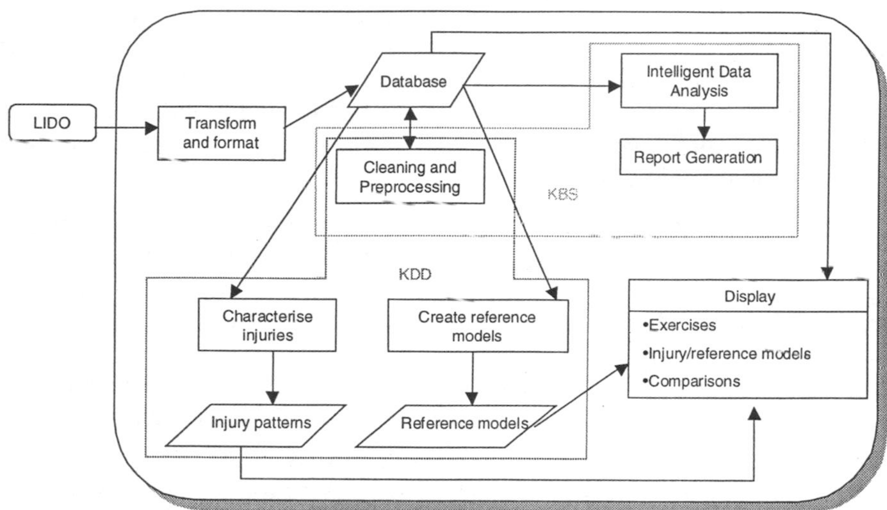

Figure 1. I4 system architecture.

The transformed and formatted data are stored in a database for later processing. Also, the exercises stored can be displayed either individually or jointly in graphical format by the visualisation module. So, this module can be used to analyse an individual exercise, compare the exercises performed with the left and right legs, any two exercises performed at the same angular speed or an exercise with a pattern or model that is representative of a particular group.

The data stored in the database are automatically processed by the data cleaning and pre-processing module in order to correct and remove any inconsistencies produced when the isokinetic tests were run. These data are processed on the basis of the expert knowledge stored in the KBS.

The intelligent analysis model is the kernel of the KBS. Its job is to intelligently interpret the isokinetic data of the database on the basis of the system expert knowledge after they have been processed by the above module. It aims to provide an assessment of the numerical parameters and morphology of the isokinetic curves. The report generator module is in charge of editing and printing the reports that describe the KBS inference process on the processed exercises.

The above three modules -data cleaning and pre-processing, intelligent data analysis and report generation- are what make up the system's KBS architecture.

Exercises in the database that are indicative of any sort of injury are processed by the characterise injuries module. Its goal is to discover sequential models in time series in order to detect patterns repeated across more than one isokinetic exercise. These can then be used to class the injuries that occur. The output models are displayed by the visualisation module discussed above.

Finally, the create reference models module processes all the exercises proper to a given patient population and gets a reference curve for the group. To do this, it is necessary to assure the similarity of the curves of the patient population and discard the atypical curves. The fast Fourier transform is used for this purpose to convert the curves into a frequency domain, thus leading to a more efficient search for similarities. The resulting reference models can be displayed by the visualisation module.

The above two modules (characterise injuries and create reference models), together with the cleaning and pre-processing module are the basic components of the knowledge discovery in databases (KDD) architecture.

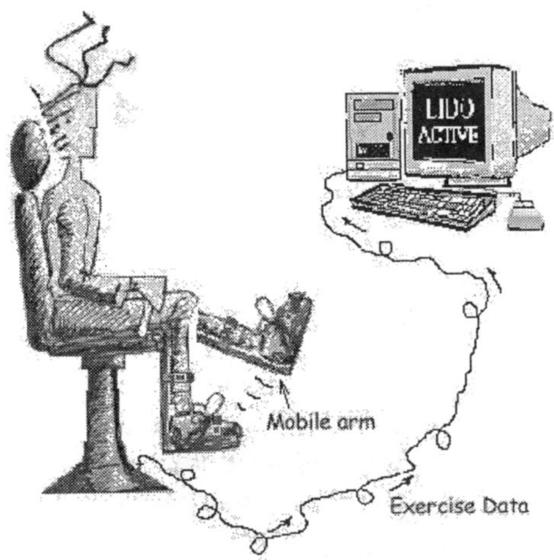

Figure 2. Diagram of isokinetics machine use.

16.2.2 Evaluation of the System as a KBS

As the project required the development of an expert system (ES) to debug invalid data and intelligently interpret the errors produced by the isokinetics machine, the first thing that we did was to check whether the requirements for ES development were met. For this purpose, we ran a test that measured four main aspects or dimensions (Gómez, et al., 1997):

- Plausibility: an ES can be developed and built if there are real experts;
- Justification: ES construction is justified if there is a shortage of human experts;
- Fitness: it is right to build an ES if the problem basically involves symbolic manipulation, is solved by heuristic rules and the knowledge required is not elementary;
- Success: the ES will be successful if managers are convinced of the importance and efficiency of this technology.

A series of characteristics that it would be essential (vital for task performance) or desirable (positive for task performance) for managers and/or users, experts and the task to have are defined for each dimension (García and Zanoletty, 1998).

Each characteristic was evaluated using Boolean, numerical (on a scale of 0 to 10) or fuzzy values (absolutely, very, fairly, not very, not at all) to rate whether or not the characteristic was present in the application. These characteristic values were represented in fuzzy intervals, entering the four interval points to represent each value. For example, the Boolean value *no* is represented as (0,0,0,0) and the value *yes* as (10,10,10,10). Each dimension is evaluated by calculating the arithmetic and harmonic means of the set of fuzzy intervals of its characteristics separately, and then taking the arithmetic mean of the two intervals obtained. That is:

$$V_{ci} = \frac{1}{2}\frac{\sum_{k=1}^{ri} W_{ik}}{\sum_{k=1}^{ri} \frac{W_{ik}}{V_{ik}}} + \frac{1}{2}\frac{\sum_{k=1}^{ri} W_{ik} * V_{ik}}{\sum_{k=1}^{ri} W_{ik}}$$

where: V_{ci}: total value of the application in a given dimension

V_{ik}: value of characteristic k in dimension i

W_{ik}: weight of characteristic k in dimension i

ri: number of characteristics in dimension *i*

The above formula produced four fuzzy intervals (one for each dimension), whose arithmetic mean outputs a fuzzy value, which will be the final result of the evaluation. The task meets the requirements of an ES if the result is over 5.

The results obtained for the I4 system were:

- Plausibility and Fitness: their fuzzy values were very high, falling between the linguistic values "very" and "absolutely", and having an associated numeric value of 8.59 and 8.40, respectively.
- Justification: its fuzzy value was within the "absolutely" interval with a numeric value of 9.15.
- Success: the result for this dimension was slightly lower, falling between "fairly" and "very", with a numeric value of 5.4.

The final result of the feasibility study (the arithmetic mean of the four dimensions) fell between a fuzzy value of "very" and "absolutely", with an associated numeric value of 8.3 (Figure 3), thus indicating that the development of the ES was highly feasible.

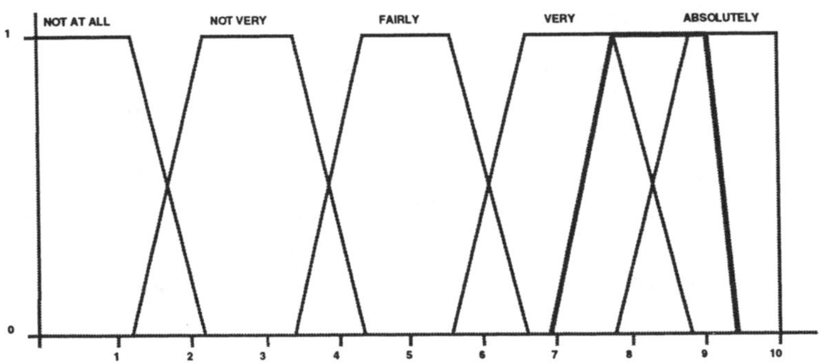

Figure 3. Global fuzzy result of the feasibility study.

16.2.3 Description of the KBS

Having demonstrated the feasibility of including a KBS within the I4 system architecture, we proceeded to develop an ES that would interpret isokinetic data. The preliminary objective of this ES was to provide an analysis of the isokinetic curves in relation to both their numeric parameters and their morphology and thus relieve the workload of specialist physicians in isokinetics, provide support for non-specialist physicians and make it feasible for physicians with impaired vision to do their job. However, the knowledge of this expert system is vital for the data cleaning and pre-processing phases in the KDD process. Therefore, we give an overview of the ES here and detail how it is applied in the KDD process, later.

The knowledge for this ES was elicited from the person who is, probably, the most experienced Spanish physician in muscle strength assessment using isokinetic systems. She has several years' experience in the muscle strength assessment of top competition athletes. This expert knowledge is represented in the system by means of three different structures: functions, rules and isokinetic models. The functions include procedural knowledge, the rules include deductive knowledge and the isokinetic models include structural knowledge, all of which goes to make up the ES knowledge.

16.2.3.1 Functions

The objectives of this representation structure are to:

- assess the morphology of each isokinetic curve
- eliminate some irregularities for which the patient is not responsible, like inertia peaks on the curves, invalid exercise extensions and flexions, etc. This is part of the KDD process and will, therefore, be described later.

The analysis of the strength curves involves the assessment of different characteristics of the extension/flexion curves morphology, which are themselves of interest to the specialist and are some of the inputs for patient assessment. Part of this analysis calls for procedural knowledge and is performed by means of functions that evaluate these curve characteristics. The functions implicitly contain the expert knowledge required for this task. The aspects evaluated by the functions are:

- *Uniformity.* Estimates uniformity, meaning how similar repeated extension and flexion exercises are.
- *Regularity.* Estimates the regularity of the exercise, that is, whether the curve has a smooth contour or a lot of peaks.
- *Maximum peak time.* Outputs a qualitative value of the time it takes to reach the maximum peak for both extensions and flexions. This time is estimated on the basis of the slope up to the maximum peak.
- *Troughs.* Indicates the existence of troughs, prolonged drops and rises of the value of the moment of exercise extensions and flexions. Figure 4 shows an example of an isokinetic exercise with troughs.

- *Shape of the curve*. Evaluates the shape of the exercise curve for both extensions and flexions, by means of an exercise morphology study, taking into account the effort employed at the central angles, the flattening of the curve and the angle at which each maximum peak is reached.

The analysis of these morphological aspects of the curves may seem straightforward for any experienced physician. However, their automated assessment is important for an inexperienced physician and crucial if sight-impaired physicians are to be able to do this sort of work.

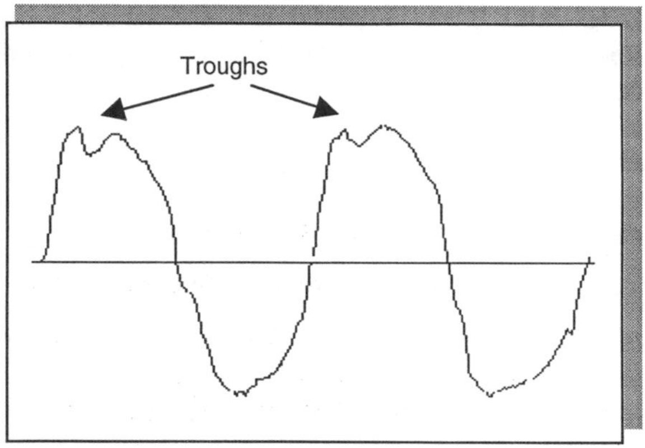

Figure 4. Troughs during extension.

Figure 5 shows the interface window that displays the expert results for the user. Additionally, they are reported to sight-impaired users by voice synthesis.

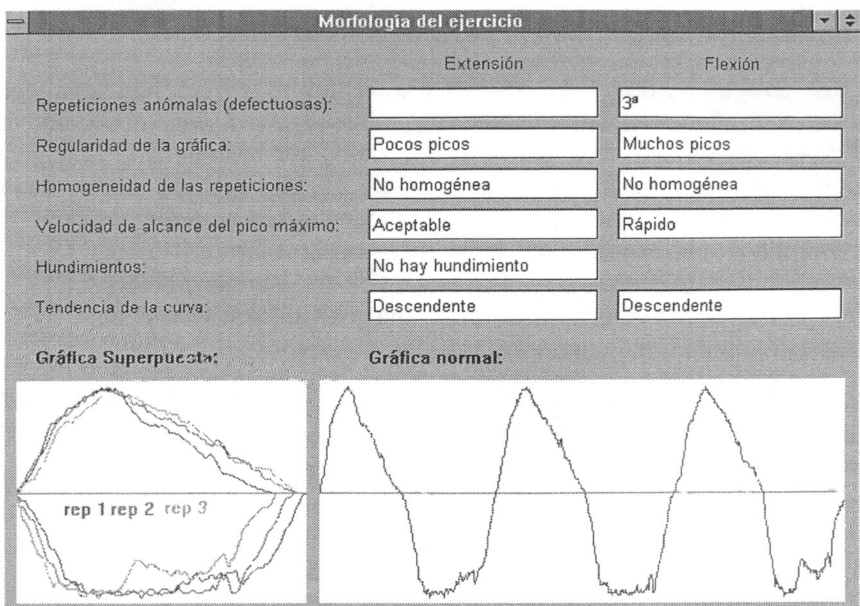

Figure 5. Window showing the morphology analysis of an exercise at 60°/second.

The design and implementation of these functions can be described as interactive human induction, that is, given a number of strength curves, the expert evaluated each one and assessed its characteristics (i.e. whether it had inputs, troughs, the shape of the curve, etc.). Then, tentative functions were implemented, whose inputs were strength curves and whose outputs were the same characteristics for the given curves. These functions were applied to a new set of tests, and the results obtained were shown to the expert for evaluation. This evaluation led to some changes in function implementation, and so on. This process ended when the methods provided the correct value in a high percentage of the cases (over 98%). It took 3 to 5 iterations, depending on the complexity of the interpretation of each characteristic.

Another important issue for function implementation was the need to assess each case according to the characteristics of the patient (male or female, age, sports, injuries, etc.). A decision table for each characteristic was elicited from the expert to solve this problem. Each decision value is stored in the respective table and entered in the functions, according to patient characteristics.

16.2.3.2 Rules

It was obvious from the very start of the design phase that functions were not enough. They represent procedural knowledge very well, especially if it involves calculations, but they are not suited for representing fine grain knowledge, like heuristic assertions, such as "If there are many invalid exercises, repeat the test". The most straightforward means of representing this knowledge is to use "If ... then ..." rules. Another important feature of this formalism is explicit knowledge representation, as it provides an intuitive representation that can be easily validated by the expert.

There are over 480 rules in the rule-based system, providing conclusions on three concerns of isokinetics analysis:

- *Protocol validation.* This part of the analysis has the mission of determining that the protocol has been correctly applied. This is very important since the expertise used for the later parts of the analysis is very sensitive to the way in which the tests are performed. These conclusions are used within the KDD process to remove the tests that do not comply with the minimum requirements for their assessment.
- *Numerical analysis of data.* Every numerical feature of the curve (maximum peak, total effort, gradients of the curve, etc.) is expertly analysed and conclusions are presented to the user. There is an individual analysis of each leg and a comparison between both legs.
- *Morphological analysis of data.* The last part of the rule-based subsystem analysis, concerned with the morphological aspects of the data, takes into account the output of the expert functions described in the previous section. That is, the rules cannot evaluate the morphology of the strength curves (this is what the functions do); the rule-based subsystem analyses the morphology of the strength curve of each leg and their comparison and tries to identify any kind of dysfunction.

Figure 6 shows the interface window for the rule-based subsystem analysis containing the results of the evaluation. There are three tags for each part of the analysis described. Morphological analysis has been selected, and there are icons for displaying the conclusions regarding each leg, its flexion and extension. The bottom window shows an overall analysis for the right leg. It points out some problems with the right flexors and extensors and suggests that this could be caused by some sort of dysfunction in the knee joint.

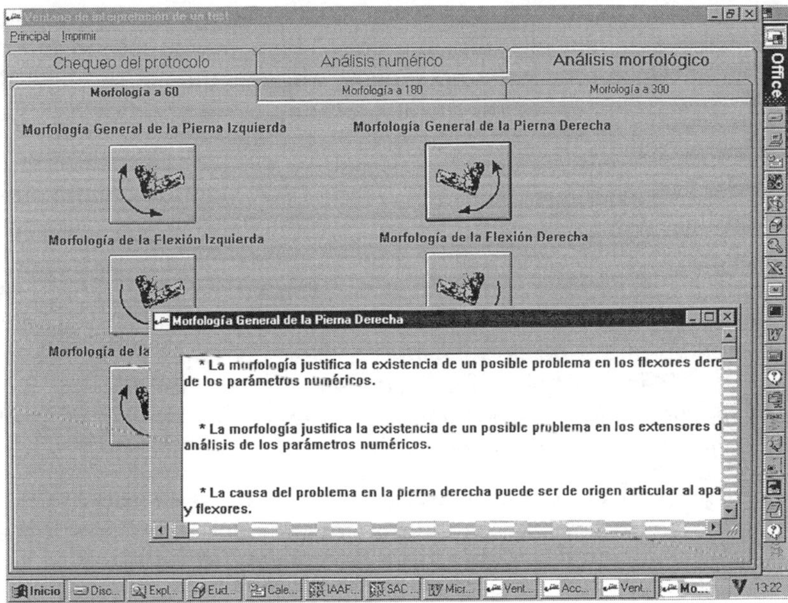

Figure 6. Window showing results from the rule-based subsystem.

16.2.3.3 Isokinetic Models

One of the processes most commonly performed to evaluate patient strength is to compare the results of their test against a standard. Yet another structure had to be built to represent expertise and assist physicians with this task. This third structure, which has been named isokinetic model, is composed of a standard isokinetic curve and a set of attributes. The curve is automatically calculated given a set of tests. The user selects a group of tests, usually belonging to patients of similar ages, the same sex, similar sport if any and or same injury, and the system calculates the reference curve for that group. This requires some sort of pre-processing (to discard bad exercises, standardise the curve, etc.), for which purpose functions are used. It also requires the detection of the extensions and flexions that are most representative of each exercise, the only ones that will be used to calculate the reference curve. Then the isokinetic curve is calculated.

Of course, this is a poor representation of the strength of the group of patients, since some of the significant irregularities are softened or even eliminated when calculating the average curve. Therefore, a set of attributes had to be added to return the information needed to compare a new patient against an isokinetic model. Some of the attributes are calculated automatically from the set of tests performed on the group in question, like its principal irregularities, whereas others, like how close the new curve should be to the model (in terms of standard deviation) for it to be considered as normal, are defined by the expert.

In order to compare an isokinetic model curve and the patient curve, both curves are translated to a frequency domain using the discrete Fourier transform[1] (Berndt and Clifford, 1996), which enables a more efficient search for similarities between the curves. This comparison is highly interesting for users, as the similar parts in the model and patient curves are marked and a global measure of similarity is presented. Additionally, the user can compare the complete curve, flexions or extensions individually and even selected regions interactively, as well as symbolically define the accuracy of the comparison.

Isokinetic models play an important role in the isokinetic assessment of patients, as they allow physicians to compare each new patient with standard groups. For example, it is possible to compare a long jump athlete with a group of elite long jumpers, compare a promising athlete with a set of models to determine which is the best suited discipline, assess strength dysfuntions in apparently normal patients, etc.

The models obtained by means of this procedure turned out not to be very useful, however, as all the tests of the group were used to calculate the reference curves and, obviously, these could be very different from each other. This obliged us to include in the process of reference model construction a stage that searched for similarity among the preliminary tests and discarded any that were too far away from the norm. This KD process is described later.

16.2.3.4 Co-Operation Between the Three Formalisms

One of the reasons for implementing the ES with three different structures is that each comprises the different types of knowledge provided by the expert more intuitively. The individual tasks involved in a full isokinetic analysis of the patient required different knowledge representation structures. The knowledge comprised in each structure (functions, rules or models) can be used separately to provide conclusions on particular issues and can also be employed together to provide more general conclusions.

---

[1] The discrete Fourier transform is used mainly to compare curves with reference models and other curves. The fast Fourier transform, as we will see later, is used to make massive comparisons within test groups.

As we have already mentioned, these three types of knowledge are related and are complementary to each other: the rule-based subsystem needs the results supplied by running the expert functions on the curves. The output of these functions is an important input for the rule preconditions. Functions also play a major role in the creation of isokinetic models, as they provide the values of some model attributes. These attributes are intended to reflect some of the common characteristics of the strength curves that could be eliminated when calculating the average strength of the individuals of a group. The conclusions supplied by the rule-based subsystem are also important for this task.

However, the relations between these structures for representing expertise are not one way. The models also input facts to the rule-based subsystem for assessing comparisons between a patient and a model. Numerical (e.g., a patient is 20% stronger than the reference group) and morphological comparisons are inputs to the rule-based subsystem, which provide a higher level conclusion than a diagnosed dysfunction or any other relevant conclusion.

Therefore, the definition of three different structures for representing isokinetic expertise is important, for two main reasons:

- The isokinetic domain (like most domains) contains different sorts of knowledge, each of which is better suited to a particular knowledge representation structure.
- The co-operation between the three knowledge representation structures is able to supply higher level conclusions that would be difficult to achieve using only one knowledge representation structure.

So far we have described the KBS devoted to the interpretation of the isokinetic tests. This system also fulfils a mission within I4: analyse the isokinetic curves and provide physicians with all the data and expert findings necessary to reach a diagnosis. This is very useful for specialist physicians, as it relieves part of their workload. However, it is essential for non-specialist physicians or physicians with impaired vision.

Nonetheless, this system has some limitations, due, on the one hand, to the shortage of expertise in given issues of isokinetic analysis and, on the other, to the need to improve the processing of some tasks. Particularly, expert knowledge for characterising muscle or joint injuries and assessing recovery has been found to be missing. Additionally, any atypical elements of the group, whose inclusion would distort the model, have to be discarded when creating the reference models for given groups of individuals. A KD process, discussed in the following sections, was developed to perform these tasks.

16.3 Understanding the Data

Although we can get a fairly close idea of the sort of data to be handled from the preceding section, we detail some of the issues as yet unmentioned and describe the collection of initial data below.

16.3.1 Data Description: The Isokinetic Test

Isokinetic systems were conceived to analyse the muscular fitness of patients who are members of any population group. During a standard session, patients must perform a set of exercises, for example, ten seconds extending and flexing their leg with the machine moving at a constant speed of 90°/s. The number of exercises and speed at which they must be performed are determined by the isokinetic protocol currently in use (López-Illescas, 1993). This protocol defines the number of exercises to be performed and at what speeds. Obviously, the protocol must always be the same, if we are to be able to analyse some patients against others, as differences in the number, order and speed of the exercises would significantly alter the isokinetic curves obtained. All of the exercises performed in a session are called an isokinetic test and, in this case, this is composed of 6 exercises for each leg at given constant speed (60, 180 or 300°/s). Each exercise is characterised by the speed and the leg used (left or right), and the angle[1] and the strength applied every 2/100 s by the patient is recorded. The graphic representation of these data (strength over time) resembles a sinusoidal curve, containing a lot of small peaks and other irregularities, as shown in the previous section. The amplitude, total area and irregularities are the main parameters in the analysis of the tests.

16.3.2 Collection of Initial Data

In the case with which we are concerned, isokinetic tests have been used to assess the physical capacity and injuries of top competition athletes since the early 90s. An extensive collection of tests and exercises has been gathered since then, albeit unmethodically. Hence, we had a set of

---

[1] Although the angle and time should be equivalent at constant speed, the angle is recorded because minor deviations from constant speed are very significant.

heterodox, unclassified data files in different format, which were, partly, incomplete. The reasons was that:

- Every time an isokinetic test is run, a series of isokinetic system database registers are created. These were kept in this database until the hard disk was full and were then dumped to diskettes. The tests were saved on different diskettes, depending on the sport in question, and in the internally coded format of the isokinetic system, which uses the imperial system of measures. Therefore, most of the data were stored and coded across a set of diskettes.
- The sex of the patient was not defined in any of the tests and personal particulars were missing in many, because they are of no interest for muscle analysis. Additionally, some tests do not include all the exercises defined in the protocol for a variety of reasons.

Obviously, this was a far from ideal situation for applying automatic information processing, where only rigorous planning of the objectives and milestones allowed us to keep up spirits and make progress toward database creation.

On the positive side, the quality of the strength data within each exercise was unquestionable, as the protocols had been respected in the huge majority of cases, the isokinetic system used was of proven quality and the personnel who operate it had been properly trained.

This collection of data was composed of close to 1580 isokinetic tests (this number grew throughout the project life cycle). In order to calculate the volume of information, it is important to take into account that the tests are formed by the personal particulars of the patient and 6 isokinetic exercises. Each exercise is a series of from 350 to 600 triplets of real numbers (strength, angle, time). All this amounted to just over 103 Mbytes of information at the start.

16.4 Preparing the Data

A series of tasks, detailed in this section, had to be carried out before the available data set could be used (not only for KD tasks but also for expert analysis itself). Although the planning of objectives and milestones was very important in this domain, it was very difficult to establish a long-term plan from the start, as it was hard to foresee the final outcome of some of the phases. Instead we set short-term milestones which, when achieved, were used as a basis for planning the next steps.

Figure 7 shows a diagram of the main data preparation tasks. Each of these is described in detail below.

16.4.1 Data Analysis and Decoding

The data came from a commercial application (the isokinetic system) that has its own internal data format, which are compressed and coded using special methods. Therefore, the current isokinetic system database could not be used (after loading the information from all the diskettes) to process the data, and each test had to be exported to text format. Apart from this being hard work, there was an added difficulty, as the format of this text file had to be decoded. This was not immediate, as the use of the imperial system of measures caused some confusion.

The milestone established at this stage was to be able to display an isokinetic test in a general-purpose graphic package. Not until this objective was achieved could we start to plan further project phases, as there was no guarantee that the data could be automatically processed until then.

16.4.2 Creation of the I4 Database

Chronologically, this was when we decided to analyse the possibility of building the ES that would analyse the isokinetic curves. The feasibility of this system was discussed in section 2.2 and the ES was described in section 2.3.

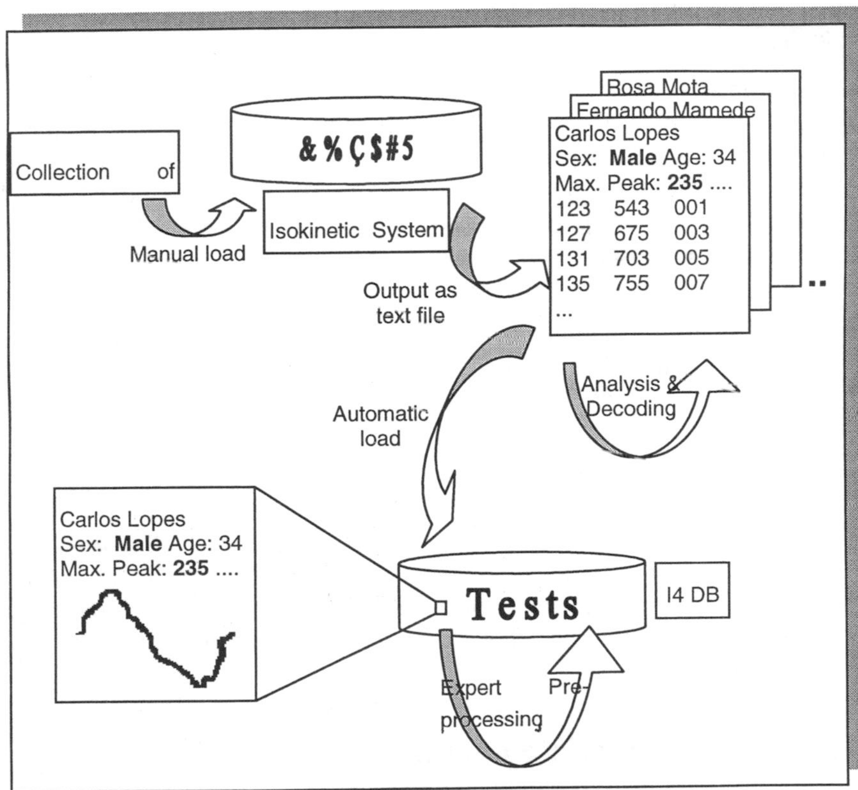

Figure 7. Database construction process and data pre-processing.

The creation of the I4 database, which was to organised and store the isokinetic tests run and would allow these and future tests to be used rationally, was a must for the success of this ES. This would make it possible to validate its knowledge and use it *a posteriori* in tests run in the past. However, another point that led us to create this database surfaced during the early phases of ES construction. This was the dearth of thorough knowledge in this field and its relative youth, which meant that expert knowledge on some points was limited and, therefore, some tasks, like, for example, characterising the isokinetic curves of patients with some sort of injury, were not practicable.

In view of these circumstances, it is not hard to imagine that the process of database creation was long and laborious. Once all the isokinetic tests run had been transferred to text files, they had to be entered in the I4 database. As discussed above, the tests were classified neither by patient nor by any other means and contained some incomplete data. An automatic loading tool was designed to transfer all the tests to the I4 database, automating this task to the utmost. Its functionalities were as follows:

- The database can be loaded with an unlimited set of exercises located in a particular directory. The exercises performed in one session (exercises that are part of one test) must be detected (depending on the date, patient, leg and speed) to allocate the same test code to the exercises that are part of the same test. This is a means of structuring separate exercises. Additionally, the test object is created containing the data common to exercises.
- With regard to incomplete data in tests and exercises, these will be included automatically when they can be calculated and, otherwise, the user is interactively asked for their value.
- Patient gender is a particularly interesting case, which was not defined in any of the exercises. This datum is very important, as it conditions any assessment of the exercises considerably (there is a discrepancy among the strength values of men and women). The loader was equipped with a name recognition feature to enable this datum to be added to the tests. This allows the sex to be identified depending on the patient's name, and the user is asked to enter this particular only if in doubt.

16.4.3 Expert Cleaning of Data

Once we had a standardised database with organised and complete information, the curves had to be evaluated to identify any that were invalid for assessing patient muscle capacity and to remove any irregularities entered by mechanical factors of the isokinetic system. Expert knowledge was needed to perform these pre-processing tasks. Therefore, the data cleaning phase called for the use of the ES functions and rules to apply the knowledge it contained.

Two data cleaning tasks were performed:

- *Removal of incorrect tests.* This pre-processing task has the mission of determining that the isokinetic test protocol has been correctly applied. Any difference in the performance of the exercises has a significant effect on strength data. All the exercises defined in the protocol must have been completed successfully in the correct order. Additionally, the strength values must demonstrate that patients exerted themselves during the exercises and, therefore, tired to some degree.

Only if this protocol validation is correct will it be possible to use the data.

- *Elimination of incorrect extensions and flexions.* Even if the isokinetic protocol has been correctly implemented, some of the extensions and/or flexions within an exercise may be of no use, owing mainly to lack of concentration by the patient at a particular time during the exercise. I4 detects exercise extensions and flexions that are invalid because much less effort was employed by the patient than was in others, as well as movements that can be considered atypical as their morphology is unlike the others.

16.4.4 Expert Pre-Processing

Having validated all the exercises as a whole and each exercise individually, they have to be filtered to remove irregularities that are not caused by patients. Again expert knowledge had to be used to be able to automatically identify the irregularities caused by the strength employed by patients and any that are due to the isokinetic machine. So, the strength curves are pre-processed in order to eliminate flexion peaks, that is, maximum peaks produced by machine inertia. This is detected when the angle at which the maximum peak is produced deviates a lot from the norm. Figure 8 shows a graph with peaks and the same graph after they have been removed.

16.5 Data Mining

Data mining techniques were required to analyse isokinetic exercises in order to discover new and useful information for later use in a range of applications. Patterns discovered in isokinetic exercises performed by injured patients were very useful, in particular for monitoring injuries, detecting potential injuries early or discovering fraudulent sickness leaves.

Another very useful question was to create reference models for different population groups. Thus, athletes can be classed according to their muscle power, their sport or even their age. This is a means of determining, for example, whether young athletes should opt for one sport or another or how they are likely to develop. Two algorithms have been built into I4 to perform these tasks.

16.5.1 Detecting Injury Patterns in Isokinetic Exercises

Data mining algorithms can only be applied to the isokinetic exercises stored in the database if they are represented in a suitable format for processing. Therefore, an isokinetic exercise was considered as a sequence of numbers that represent values at a point of time. One of the most important potential applications of data mining algorithms for this sort of time series is to detect any parts of the graph that are representative of any irregularity. As far as isokinetic exercises are concerned, the presence of this sort of alterations could correspond to some kind of injury, and correct identification of the alteration could be an aid for detecting the injury in time. So, the identification of patterns, that is, portions of data that are repeated in more than one graph, is of vital importance for being able to establish criteria by means of which to classify the exercises and, therefore, patients.

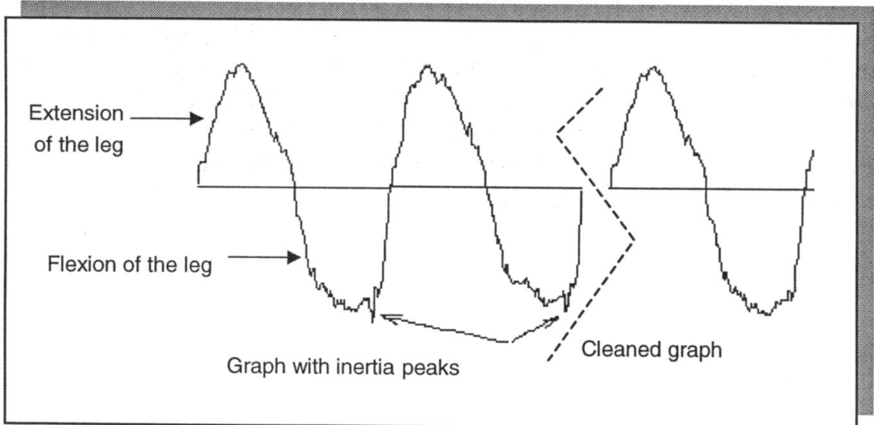

Figure 8. Exercises at 60°/s with inertia peaks and their elimination.

Isokinetic exercises have a series of characteristics that cannot be overlooked when designing an algorithm to identify patterns. Remember that each datum in an isokinetic exercise is a measurement of strength at a particular time. Owing to the special characteristics of the individuals who complete an exercise of this sort, the graphs can have different amplitudes and be removed in time, even if the same pattern is observed. Therefore, some sort of distance has to be used to take into account not only the parts that are repeated exactly but also any that are approximately the same.

Another particular to be considered in the search for patterns is that there is no expert knowledge about the possible patterns and their length. Therefore, all the exercises have to be run through to get patterns of different lengths. The memory consumption and execution time of this process can be very high, and these are both factors to be considered when designing the algorithm.

As mentioned above, an isokinetic exercise will be represented as a series of real numbers. That is, an exercise Si can be represented as

$$S_i = \{s_{i1,} s_{i2}, \ldots, s_{in}\} s_{ij} \in \Re \, \forall j$$

A pattern will be a sequence of numbers that is repeated in enough exercises. The number of repetitions is known as frequency, and this frequency, divided by the total number of exercises, is called pattern confidence. Formally, the frequency of a pattern *p* is defined as

$$\text{frequency(p)} = \{S_i \mid 1 \leq i < m \text{ where p appears in } S_i\}$$

$$\text{confidence(p)} = \frac{\text{frequency(p)}}{m}$$

where *m* is the total number of exercises.

The length of a pattern is called period. A pattern *p* of period *l* is said to be a frequent periodic pattern of period *l* if its confidence is greater or equal to a given threshold ε. The objective of this algorithm is to find periodic patterns in the isokinetic exercises in the database. The Euclidean distance, defined as

$$D(R,S) = \left(\sum_{i=1}^{i=n} (R_i - S_i)^2 \right)^{1/2}$$

where R and S are two isokinetic exercises, will be used as a measure of the distance.

As mentioned above, the main problem of searching for what are originally unknown patterns is the exhaustive use of memory and the amount of time it can take an algorithm to run through all the isokinetic exercises stored in the database. One way of making the search space smaller is to use the property known as *A priori* (Agrawal, et al., 1993). This states that if a pattern is not frequent, that is, if its confidence is not over the threshold value, no pattern of a longer period that contains it will be able to be frequent. This means that rather than checking all the patterns, only patterns containing infrequent sub-patterns have to be inspected, that is, the patterns of period i will be used as filters for the candidates of period i+1.

16.5.1.1 Proposed Method

The process of developing a data mining algorithm that detects patterns in isokinetic exercises and identifies patterns that potentially characterise some sort of injury was divided into two phases:

a) Develop an algorithm that detects patterns in exercises.

b) Develop an algorithm that uses the algorithm developed in point a) and is capable of detecting any patterns that appear in exercises done by patients with injuries and do not appear in exercises completed by healthy patients.

A pattern search tree was built in order to speed up pattern-searching algorithm operation by applying the A priori property. Each depth level of this tree coincides with the period of each pattern, that is, a branch of depth 2 corresponds with a given pattern of period 2. An example of this sort of trees is given in Figure 9. Each branch of the tree will contain a counter that will specify the number of exercises in which the pattern appears. Further appearances of one pattern within the same exercise will not be taken into account. This counter can be used to prune any branches under the threshold in question, and the pattern will be ignored in the future. The patterns are formed by running through the exercises using a window of the same size as the period under consideration. So, the algorithm will be capable of forming all the patterns of any period, ending when there are no more branches to run through or when the period of the pattern is greater than the length of the longest isokinetic exercise.

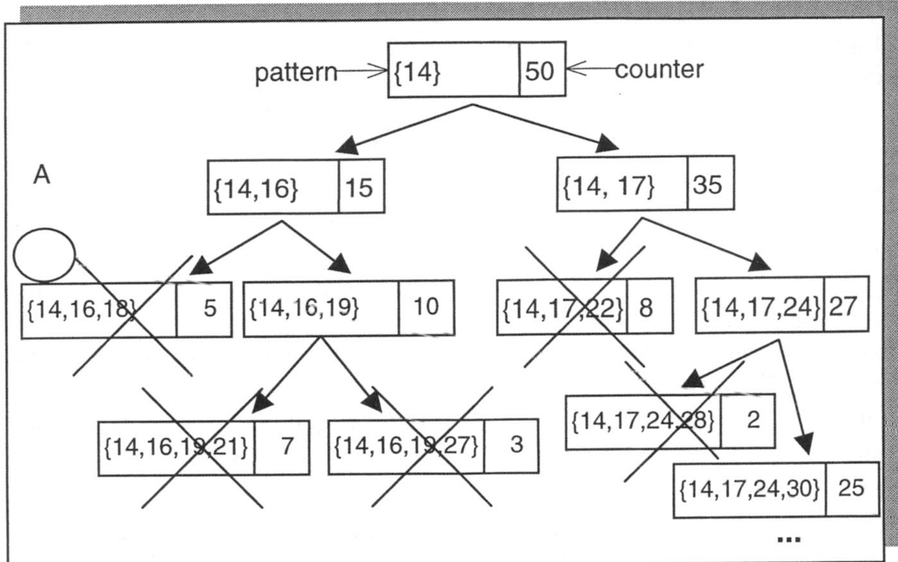

Figure 9. Pruning tree.

For example, if a frequency of 10 were established for the tree shown in Figure 9, branch A would be pruned, because pattern {14, 16, 18} was only found in five exercises, which does not meet the minimum requirement. Any pattern {14, 16, 18, x_i, ...,x_j} will be ignored in the future.

Below we will present two pattern-searching algorithms, which we applied in the research. One considers identical sequences as patterns and the other adds the Euclidean distance to compare patterns. The difference between the two is significant and has a very considerable impact on algorithm performance. In the algorithm that does not consider distance, each pattern corresponds to one and only one branch of the search tree. Therefore, the pattern search in the tree ends when the respective branch is found. This is not possible in the algorithm that takes into account distance, as a pattern has more than one correspondence in the search tree. For example, pattern {12, 14, 16, 18} and pattern {12, 14, 16, 19} would be considered as similar at distance 1, and the tree should increase the counter of the respective branches for both patterns.

Algorithm 1. Exact pattern search

The algorithm runs through the exercises in the database and forms patterns of different periods, which are inserted in the search tree and their counter is increased. The process is iterative, starting with patterns of period 1 up to the patterns with the maximum period, corresponding to the length of the longest exercise. This is a very similar process to the one presented in (Han et al., 1998).

The search tree must be pruned before moving on to a longer pattern. In accordance with the A priori property described above, all the branches corresponding to patterns whose confidence is not over the threshold will be pruned. This means that the algorithm ignores patterns that cannot possibly be frequent.

Basically, the algorithm starts with the first exercise in the injuries database and forms patterns of period 1 with a window of the same size. As they are formed, they are inserted in the search tree, and the counter is set at one. This is meant to reflect that the above pattern appears in at least one series. This window moves through the exercise forming all the patterns. The same process is carried out on the other exercises in the database. The counter will merely be increased for exercises already entered in the search tree, and any not entered for any previous exercise are inserted with the counter at 1.

Having finished the search for all the patterns of period 1, any patterns that cannot possibly be frequent will have to be pruned. Any patterns of less than the desired frequency will not be run through again, and their branch will be pruned. The process will now be repeated with patterns of period 2, except that patterns which are part of a pruned branch will not be inserted, and the window will immediately move to the next pattern. This rules out having to run through the tree to enter a pattern that is not going to be frequent. The algorithm ends when the window is longer than the maximum period in the tree.

At the end of algorithm execution, we will get all the patterns that have the required confidence. Although it can be useful to find patterns that are exactly repeated in the isokinetic exercises, these patterns are not sufficient in most applications. The differences in the values measured in most isokinetic exercises can cause two similar patterns not to appear as such when the algorithm is executed, losing a lot of useful patterns that should be identified. This is why we had to develop another algorithm that enhances the potential of the one described above, using the notion of distance among patterns for this purpose.

Algorithm 2. Similar pattern search using Euclidean distance

After adding the pattern search distance, the algorithm becomes more complicated and has to be modified. Just one run through the tree could form all the patterns of a given period before. However, the number of appearances of a pattern can now change owing to other similar patterns appearing. Therefore, the tree has to be run through again to add the actual number of times a pattern appears, that is, not only the exact appearances but also occurrences of other similar patterns.

Also special care has to be taken not to prune patterns, which, although not frequent themselves, play a role in making another pattern frequent. If this sort of patterns were pruned, the algorithm would not be complete, that is, would not find all the possible patterns. Therefore, the pruning condition must be modified. Any patterns that are not frequent and whose minimum distance from the other patterns is further than the required distance will be pruned. When the patterns are presented, only the frequent ones will be displayed, although not all the patterns in the tree are frequent owing to the above pruning condition.

The form chosen for the new algorithm was to use a variant on the above, which retained both the number of series in which a pattern appeared and a reference to the series in which it appeared. The series are run through using a window, which forms patterns, alters the counter and enters the series in which they appear. Before moving on to the pruning phase, the patterns must be run through again, this time to count the appearances attributed to similar patterns. The presence of the series entered by each pattern is helpful in this respect. For each pattern, all the patterns in the tree that are at a lesser distance than the threshold d are searched, and as they are considered similar patterns, the counters of both must be increased. Figure 10 shows a formal description of this algorithm.

The algorithm is applied directly to detect irregularities in the graphs that possibly identify the presence of injuries. All the series of the databases are used for this purpose, and series that indicated a given injury are separated from any that did not. The above algorithm was simply applied to the two sets, getting two collections of patterns. Any patterns that appeared in the graphs of injured patients and did not appear in the graphs of healthy patients were identified as injury patterns and, after assessment by the expert, were used to indicate an injury. The graphs obtained from subsequent isokinetic tests will then be able to be searched for these patterns to check whether or not there is an injury.

```
Input:
        ε: minimum confidence
        m: number of time series
        s[m:i]: collection of time series
        d: minimum distance
Code:
        Begin {
        l= 0;
        While ((the tree has unpruned branches) or (l>i))
        {
                l = l + 1;
                for (i=0 to i=m)
                {
                        run through s[i] forming patterns of length = l;
                        insert the pattern in the tree;
                }
                calculate distance(l);
                prune branches;
        }
        run through the tree forming patterns;
        }end
insert pattern in the search tree
        input:
                tree: search tree
                i: number of the time series that aims to insert pattern
                pattern: pattern to be inserted
            begin {
                if the pattern was not inserted
                        insert it, place i in the collection of appearances;
                }end
calculate distance
        input:
                tree: search tree
                l: length
                d: minimum distance
            begin {
                For each pattern p of length=l
                        For each pattern q of the same length
                                if distance(p,q)<d
                                        unite the collection of p and the collection of q and
                                        place it in the new collection
                        Keep the same distance for the other patterns
            }end
                }end
prune branches
        input:
                tree: search tree
            begin {
                Prune each branch:
                (conf(p)<ε) AND (minimum distance < d)
            }end
```

Figure 10. Pattern Search Algorithm using Euclidean distance.

Figure 11 shows three real examples of isokinetic exercises stored in the database. Possible patterns can best be viewed by representing the exercises alongside each other. The algorithm that does not include the Euclidean distance is incapable of finding any pattern in these exercises. However, depending on the application to which they are put, several similarities can be found. For example, using ε=0.8 and a threshold of 50 for the distance, algorithm 2 finds the pattern shown in Figure 12.

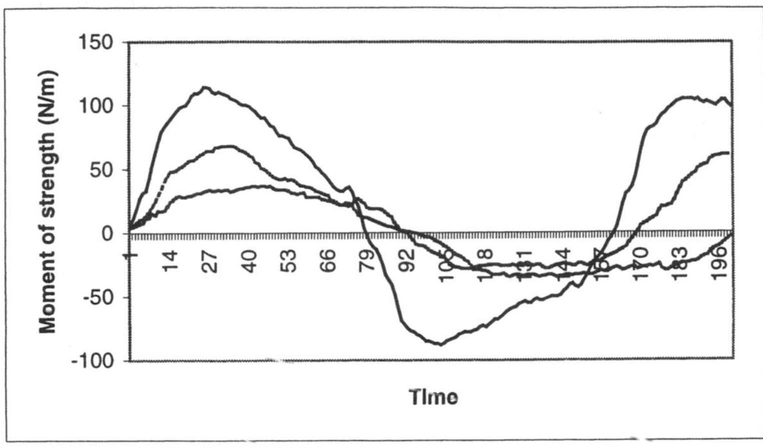

Figure 11. Isokinetic exercises.

The pattern shown in Figure 12 is a magnification of a region common to the three graphs, specifically the region between the times 100 and 161. It is important to note that although the pattern appears more or less in the same region of the three exercises in this example, this is not generally the case. Additionally, the pattern does not necessarily have to appear in all the database exercises, but it must appear in enough to comply with the required confidence.

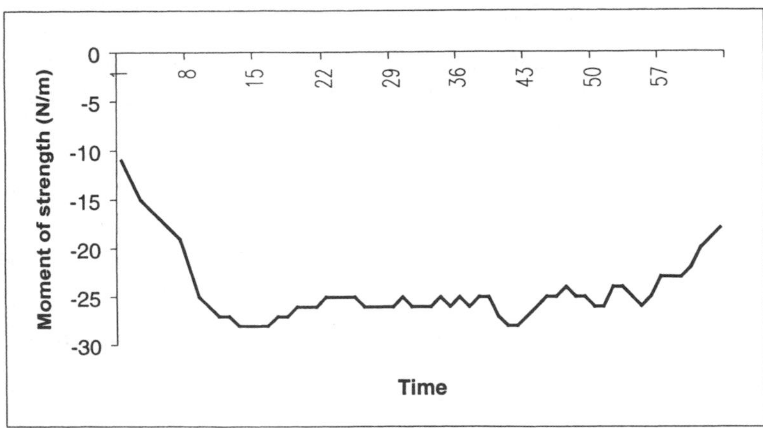

Figure 12. Magnification of the pattern found.

16.5.2 Creation of Reference Models for Population Groups

One of the most common tasks involved in the assessment of isokinetic exercises is to compare a patient's test against a reference model created beforehand. These models represent the average profile of a group of patients sharing common characteristics.

All the exercises done by individuals with the desired characteristics of weight, height, sport, sex, etc., must be selected to create a reference model for a particular population. However, there may be some heterogeneity even among patients of the same group. Some will have a series of particularities that make them significantly different from the others. Take a sport like American football, for instance, where players have very different physical characteristics. Here, it will make no sense to create a model for all the players, and individual models would have to be built for each subgroup of players with similar characteristics. Therefore, exercises have to be discriminated and the reference model has to be created only with exercises among which there is some uniformity.

It was the expert in isokinetics who used to be responsible for selecting the exercises that were to be part of the model. Discarding any exercises that differ considerably from the others is a job that is difficult to do manually. This meant that it was mostly not done. The idea we aim to implement is to automatically discard all the exercises that are different and create a model with the remainder.

The problem of comparing exercises can be simplified using the discrete Fourier transform to transfer the exercises from the time domain to the frequency domain (Agrawal, et al., 1993). The fact that most of the information is concentrated in the first components of the discrete Fourier transform will be used to discard the remainder and simplify the problem. The advantage of the discrete Fourier transform is that there is an algorithm, known as the fast Fourier transform, that can calculate the required coefficients in a time of the order of O(n log n).

The discrete Fourier transform of an exercise $s_i = \{s_{i1}, s_{i2}, \ldots, s_{in}\} s \in \Re$ is given by

$$S_{if} = \frac{1}{\sqrt{n}} \sum_{t=0}^{n-1} s_{it} \exp(-j2\pi ft/n) \quad f = 0,1,\ldots,n-1$$

Each of these components will be a complex number and, hence, some useful properties can be defined. For a complex number c=a+jb=A exp(jϕ), the following concepts can be defined:

The conjugate c* of c = a + jb is defined as a – jb.

The energy E(c) of a complex number c is defined as the product of c and its conjugate, that is, *E(c) = cc**. The energy of a series is maintained in the time and in the frequency domain, and this characteristic can be used to simplify the process.

The discrete Fourier transform has the plus that it accumulates almost all its energy in the first components, which means that the first coefficients can be used for the purpose of comparison. In practice, it has been demonstrated that 2 or 3 coefficients are sufficient in most cases (Agrawal et al., 1993). Also Parseval's theorem can be used towards our goal:

Let $\vec{X}$ be the discrete Fourier transform of the sequence $\vec{x}$. Then we have that

$$\sum_{t=0}^{n-1} |x_t|^2 = \sum_{f=0}^{n-1} |X_f|^2$$

That is, the energy in the time domain is the same as the energy in the frequency domain and, therefore, the Euclidean distance between two data series in the time domain is the same as the Euclidean distance in the frequency domain.

The number of comparisons to be made is drastically reduced using this technique, a very important factor in this case, since there are a lot of exercises for comparison in the database and comparison efficiency is vital.

Once the user has selected all the tests of patients of which the model will be composed, the process for creating a new reference model is as follows:

- Calculate the discrete Fourier transform of all the exercises.
- Class these exercises, using some sort of indexing to rapidly discard all the exercises that are different from the one that we are searching for. Trees of the B family (like B+) or R trees are the best suited. R* trees (Beckmann et al., 1990), which divide the n-dimensional space geometrically into rectangles of n dimensions, are proposed in (Agrawal, et al, 1993) as a very suitable indexing method for the problem. The system creates an R* search tree with the exercises of each class. So, they are grouped in classes, and the groups of similar exercises are clearly identified.
- Normally, users mostly intend to create a reference model for a particular group, there is a clearly majority group of similar exercises, which represents the standard profile that the user is looking for, and a

disperse set of groups of 1 or 2 exercises. The former are used to create a reference model, in which all the common characteristics of the exercises are unified.

- Given an isokinetic exercise, or a set of isokinetic exercises, for a patient, they will later be able to be compared with the models stored in the database taking advantage of the above discrete Fourier transform. Thus, we will be able to determine the group of which patients are members or should be a members and identify what sport they should go in for, what their weaknesses are with a view to improvement or how they are likely to progress in the future.

This algorithm was implemented in I4 and is used in several kinds of isokinetic curve comparison. Therefore, its contribution is not merely confined to model creation.

Figure 13 shows an example of how the algorithm is applied to search for similarities between graphs. Particularly, it shows the results of the comparison between an isokinetic exercise and a given reference model. Similar regions are highlighted for rapid location. Using the Fourier transform algorithm, both exercises are transferred from the time to the frequency domain. As explained earlier, the comparison is more efficient in this domain, and partial or total comparisons can be done in a simpler way.

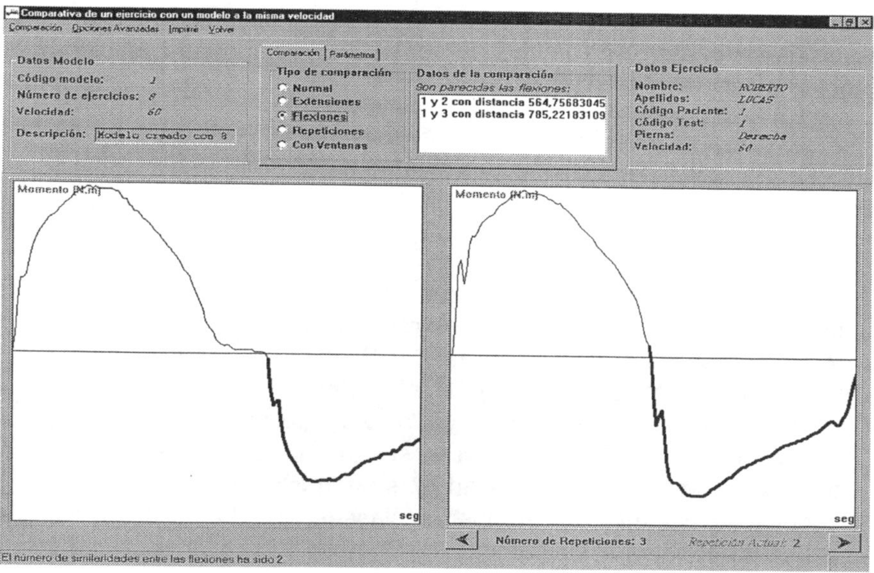

Figure 13. Comparison of graphs.

16.6 Evaluation of the Discovered Knowledge

It was not easy to evaluate the results obtained by means of the above methods. Remember that the entire discovery process was motivated by the dearth of prior knowledge concerning the behaviour of most of the populations under study. This is an obstacle for evaluating the quality of the results, as it rules out a comparison with well-known widely accepted models.

However, this was not the only problem we faced. The fact that there was no well-defined preliminary goal or rather that we had a wide range of possible uses to which the results could be put, especially for characterisation knowledge, further complicated the planning of the validation tests to be run.

Bearing this in mind, the entire evaluation process had to concentrate on the following goals:

- Verify whether the models obtained actually represented the populations for which they had been created and validate how representative the models were.
- Validate their fitness for achieving the selected goals: pattern-based injury detection and model-based population characterisation. Then select other possible goals and test the models to predict their potential for application.

The sources of knowledge for both evaluations were confined to the experts, the cases database, the preliminary models and everyday practice. So, the whole process had to be carefully planned as a long-term evaluation, which is still on going. A five-step procedure was used for both evaluation goals:

1. Subjective appraisal of the results by the expert. The aim of this step was to get a rough idea of the possible quality of the results in order to plan new decision-making (DM) tasks, if required. Therefore, it was carried out in parallel to the DM process.
2. Statistical tests comparing the results with previous known cases. All we had to go on for this task were the cases themselves and the preliminary models described in section 2. These tests had, therefore, some limitations.
3. Turing Test-based validation tests, in which the effectiveness of the discovered knowledge was compared against the expert using the

KBS. This task was planned to get a neat idea of the strength of the results when applied in everyday practice.

4. Continuous daily evaluation with real–life cases. This is a corrective stage and will continue throughout the research project life cycle.
5. Evaluation of satisfaction. This is an important part of any applied KD process evaluation, which is often overlooked. Its goal is to gain an understanding of the feelings of the practitioners when the new technology derived from the DM is transferred to everyday practice. The information obtained here is indispensable for defining new tasks or research lines and for getting accurate data about the potential of technology of this sort within the target domain.

The last two stages have a lot to do with the daily use of the discovered knowledge and will be discussed in the next section. Hence, we will concentrate on the first three stages here.

As mentioned above, the first evaluation step took place during the actual KDD process. The goal was to detect any significant deviation of the partial results obtained during DM from the results expected by the practitioners. A clear distinction must be made between the two problems we faced in order to understand the results and the importance of this evaluation.

With regard to the creation of population reference models, there was little background knowledge, so it was very difficult for the experts to determine in advance whether the models were representative for the populations under study. Hence, the efforts focused on testing the quality of the partial models using a small set of carefully selected cases. These contained typically representative cases of the population under study, plus a small group of atypical occurrences and some instances that did not even belong to the population. The results of the tests were optimal. Every typical case was well characterised by the reference models, and not one single example that was not a member of the class came close to its model. The outcomes for the atypical cases were inconclusive. About 50% of the cases were similar to some reference model and the remainder were not. However, it is important to note that the real objective of these tests was to check whether the process was good for the intended goals. The results cannot as yet be considered conclusive in this respect.

This early evaluation was much more fruitful as far as the injury detection problem was concerned. In this case, the method used was to give the injury patterns to the experts and ask them for a documented opinion about their quality. If they felt they were fine, they were asked to provide at least five examples that confirmed the pattern; whereas if they did not agree with the result, they had to come up with the same number of negative examples.

Thanks to exercises of this sort, we were able to identify some strengths and weaknesses of the DM methods. The first outcome was related not with the DM methods, but with the detection process as a whole. The planned procedure involved comparing any new case against the injury patterns discovered by the system. If the case matched any pattern, then an injury had been detected. The problem with operations of this sort is that not every single injury has a pattern, so a few injury cases were detected as perfectly normal. There are two possible explanations for this effect. The most immediate one is to consider that the results are not final and a lot of knowledge still remains to be discovered. The more critical one is to think that the above injury patterns will never be discovered or will even be discarded by the system, because they belong to rather atypical or infrequent cases.

These exceptional cases are just ignored in some domains (like the characterisation domain, for example) and nothing happens. In a diagnosis domain, however, this problem (hereinafter referred to as the minorities problem) can be an extremely tricky matter. At this stage, two possible solutions were suggested to overcome the minorities problem.

The first was to adapt the DM method so that it would be able to detect exceptional cases. This solution was absolutely unworkable at this stage, because it would have delayed the achievement of more significant results. Moreover, many of the commonly used DM methods had no such problem with exceptional cases. Hence, this possibility was left for a future research line.

The second solution was to change the actual pattern application procedure. Apart from finding patterns for cases with injuries, another disjunct set of patterns for normal cases were to be found, as described in section 5, and any new case was to be compared with both sets. If the case matched any injury pattern, then a possible injury would exist. If the case matched any normal pattern, then the hypothesis would be that no injury is present. If it matched neither, a possible exceptional case would be identified. This procedure met the needs of the experts and, hence, was chosen. So, the DM stage was expanded to also locate normal patterns.

Another potential problem that was detected early on was a consequence of the DM method used and had to do with the two parameters d and ε. As no background knowledge was available for use, the optimal values for both parameters in this domain had to be determined empirically, and the quality of the results would depend on this. However, this obstacle could not be overcome at this stage.

The objectives of the second evaluation step were to empirically check the results and, at the same time, determine the best values for the above-mentioned parameters. Five scenarios were defined using the same database. Twenty per cent of the cases in each scenario were randomly chosen for testing, while the other 80% were used to create the patterns. For each scenario, 25 different sets of patterns were generated for each combination of values of ε (0.60, 0.70, 0.75, 0.80 and 0.90) and d (100, 150, 175, 200, 250) for series of period 500. It must be mentioned that the thereshold d depends of the period of the series, and longer series need for higher values of d. The best scenarios prove to be those where ε is 0.75 or 0.80 and d is 175 or 200 (for period 500). In these cases the results where very similar, and about 85% of the test cases where found to present the corresponding patterns.

For the reference model domain, tests were run in two stages. Cross-validation was used in stage 1 to analyse the quality of the discovered models. During stage 2, the models were compared against those built by the KBS as described in section 2. The results were extremely good in both cases. During cross-validation, 98% of the test cases that were classed as belonging to the target population were correct, and the goal was achieved. The other 2% are cases that were not initially classed as belonging to the population, but, after the expert's analysis, happened to share all the characteristics typical of the population. This happens because many features of athletes from different sports are the same (for instance, a volleyball player may be very similar to a basketball player). About 4% of the cases that were not recognised as belonging to the population were in fact members of it. They were all representative of minorities within the population and did not share its typical characteristics. This was the expected behaviour. The results far surpass the preliminary models.

The third step of the evaluation process was to use the KBS to compare the effectiveness of the discovered knowledge against the expert's. The most straightforward means of carrying out such a comparison is to use an approach based on the Turing Test. The Turing Test (Gupta, 1991) is a well-known validation method, commonly used in KBS development, which involves having the expert and the system solve the same real case simultaneously and then compare the results. If any other specialist is unable to distinguish the solutions provided by the expert and the computer, then the evaluation is optimal.

The information supplied to both the system and the experts was exactly the same (an isokinetic test) in order to assure that the test was meaningful. This test was repeated for 25 occurrences in the injury problem (15 with common injuries, 5 with rare injuries and 5 without injuries at all), and 50 in the reference model problem (30 belonged to different kinds of the population, 10 did not and 10 had not been classified at all). In both cases, the examples had not been used during DM, and the comparison was made between our expert, a less experienced specialist and the system.

The results were as follows in the injury detection scenario. Both the system and the expert identified the 15 common injuries, while the novice omitted 2. The expert identified the five cases without injuries, while the system found one that matched neither the normal nor the injury patterns, and the novice found three of the five possible injuries. Finally, for the five cases of rare injuries, the system was unable to find any match to normal or injury patterns (which was the expected behaviour). Meanwhile, the expert found 2 normal patterns, 2 injury patterns and could not make a decision on the other, and the novice found two injuries and was unable to make a decision on the others. It is important to note that the experts were unable to use any information apart from the isokinetic data.

The results were even more remarkable for the reference model problem. Of the 30 members of the population, 26 were identified by the system. The four mistakes were in respect of minorities. This was considered a high error margin until it was compared with the performance of the expert. Again, the only information supplied to the experts and the system were the isokinetic data of the individuals. With the above information, the expert made 9 mistakes and the novice 21. The system, the expert and the novice made exactly the same decisions on the 10 examples that did not belong to the population. And, finally, for the 10 unclassified cases, the system made no mistakes, while both the expert and the novice made 2 each.

Some important conclusions can be drawn from the results of these three evaluation phases:

- Firstly, the importance of early evaluation has been demonstrated. The main problems were detected in a phase in which they could be easily prevented, corrected or, at least, identified for further testing and research.
- The minorities problem is crucial for diagnosis domains. Although the I4 approach finds a way around and thus solves the problem, a DM method able to detect and find patterns or models within minorities would be important.
- The values of the above-mentioned empirical parameters are valid for this particular domain, but if the method is used for other similar problems, their values should be recalculated in similar way as for the injury problem.

- The results are not error free, but the number of mistakes found during testing is considerably lower than the threshold that is acceptable to practitioners.

16.7 Using the Discovered Knowledge

The knowledge discovered in the previous phases is currently being used in the I4 project. I4 has been designed using an object-oriented ES development methodology (Alonso et al., 1998a), and its first phase is now fully operational. The project has produced two applications (Alonso et al., 1998b), which are quite similar, except for the interface. One, called ES for Isokinetics Interpretation (*ISOCIN)*, was designed for use by sight-impaired physicians, so the interface includes complete voice synthesis of every piece of information presented to the user. That is, it includes information on how to use the system, the options open at any time and, of course, the isokinetic data and their interpretation. The system can be used without a display. *ISOCIN* is currently being used by blind physicians at *EFONCE* to analyse injuries and assess their evolution, adapting the physiotherapy administered and rehabilitation process.

The other application, an ES for Interpreting Isokinetics in Sport (*ISODEPOR)*, is being used at the National High Performance Centre to evaluate the muscle strength of Spanish top-competition athletes.

As mentioned in section 6, two important evaluation tasks remained to be performed during and after technology transfer. The first one concerned continuous evaluation of the results provided by the system. So far, no significant errors have been reported by the physicians, hence confirming the results obtained during off-field evaluation.

The second evaluation task was related to user feelings about the new technology and user satisfaction. Members of the centre's staff claim that this system has improved the work of physicians working in the field of isokinetics and list the system's prominent features as follows:

- Physicians who are not specialists in isokinetics can use and exploit the system, thanks to the help provided by the intelligent interpretation, patterns and models.
- Analysis of the full isokinetic strength curve is possible, from which the complex or specific strength parameters that are of use for interpreting the tests can be inferred more correctly and completely.

- I4 increases the power of isokinetic systems. Population modelling (by sports, specialities, diseases, etc.), used to detect both coincidences with and slight deviations from group norms. It is now planned to use the models for the early evaluation of the capabilities of young athletes and detect what likelihood elite athletes have of suffering certain injuries.
- Intelligent analysis of the strength curves obtained from the isokinetic tests provided by I4 has improved evaluation procedures. The isokinetic system features are better exploited thanks to the automatic extraction of improved information concerning injuries.
- I4 has provided friendly access for medical practitioners to the isokinetic parameters and an improved graphical presentation of the results of isokinetic tests, making reports easier to understand and more useful.

Furthermore, the I4 system will provide more knowledge of the characteristics of athletes' strength, which has implications for the development and evaluation of training and rehabilitation programs. The deployment of the I4 system is a major advance in isokinetic data processing, as it means that muscle strength measurement systems can be better exploited. These issues make it highly relevant in the field of top-competition sport.

Additionally, as there are few specialists in isokinetic assessment of muscle strength data, this system will be extremely valuable as an instrument for disseminating isokinetic technology and encouraging non-expert medical practitioners to enter this field.

16.8 Conclusions

The development of an ES and its later refinement is mainly based on eliciting and entering experts' present knowledge of the subject into the system. At later stages, more domain knowledge of the problem was added to the system on the basis of the experience gained by the experts in the meantime.

Thanks to data mining techniques, a more efficient and objective process can be applied that is complementary to the above for developing an ES, provided enough data are available from which new knowledge can be discovered.

The I4 project, described in this chapter, is an example of this approach applied to the expert processing of isokinetic data. Initially, the expert knowledge of the isokinetic physician was entered into the system in order to conduct an intelligent analysis of the numerical parameters and morphology of the strength curves produced by the isokinetic tests. Later and considering the volume of tests there were, data mining techniques were applied, based on time series processing to discover patterns, injuries and reference models. This new knowledge, evaluated and validated by the expert, was entered into the system and produced a system that performed better and was more efficient than the one directly elicited from the expert. This has meant that it has been able to be applied at the Spanish National Centre for Sports Research and at the School of Physiotherapy of the Spanish National Organisation for the Blind.

With regard to the application of a methodological KDD process for extracting the knowledge from the data, it is noteworthy that the data preparation was so domain dependent that we were unable to set out a general-purpose methodological approach that could be extrapolated to any other system.

The same conclusion is applicable to the selection and design of the DM techniques best suited to the problem. Domain dependency is total, with regard to both the data in question and the planned use to which they are to be put. Therefore, it is impossible to generalise a mechanism of selection. In the examples described here, we examined a case (injuries) in which any error whatsoever could be serious and another (identification of population models) in which the lack of knowledge did not entail disastrous consequences. These two cases had necessarily to be processed differently, and this treatment was founded on the characteristics of each particular problem.

What is clear in this regard is that it will be necessary in many situations to use DM techniques of different sorts in combination to assure fuller data processing. In the case of the problem detected concerning minorities (a problem that can arise in a host of different application domains), it appears to be necessary to include techniques by means of which to detect and process these situations, according to a similar approach as outlined in (Caraça-Valente and Montes, 1998).

On the other hand, we were able to demonstrate the importance of carrying out an early evaluation of any results obtained, by means of which to identify as soon as possible any problems in the final results that could affect the success of the KDD.

Furthermore, the participation of experts throughout the entire KDD process was fundamental, not only as a vital source of knowledge but also to get them to identify with the project, thus overcoming their traditional rejection of technologies of this sort.

Acknowledgements

We would like to thank África López-Illescas for her co-operation in the I4 project. The I4 project was partly funded by CICYT project no. TIC98-0248-C02-01. This paper was written in co-operation with CETTICO (Centre of Computing and Communications Technology Transfer).

References

Agrawal, R., Faloustsos, C. and Swami, A. 1993. Efficient similarity search in sequence databases. In: *Proc. Foundations of Data Organisations and Algorithms (FODO Conference.*

Alonso Amo, F., Barreiro, J., Fuertes, J.L., Martínez, L. and Montes, C. 1998a. Incremental Prototyping Approach to Software Development in Knowledge Engineering. In *Proc. 5th International Conference on Information Systems Analysis and Systemics*, Orlando.

Alonso, F., Barreiro, JM., Valente, JP. and Montes, C. 1998. Interpretation of Strength Data. In Proc. *11th International Conference on Industrial and Engineering Applications of Artificial Intelligence and Expert Systems*, Benicassim, LNAI no. 1415, vol. I, Spain.

Beckman, N., Kriegel, H.-P., Schneider, R. and Seeger, B. 1990. *The R*-tree: an efficient and robust method for points and rectangles. ACM SIGMOID*, 322-331.

Berndt, D. and Clifford, J. 1996. Finding patterns in time series in advances. In: U. Fayyad et al. (eds.) *Knowledge Discovery and Data Mining.* MIT Press.

Brachman, R. And Anand, T. 1996. *The process of knowledge discovery in databases: A human centered approach.* AKDDM. MIT Press, 37-59.

Caraça-Valente, J. P. and Montes, C. 1998. Improving Inductive Learning in Real-World Domains through the Identification of Dependencies: the TIM Framework. *Lecture Notes in Artificial Intelligence. Proceedings of the IEAQ-98-AIE*, vol. II. Springer, 458-468.

Fayyad, U., Piatetsky-Shapiro, G. and Smyth, P. 1996. *Knowledge Discovery and Data Mining: Towards a Unifying Framework. Proceedings of KDD-96.* AAAI Press, 82-88.

García, C. and Zanoletty, D. 1998. ISOCIN. Sistema experto para la interpretación de isocinéticas. Technical report, Facultad de Informática de Madrid, Madrid.

Gleeson, N.P., and Mercer, T. H. 1996. The utility of isokinetic dynamometry in the assessment of human muscle function. *Sports Medicine*, 21(1).

Gómez, A., Juristo, N. and Pazos, J. 1997. *Ingeniería del conocimiento. Diseño y construcción de sistemas expertos.* Madrid: Ceura.

Gupta, U. 1991. (Ed.). *Validating and Verifying Knowledge Based Systems.* IEEE Computer Society Press.

Han, J., Dong, G., and Yin Y. 1998. Efficient mining of partial periodic patterns in time series database. In *Proc. Fourth International Conference on Knowledge Discovery and Data Mining*. AAAI Press, Menlo Park. 214-218.

Kannus, P. 1994. Isokinetic evaluation of muscular performance: implications for muscle testing and rehabilitation. *Int. J. Sports Medicine* 15(Suppl 1).

López-Illescas, A. 1993. Estudio del balance muscular con técnicas isocinéticas. In: *Proc. I Curso de Avances en Rehabilitación*, Seville.

Studies in Fuzziness and Soft Computing

Vol. 26. A. Yazici and R. George
Fuzzy Database Modeling, 1999
ISBN 3-7908-1171-8

Vol. 27. M. Zaus
Crisp and Soft Computing with Hypercubical Calculus, 1999
ISBN 3-7908-1172-6

Vol. 28. R.A. Ribeiro, H.-J. Zimmermann, R.R. Yager and J. Kacprzyk (Eds.)
Soft Computing in Financial Engineering, 1999
ISBN 3-7908-1173-4

Vol. 29. H. Tanaka and P. Guo
Possibilistic Data Analysis for Operations Research, 1999
ISBN 3-7908-1183-1

Vol. 30. N. Kasabov and R. Kozma (Eds.)
Neuro-Fuzzy Techniques for Intelligent Information Systems, 1999
ISBN 3-7908-1187-4

Vol. 31. B. Kostek
Soft Computing in Acoustics, 1999
ISBN 3-7908-1190-4

Vol. 32. K. Hirota and T. Fukuda
Soft Computing in Mechatronics, 1999
ISBN 3-7908-1212-9

Vol. 33. L.A. Zadeh and J. Kacprzyk (Eds.)
Computing with Words in Information/ Intelligent Systems 1, 1999
ISBN 3-7908-1217-X

Vol. 34. L.A. Zadeh and J. Kacprzyk (Eds.)
Computing with Words in Information/ Intelligent Systems 2, 1999
ISBN 3-7908-1218-8

Vol. 35. K.T. Atanassov
Intuitionistic Fuzzy Sets, 1999
ISBN 3-7908-1228-5

Vol. 36. L.C. Jain (Ed.)
Innovative Teaching and Learning, 2000
ISBN 3-7908-1246-3

Vol. 37. R. Słowiński and M. Hapke (Eds.)
Scheduling Under Fuzziness, 2000
ISBN 3-7908-1249-8

Vol. 38. D. Ruan (Ed.)
Fuzzy Systems and Soft Computing in Nuclear Engineering, 2000
ISBN 3-7908-1251-X

Vol. 39. O. Pons, M.A. Vila and J. Kacprzyk (Eds.)
Knowledge Management in Fuzzy Databases, 2000
ISBN 3-7908-1255-2

Vol. 40. M. Grabisch, T. Murofushi and M. Sugeno (Eds.)
Fuzzy Measures and Integrals, 2000
ISBN 3-7908-1255-2

Vol. 41. P. Szczepaniak, P. Lisboa and J. Kacprzyk (Eds.)
Fuzzy Systems in Medicine, 2000
ISBN 3-7908-1263-4

Vol. 42. S. Pal, G. Ashish and M. Kundu (Eds.)
Soft Computing for Image Processing, 2000
ISBN 3-7908-1217-X

Vol. 43. L.C. Jain, B. Lazzerini and U. Halici (Eds.)
Innovations in ART Neural Networks, 2000
ISBN 3-7908-1270-6

Vol. 44. J. Aracil and F. Gordillo (Eds.)
Stability Issues in Fuzzy Control, 2000
ISBN 3-7908-1277-3

Vol. 45. N. Kasabov (Ed.)
Future Directions for Intelligent Information Systems on Information Sciences, 2000
ISBN 3-7908-1276-5

Vol. 46. J.N. Mordeson and P.S. Nair
Fuzzy Graphs and Fuzzy Hypergraphs, 2000
ISBN 3-7908-1286-2

Vol. 47. E. Czogała† and J. Łęski
Fuzzy and Neuro-Fuzzy Intelligent Systems, 2000
ISBN 3-7908-1289-7

Vol. 48. M. Sakawa
Large Scale Interactive Fuzzy Multiobjective Programming, 2000
ISBN 3-7908-1293-5

Vol. 49. L.I. Kuncheva
Fuzzy Classifier Design, 2000
ISBN 3-7908-1298-6

Vol. 50. F. Crestani and G. Pasi (Eds.)
Soft Computing in Information Retrieval, 2000
ISBN 3-7908-1299-4

Vol. 51. J. Fodor, B. De Baets and P. Perny (Eds.)
Preferences and Decisions under Incomplete Knowledge, 2000
ISBN 3-7908-1303-6

Vol. 52. E.E. Kerre and M. Nachtegael (Eds.)
Fuzzy Techniques in Image Processing, 2000
ISBN 3-7908-1304-4

Vol. 53. G. Bordogna and G. Pasi (Eds.)
Recent Issues on Fuzzy Databases, 2001
ISBN 3-7908-1319-2

Studies in Fuzziness and Soft Computing

Vol. 54. P. Sinčák and J. Vaščák (Eds.)
Quo Vadis Computational Intelligence?, 2000
ISBN 3-7908-1324-9

Vol. 55. J.N. Mordeson, D.S. Malik
and S.-C. Cheng
Fuzzy Mathematics in Medicine, 2000
ISBN 3-7908-1325-7

Vol. 56. L. Polkowski, S. Tsumoto and T.Y. Lin
(Eds.)
Rough Set Methods and Applications, 2000
ISBN 3-7908-1328-1

Vol. 57. V. Novák and I. Perfilieva (Eds.)
Discovering the World with Fuzzy Logic, 2001
ISBN 3-7908-1330-3

Vol. 58. Davender S. Malik and John N. Mordeson
Fuzzy Discrete Structures, 2000
ISBN 3-7908-1335-4

Vol. 59. Takeshi Furuhashi, Shun'Ichi Tano and
Hans-Arno Jacobsen
Deep Fusion of Computational
and Symbolic Processing, 2001
ISBN 3-7908-1339-7

Druck: Strauss Offsetdruck, Mörlenbach
Verarbeitung: Schäffer, Grünstadt